The Jordan Report
20th Anniversary
Accelerated Development of Vaccines 2002

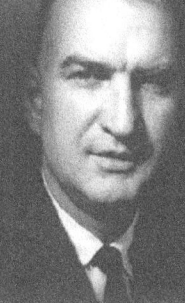

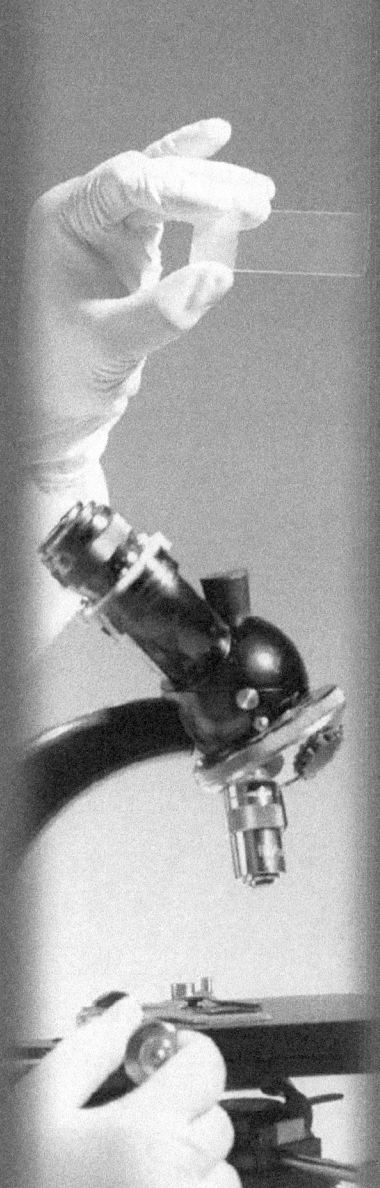

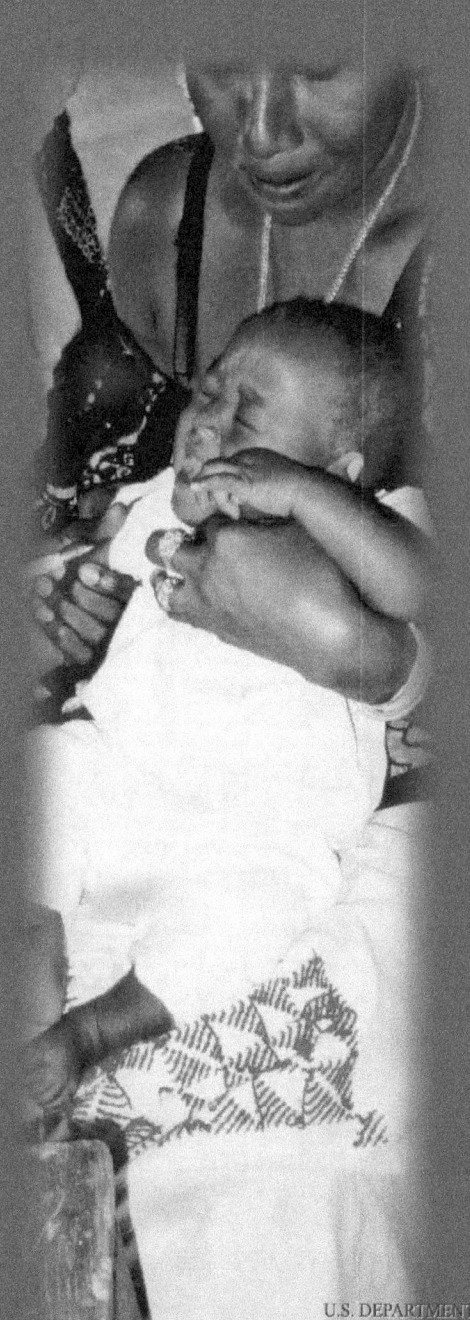

U.S. DEPARTMENT OF HEALTH AND HUMAN SERVICES
National Institutes of Health

National Institute of Allergy and Infectious Diseases

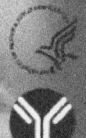

The Jordan Report

20th Anniversary

Accelerated Development of Vaccines 2002

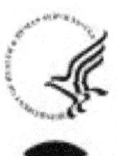

U.S. DEPARTMENT OF HEALTH AND HUMAN SERVICES
National Institutes of Health

National Institute of Allergy and Infectious Diseases

Preface

In 1982, the National Institute of Allergy and Infectious Diseases (NIAID) established the Program for the Accelerated Development of Vaccines. For 20 years, this program has helped stimulate the energy, intellect, and ability of scientists in microbiology, immunology, and infectious diseases. Vaccine research has certainly benefited. The status report reflecting this progress in vaccine research has come to be known as the Jordan Report *in recognition of Dr. William Jordan, past director of NIAID's Division of Microbiology and Infectious Diseases (DMID) and the program's earliest advocate.*

This anniversary edition of the *Jordan Report* summarizes 20 years of achievements in vaccine research driven by the explosive technological advances in genomics, immunology, and molecular biology. Increased knowledge of the immune system has helped to define the mechanisms needed for successful immunization. Genomic tools are helping researchers identify and fine-tune the targets most appropriate for use in developing candidate vaccines. The payoffs from genomics are just beginning. Using tuberculosis as an example, in just 6 years researchers have sequenced the genome, have identified new targets for vaccine development, are working to analyze the function of more than 400 proteins, and are poised to conduct clinical evaluations of the first new candidate vaccines in 80 years. This year the *Anopheles gambiae* and *Plasmodium falciparum* genomes have been sequenced and, together with the human genome data, will allow researchers for the first time to listen in on immunologic conversations of vector, pathogen, and host.

Along with these technological advances, there has been a heightened awareness of the importance of vaccines for global health and security. Acquired immunodeficiency syndrome (AIDS), malaria, and tuberculosis have demonstrated to the world the importance of public health in economic development. Most recently, the threat of bioterrorism has reminded many Americans of the value of vaccines as public health tools.

Articles by outside experts in this edition highlight many of the scientific advances, challenges, and issues of vaccine research during these two decades. As we look to the decade ahead, the payoffs from basic research will continue to invigorate vaccine development, but economic, risk communication, and safety challenges are likely to influence the licensing of new vaccines. The "easy" vaccines have been developed; many challenges lay ahead for new and improved vaccines. The emergent tools and enhanced interest, commitment, and resources that have been developed in the preceding decades will be required to meet these challenges.

Carole Heilman, Ph.D.
Director
Division of Microbiology and Infectious Diseases
National Institute of Allergy and Infectious Diseases
National Institutes of Health

Acknowledgements

This report was prepared under the supervision of the Division of Microbiology and Infectious Diseases (DMID), National Institute of Allergy and Infectious Diseases (NIAID), National Institutes of Health (NIH).

Dr. Carole Heilman   Dr. Pamela McInnes   Ms. Sarah Landry
Director   *Deputy Director*   *Editor*

In addition to those who wrote special articles, sincere thanks and appreciation are expressed to the staff of DMID for updating the scientific sections and the material presented in Appendix C; to Ms. Alice Knoben, U.S. Food and Drug Administration, for reviewing and updating the material presented in Appendix D; to the staff of the Division of Acquired Immunodeficiency Syndrome for assembling the information in Appendices E and F; and to Dr. William Jordan for his continued enthusiasm for this important document.

A special thanks to Steve O'Krepky, Becky Lau, Louise Dickerson, Judy Reemes, Bruce Dennis, Ann Hennigan, and Judy Zukoski at Analytical Sciences, Inc., for their help in designing, compiling, and editing the report.

Images, unless otherwise noted, were provided by the Centers for Disease Control and Prevention (CDC) image database.

EXPERT ARTICLE CONTRIBUTING AUTHORS

Dr. Carl R. Alving   Dr. Maurice R. Hilleman

Dr. Norman W. Baylor   Dr. William Jordan

Dr. Ann Bostrom   Dr. Margaret A. Liu

Dr. Brenda Candries   Dr. Loris D. McVittie

Dr. Susan S. Ellenberg   Dr. Julie Milstien

Dr. Geoffrey Evans   Dr. Derek O'Hagan

Dr. Anthony S. Fauci   Dr. Stanley A. Plotkin

Mr. Gregory K. Folkers   Dr. Jeffrey B. Ulmer

Dr. Mary A. Foulkes   Dr. Frederick R. Vogel

Table of Contents

APPENDICES

Selected Topics in Vaccine Development

History
and
Commentary

History and Commentary

William Jordan, M.D.

One weekend in early 1980, Dr. John R. Seal, Deputy Director of the National Institute of Allergy and Infectious Diseases (NIAID), sat at his desk in the basement office of his home in Bethesda, Maryland, and drafted a hand-written proposal for the launching of a new initiative that led, with few modifications, to the creation of the Program for the Accelerated Development of Vaccines and established NIH as the lead Federal agency for vaccine research and development. The Microbiology and Infectious Diseases Program (MIDP), the division I became the director for in 1976, assumed responsibility for implementation of the program. During my tenure, I reported annually to NIAID's Advisory Council on the status of vaccine development. In 1992, for the 10th anniversary of this update, Dr. John La Montagne, my successor as the director of what is now the Division of Microbiology and Infectious Diseases (DMID), named this report the Jordan Report. Although I retired in 1987, I have been able to keep in touch with the staff of this division thanks to the kindness of Dr. Anthony Fauci, Director of NIAID, and have been doubly honored by the request that I write my personal historical perspective for this 20th anniversary report. I beg the indulgence of the reader for what follows is, of necessity, somewhat autobiographical, and the "introduction" has evolved into an accounting of 20 years of effort to develop new and improved vaccines.

How was it that I came to discuss vaccines with Dr. Seal? Without conscious effort, I was prepared to do so, beginning with Dr. Hans Zinsser's bacteriology course at Harvard Medical School and Dr. Leroy Fothergill's elective in immunology. My laboratory instructor was Dr. John Enders. For the thesis required by the Department of Parasitology, I chose to write about the epidemic of eastern equine encephalomyelitis in humans that occurred in New England in August 1938, the month before I entered medical school. I wrote that Fothergill and Dr. John Dingle (unknown to me at the time) had recovered the virus from brain tissue, and that the latter had shown that the virus produced a fatal disease in pigeons (1). In 1940-41, during my medical clerkship on the Harvard service of Boston City Hospital, I functioned as an intern (striker) because so many of our house officers had joined military service. My attendants included Dr. Maxwell Finland, Dr. Chester Keefer, and Dr. Dingle. I sat by the bedside of a patient with pneumococcal pneumonia who was experiencing a crisis induced by type-specific immune serum. One year later, as an intern on the same service, I was successfully treating patients, under the direction of Dr. Finland, with sulfonamide drugs for similar infections. About this time, Dr. Dingle and Dr. Lewis Thomas confirmed Dr. Harry Dowling's report that sulfadiazine was highly effective in the treatment of meningococcal meningitis.

After Pearl Harbor, most of my able-bodied classmates joined either the Army or the Navy. Just before I left for active duty in the Navy, I was an assistant resident and treated a patient critically ill with staphylococcal bacteremia secondary to a huge carbuncle with penicillin, a new antibiotic rationed by a committee chaired by Dr. Keefer. My chief resident, Dr. Carlton Chapman, kindly mailed the patient's discharge summary to me at my first duty station at the Naval Operations Base in Reykjavik, Iceland. After enjoying this capital city for some months, I was assigned as medical officer to a remote tank farm—run by the Seabees and guarded by the Marines—that served as the North Atlantic fuel depot for the United States and British fleets. Shortly after we had been frozen in for some days, a liberty party made it to Reykjavik and back, bringing influenza virus to the base. I was able to track the spread of illness from Quonset hut to Quonset hut while rejoicing that there were no serious illnesses even among the older Seabees. I was so pleased with the report on the epidemic that I prepared for the Navy that I sent a copy to Dr. Finland. I was later to learn that Dr. Thomas Francis, with the help of Dr. Jonas Salk, had recently developed an inactivated influenza virus vaccine that was highly effective in young military recruits.

Shortly after D-day in the summer of 1944, I flew home on leave before my next duty assignment. My home was in Fayetteville, North Carolina, just 10 miles from Fort Bragg, an Army base whose mission included the basic training of new recruits. It also housed the laboratory of the Commission on Acute Respiratory Diseases (CARD) under the auspices of the Armed Forces Epidemiological Board (AFEB). Dr. Dingle was now Director of CARD, with a staff that included Dr. T. J. Abernathy, Dr. George Badger, Dr. Alto Feller, Dr. Alex Langmuir, Dr. Clayton Loosti, Dr. Irving Gordan, Dr. Charles Rammelkamp, and Dr. Hugh Tatlock. That group was to define an epidemic respiratory disease syndrome distinct from influenza—acute respiratory disease (ARD) for military recruits—and to show by volunteer studies that it was etiologically distinct from the common cold and primary atypical pneumonia, despite the inability to culture any of the agents (2). Some years later, Dr. Maurice Hilleman, then at Walter Reed Army Institute of Research (WRAIR), isolated an agent (RI 67) during an epidemic of ARD at Fort Leonard Wood that was shown to belong to the family of adenoviruses first identified by Dr. Robert Huebner and Dr. Wallace Rowe of NIAID's intramural laboratories (3). Even later, Dr. Robert Chanock, working in the same laboratories with adenoviruses type 4 (RI 67) and type 7, developed a live, oral vaccine that was shown to be highly effective in marine recruits (4). A manufacturer, Wyeth, devised a way to stabilize the live virus in tablets and created a bivalent adenovirus vaccine that was soon being administered to all military recruits. ARD essentially disappeared. Curiously, attempts to find adenovirus 4 at the military academies and in civilian populations failed, limiting the market for the vaccine. This fact was to have serious consequences in recent years when the manufacturer stopped making the vaccine for the Department of Defense, and ARD returned to recruit camps. As for another of the three entities identified by CARD, atypical pneumonia, NIAID's Dr. Chanock was among the first to show that it was not caused by a virus, but by an antibiotic-sensitive mycoplasma, Mycoplasma pneumoniae (5), subsequently shown to be the cause of 25 percent of all cases of pneumonia requiring hospitalization. Attempts to develop a vaccine have not been successful to date.

My next duty assignment was to the Tropical Disease Service of the Hospital of the National Naval Medical Center in Bethesda, Maryland, where the wards were full of marines back from the South Pacific with P. vivax malaria and filariasis. We were able to report to a committee headed by Dr. James Shannon, destined to become Director of NIH, that a new drug, chloroquine, was effective for the treatment of malaria. Also, my rudimentary knowledge of immunology was boosted by a study of the use of the antigen of the dog worm, Dirofilaria immitis, for a skin test in humans. Thanks to the kindness of my two senior officers, this resulted in my first scientific publication (6). Next followed 16 months of sea duty in the Pacific, culminating in ferrying troops to Japan and waiting to bring them home. I learned that respiratory infections disappeared after a week at sea.

In August 1946, I returned to Boston City Hospital as Assistant Resident and reestablished contact with Dr. Finland and Dr. Dingle. The latter had accepted the invitation of the dean of the School of Medicine of Western Reserve University (now Case Western Reserve University) in Cleveland, Ohio, to create a new Department of Preventive Medicine with responsibility for the care of patients with infectious diseases in University Hospital. Dr. Dingle accomplished this by bringing along three members of the senior staff of the CARD laboratory at Fort Bragg and adding others, including Dr. Harold Ginsberg, who had been Chief of Medicine at Fort Bragg's hospital and had done postwar research at the Rockefeller Institute, and Dr. Richard Hodges, a pediatrician who had conducted the pioneering study of pneumococcal polysaccharide vaccine with Dr. Colin McLeod at an Army air base in Sioux Falls, South Dakota. Development of this effective vaccine was made possible by the basic research of Dr. O. T. Avery, Dr. Michael Heidelberger, Dr. Maclyn McCarty, and Dr. McLeod. It led to the successful studies of Dr. Robert Austrian involving South African gold miners, which became the basis for the current 23-valent polysaccharide vaccine recommended for use in adults. Dr. Dingle, now adept at soliciting grant and contract funds, asked me to join his Department of Preventive Medicine in the summer of 1947, with a joint appointment in medicine.

My first assignment was to Division 30 in University Hospital, a unit with airflow designed to limit the spread of microbes. This clinical setting provided the opportunity for me to observe multiple cases of cold agglutinin positive (the only diagnostic test that was available until M. pneumoniae was discovered) primary atypical pneumonia in a number of families and to confirm the previously reported incubation period before antibiotic therapy altered the epidemiology. Patients with pneumococcal pneumonia became the source of convalescent sera for a study of the effect of penicillin treatment on the immune response to the infecting pneumococcus. Most importantly, this continuous clinical activity introduced me to the young and senior physicians of the staff so that when the polio epidemic of 1952 struck, I was asked to chair the hospital's polio team. It was a brutal introduction to paralysis and tracheostomies when city and university hospitals faced a shortage of respirators. A fated care of love bird-related psittacosis led to the identification of a family epidemic with the help of serologic studies done by Dr. Hillerman's laboratory at WRAIR (7). Division 30 also gave me access to beds for two patients suffering a late complication of syphilis—paroxysmal cold hemoglobinuria. With the help of a fine protein chemist, Dr. Louis Pillemer, I was able to describe the role of complement components in the hemolysis of the Donath-Landsteiner reaction (8).

At Western Reserve University, I joined in the teaching of preventive medicine, including the use of vaccines, and soon became involved in two major research activities: Examination and experimental revision of the medical school curriculum, and planning and participation in a longitudinal study of illness in a group of young families living in the Cleveland suburbs close to the medical school. This 9-year (1948-1957) study of a defined population of civilians became known as the Cleveland Family Study (9). It described the incidence and behavior of undifferentiated common respiratory diseases, streptococcal infections, influenza, infectious gastroenteritis, and all other illnesses using the laboratory tools then available. The plethora of new respiratory and enteric viruses "searching for diseases" became available just as the project ended. But I did have the opportunity to study epidemics of H_1N_1 influenza in 1950, 1951, and 1953 and to show that prior familial contact with the virus effected an approximate 70-percent reduction in rates of influenza-like diseases after an interval of either 1 or 2 years. The study continued through the pandemic of H_2N_2 (Asian) influenza in 1957. In comparison with the earlier H_1 epidemics, H_2 virus infected more than three times as many families and two to three times as many persons. Little influenza vaccine was used despite its availability. The attack rate was highest in the 5- to 15-year-old age group, and school children were responsible for more than four-fifths of the introductions of virus to the homes—a good reason for immunizing children during the next pandemic.

It was now possible to grow adenoviruses. This allowed Dr. Ginsberg to test sera stored since the CARD volunteer experiments. Men infected with the ARD inocula showed antibody responses to type 4 adenovirus, confirming the observation that this virus is a cause of ARD for military recruits (10). In the spring of 1954, shortly after the identification of type 4 adenovirus, I screened sera for type 4 neutralizing antibody. None of 73 children (1 to 18 years of age) had this antibody. For the parents, 6 of 43 mothers (14 percent) and 20 of 41 fathers (49 percent) had type 4 antibodies (11). Further, the availability of sera collected at intervals in previous years permitted measurement of the time and frequency of acquisition of type-specific adenovirus antibodies in the first 5 years of life. There was a steady increase in the percentage of children with type 2 antibody such that by the age of 5 years, 51 percent of children had this antibody. The acquisition of type 1 antibody occurred at a similar rate to the 37-percent level by age 5. Except for an epidemic of nonbacterial tonsillitis and pharyngitis in the summer of 1954 that was associated with type 3 adenovirus, it was not possible to associate an illness with the viral isolation that was responsible for the acquisition of antibody. For this and other reasons, it was estimated that an effective polyvalent vaccine would result in only a 6-percent reduction in the number of illnesses experienced by children in the first 10 years of life—an observation that undoubtedly reinforced industry's lack of interest in such a vaccine. It is now known that there are more than 50 adenovirus serotypes.

As noted, during the summer and fall of 1952, the Cleveland metropolitan area experienced the highest incidence of poliomyelitis in its history. The virus most frequently isolated from clinical cases was type 1. One paralytic case of type 1 occurred in a 13-year-old boy in one of the study families. He recovered without residual. Testing of pre-epidemic sera from 158 persons showed that this group was highly susceptible (68-70 percent) to all polio types. Of 147 persons tested, there were a total of 52 isolations, of which 48 were from the throat. Type 2 predominated (12), followed by type 1 (9) and type 3 (1). There was no evidence of infection in the presence of homotypic antibody. Two years later, during the months of October and November 1954, at which time no cases of paralytic poliomyelitis were reported in the community, six strains of type 1 poliovirus were isolated from pharyngeal swabs collected at the time of respiratory illnesses in three families (12). The individuals who shed virus developed serologic incidence of infection. Because of Dr. Albert Sabin's interest in finding avirulent strains, the viruses were sent to him for testing in cynomolgus monkeys. He summarized his results as follows: "The quantitative tests…performed in monkeys with the poliomyelitis strains from families 29 and 80 indicate that they belong at the other attenuated end of the spectrum that would be expected to be nonparalytogenic for chimpanzees in the maximum dosage."

I later visited Dr. Sabin at his laboratory at Children's Hospital in Cincinnati, Ohio, with the request that he test paired sera from patients with gastroenteritis with an agent recently identified by him that he first called "human enteric virus," later classified as a reovirus. The tests were negative, but I was treated to a review of his laboratory notebooks for testing polioviruses in monkeys during the several days of my visit. One of the investigators in

Sabin's laboratory prior to joining NIAID was Dr. Robert Chanock, who had just discovered parainfluenza viruses (13); three types were later to be identified. Accordingly, sera collected throughout the Cleveland Family Study and in the fall of 1957 were tested for neutralizing antibody for each type (9). With type 1, the percentage of individuals with a detectable antibody increased with age to 50 percent by age 14 years, along with 75 percent of adults. Comparison of the 1957 antibody levels for parents with their levels in 1947-48 indicated that type 1 was highly active in this population during the 10 years of the study. With type 2, antibody was found in one-third of the children and one-half of adults. With type 3, the percentage of individuals with antibody was low at 1 year of age (9.5 percent), but rose rapidly, reaching 65 percent by 2½ years of age. By 3½ years, 85 percent of the children had the antibody. Studies by others have shown that such infections are responsible for a significant amount of morbidity, a fact that has stimulated efforts to develop a parainfluenza virus vaccine.

The gastrointestinal illnesses that prompted the visit to Dr. Sabin were among the 4,057 (16 percent) of 25,155 total illnesses observed during the 10 years of the family study. Early observations suggested that at least two types of illness—afebrile and febrile—were occurring in the population. In collaboration with Dr. Irving Gordon, then at the Division of Laboratories at the New York State Health Department in Albany and who facilitated transmission and cross-challenge studies with volunteers housed in an isolation unit at the New York State Vocational Institution, West Coxsackie, New York, evidence was obtained that at least two agents were responsible for nonbacterial gastroenteritis (14). We lacked the electron microscopy and other sophisticated technology used by Dr. Albert Kapikian to identify rotaviruses and a number of other viruses responsible for diarrheal illnesses. Many studies have now shown that such viruses cause sufficient morbidity here and abroad, particularly in developing countries, to justify the development of vaccines.

There was no difficulty making the diagnosis of streptococcal tonsillitis and pharyngitis in the well-housed Cleveland Family Study population. Fortunately, the 437 infections accounted for only 2.77 percent of 15,783 respiratory infections. The same was not true of military populations, particularly those in the Rocky Mountain area. CARD created a committee headed by Dr. Rammelkamp to attack the problem, and the Army assigned two medical officers, Dr. Floyd Denny and Dr. Lewis Wannamaker, to temporary duty at Western Reserve University to work with Dr. Rammelkamp. A field laboratory was established at Fort Francis E. Warren, an Air Force base near Cheyenne, Wyoming, for conducting epidemiological and clinical studies of streptococcal infections and rheumatic fever. It was this group that demonstrated that penicillin treatment of streptococcal infections prevented rheumatic fever (15). The committee evolved into the Commission on Streptococcal and Staphylococcal Diseases and advised the armed services regarding the use of routine bicillin prophylaxis. Another man in the "Strep Lab" was Richard

Krause, a student at Western Reserve University School of Medicine who took a year off in 1950-51 between his third and fourth years to work as a laboratory technician in Wyoming. In time, he became Director of NIAID and sent Dr. Seal to Lexington, Kentucky, to recruit me to NIH. Now with Fogarty International Center, Dr. Krause maintains an interest in streptococcal infections and is so encouraged by the work of those trying to develop a group A vaccine that he is seeking a site in India where one could be tested.

During my years in Cleveland, I had increasing contact with other investigators with similar interests through attending meetings of professional societies. My mentor, Dr. Dingle, made me a member of CARD in 1956, and I became the director of this busy commission in 1959. It was in this capacity that I first met Dr. Seal, then a naval medical officer at Great Lakes Naval Training Station. It was customary for CARD and the Commission on Influenza to hold a 1-day joint meeting before the annual fall meeting of the Central Society for Clinical Research in Chicago. Dr. Seal and others were active participants. Our contact continued during my years at the University of Virginia School of Medicine in Charlottesville. He retired from the Navy to become Scientific Director and then Deputy Director of NIAID under Dr. Dorland Davis. In this capacity, he invited me to serve as chairman of two U.S. delegations to the Soviet Union in the early 1970s while I was Dean of the College of Medicine at the University of Kentucky in Lexington.

Prior to my years in Kentucky, I served as Chairman of the Department of Preventive Medicine and Professor of Preventive Medicine and Medicine at the University of Virginia. Shortly before my move from Western Reserve University, rhinoviruses had been grown in human diploid cells, so this breakthrough was used in the study of respiratory illnesses in a large population of office workers (16). I had the help of Dr. Jack Gwaltney, a graduate of the University of Virginia Medical School who had interned at University Hospital in Cleveland and was recruited fresh out of military service at Fort Dix, as well as Dr. Owen Hendley and Dr. Gilbert Simon, EIS officers assigned by the Centers for Disease Control and Prevention (CDC) to my laboratory. Rhinovirus infections occur year round, with a peak in September and early October. There are many viruses that cause upper respiratory symptoms, but rhinoviruses are the most common. Dr. Gwaltney joined an informal consortium consisting of Dr. Vincent Hamparian, Dr. Kapikian, and others to characterize more than 100 serotypes, with no few types predominating. The prospect of developing a broadly protective vaccine given so many different serotypes is daunting, although type-specific immunity has been shown to occur.

While still in Charlottesville, I became more familiar with NIAID through service as Chairman of the NIAID Panel on Respiratory and Related Viruses and as a member of its Board for Virus Reference Reagents. At the University of Kentucky, I served as a member of the NIAID Infectious Diseases Advisory Committee and as a member of the Food and Drug Administration (FDA) Bureau of Biologics Panel on Review of Viral and Rickettsial Vaccines. I resigned as Dean of the University of Kentucky's College of Medicine in 1974 to take a sabbatical year at the London School of Hygiene and Tropical Medicine. During this time, I visited the departments of community/social medicine in all of the medical schools in the United Kingdom to study the relationship between medical education and a recent reorganization of the National Health Service. I met a number of infectious disease investigators and became familiar with the personnel and activities of the National Institute for Biological Standards and Control. I was back in Lexington writing a book about my observations when Dr. Krause, Dr. Davis' successor in 1975, had Dr. Seal invite me in 1976 to head a newly created extramural program (MIDP). By this time, I knew something about vaccines and the role of the government in their development.

Attracted by the opportunity to return to infectious diseases, I visited NIAID to learn more about the director's reorganization of the management of extramural research into two programs (now divisions): Immunology, Allergic and Immunologic Diseases and Microbiology and Infectious Diseases. Each of these programs was organized into branches. In subsequent correspondence, it was agreed that I could add a new Epidemiology and Biostatistics Branch and rename an existing one Development and Applications. The latter was to be led by an aggressive branch chief, Dr. George Galasso, with a focus on the development of vaccines and antivirals. He was assisted by a group of talented program officers, including Dr. James Hill (respiratory infections) and Dr. Frank Tyeryar (hepatitis), along with Dr. John La Montagne, who arrived with me in 1976 in time to mastermind the testing of monovalent swine influenza vaccine as Influenza Program Officer. When Dr. Hill left in 1983 to assist Dr. Kenneth Sell, Scientific Director, Dr. David Klein assumed responsibility for Haemophilus influenzae and Streptococcus pneumoniae and was to play a major role in support of the acellular pertussis vaccine trials in Sweden. Along with Dr. Pete Allen (virology), Dr. Richard Horton (mycology), and Dr. Milton Puziss (bacteriology), they did much to further my education.

Within a year, I was able to recruit Dr. Robert Edelman, again with the help of Dr. Seal, to serve as Chief of the Clinical Studies Branch. As an Army medical officer, Dr. Edelman had been assigned to Western Reserve University to assist Dr. Dingle as President of AFEB. He then was stationed at the U.S. Army Medical Research Institute of Infectious Diseases (USAMRIID) doing vaccine research there and in Southeast Asia. He later became my deputy and joined in a failed attempt to develop a vaccine for Rocky Mountain spotted fever with collaborators at USAMRIID and the NIAID Rocky Mountain Laboratory.

One of my first assignments after my arrival was to serve as Chairman of the Technical Advisory Committee for the Cholera Laboratory in Dhaka, Bangladesh, a U.S. Agency for International Development (USAID)-funded activity in which Dr. Seal had a great interest. There, I met Dr. George Curlin, who had first been sent to Dhaka by Dr. Seal and was now Chief of the Cholera Laboratory's Division of Epidemiology. He joined us as Chief of the new Epidemiology and Biostatistics Branch. Dr. Bill Blackwelder was recruited from the biostatistics program at the University of North Carolina School of Public Health and proved to be a valuable critic and designer of vaccine field trials. He and Dr. Curlin were to spend many months fostering successful trials of acellular pertussis vaccines. Others who joined the Epidemiology and Biostatistics Branch were Dr. Richard Kaslow from CDC and Dr. Alfred Saah from the University of Maryland. They later designed and implemented one of NIAID's first research efforts before the discovery of the human immunodeficiency virus (HIV), the acquired immunodeficiency syndrome (AIDS) virus: The Multicenter AIDS Cohort Study (MACS), a longitudinal study of male homosexuals that continues to provide useful guidelines for vaccine trials.

By reason of my position, I became a liaison attendee at meetings of the CDC Advisory Committee on Immunization Practices (ACIP) and the FDA Vaccines and Related Biological Products Advisory Committee (VRPAC), and became part of an unofficial interagency group concerned with vaccines. One of this group's first activities was to attend open meetings of distraught parents who were convinced that the whole-cell pertussis vaccine then in use had caused their young infants' sudden death or their children's epilepsy. This proved to be the forerunner of a national—indeed international—anti-immunization movement that began with the showing of a television program entitled "DPT-Vaccine Roulette" on April 19, 1982. For pertussis, it accelerated the effort to develop a less reactogenic acellular vaccine. As for the interagency group, there were influential spokesmen like Dr. D. A. Henderson of smallpox fame who called for an expanded and more coordinated national effort to develop vaccines. The Department of Health and Human Services (DHHS) had authorized the creation of an official interagency group in 1980, and its members worked with the legislative staff of DHHS to design the National Vaccine Program and its National Vaccine Advisory Committee later called for by Congress. As we shall see, NIAID is justified in claiming parenthood for this course of events, beginning with Dr. Seal's draft proposal.

In addition to CDC and FDA, my knowledge of the vaccine needs of the military and of children was enhanced by continuing membership on AFEB and as a liaison member of the Committee on Infectious Diseases of the American Academy of Pediatrics. With these contacts and considerable input from MIDP staff, I was prepared to present a paper requested by the Institute of Medicine (IOM) at a conference on pharmaceuticals for developing countries in January 1979. With reference to vaccines, I reported that NIH, CDC, FDA, Army, Navy, and USAID spent only $23 million in fiscal year 1978 on vaccines for 11 domestic diseases and 7 tropical diseases. NIH, mostly NIAID, spent $4.7 million, of which $871,000 was for topical diseases. Clearly, the vaccine effort needed to be expanded.

The American Society for Microbiology's Washington, DC, branch invited me to address its annual banquet in October 1979, and I used the title "Microbes, Parasites and the Health of Nations" to compare life expectancy in the United States with that in the developing world and to describe the new World Health Organization (WHO) program for research in six selected tropical diseases. I concluded with mention of "a new NIAID program that could be expanded if additional funds were available" entitled International Collaboration in Infectious Disease Research (ICIDR). The ICIDR program is a modification and extension of a prior program that supported International Centers for Medical Research (ICMR), whose studies included noninfectious diseases. The ICMR grants expired in May 1980 to be replaced by ICIDR grants, with major portions of the research being conducted overseas in collaboration with international scientists. As a complementary initiative, NIAID provided funds for the establishment of U.S.-based Tropical Disease Research Units (TDRUs). These two related programs were designed and monitored by Dr. Earl Beck, who also supervised the United States-Japan Cooperative Medical Sciences Program. Joint panels of this program, as well as the ICIDR and TDRU, deal with vaccines when appropriate: Cholera, dengue, rabies, encephalitis, tuberculosis, leprosy, and malaria. Dr. Harley Sheffield, a parasitologist, succeeded Dr. Beck. They, like me, have now retired; none can claim much success with the development of vaccines for parasitic diseases.

With a description of my personal background and of the members of the MIDP staff who wrote the early issues of this report, it is time to return to the proposal written by Dr. Seal, the hero of this story. The proposal was prepared for Dr. Richard Krause, NIAID Director, in response to a 1979 call from DHHS for new health research initiatives. Dr. Krause, along with reference to bound volumes of NIAID Advisory Council minutes, has helped me verify the sequence of events before and after Dr. Seal set pencil to paper. Dr. Krause recalls, as do I, that the draft was written in near perfect sequence on a long yellow pad. He particularly recalls how often he referred to the resulting vaccine program when testifying before congressional budget committees.

Dr. Seal and I had discussed vaccines many times over the years, and he was, of course, familiar with the extramural vaccine research being supported by MIDP. Since he had recruited many of the institute's intramural investigators when he was Scientific Director, he also knew of their work on vaccines. He had cleared my manuscript for presentation at the IOM meeting in early 1979 in agreement with the statement that the Federal Government, particularly NIAID, should do more to promote vaccine research and development.

The first mention of the call by DHHS for initiatives for health research appears in the NIAID Advisory Council minutes for January 29-30, 1981. (I elected not to explore DHHS archives.) These are the minutes that included as Attachment XI a copy of the full proposal for the Program for the Accelerated Development of Vaccines submitted to DHHS in September 1980. Curiously, there is no mention of the DHHS request in NIAID Advisory Council minutes for 1979 or 1980. But there were hints that we were at work. A virology task force had been created in the fall of 1976, and its report was reviewed at the January 31-February 1, 1980, meeting. It recommended that the areas to be emphasized and expanded should include live virus vaccines and new and improved inactivated virus vaccines. Earlier, I had worked with MIDP staff and Dr. Seal to prepare a listing of vaccines being developed by NIAID intramural and extramural scientists. This listing was included as Attachment II in the NIAID Advisory Council minutes of October 23-24, 1979. It was the basis for the tables submitted with the NIAID proposal, one of which became the prototype for the tables included in annual reports thereafter.

A copy of the proposal sent by Dr. Krause to the secretary of DHHS in September 1980 was included in the NIAID Advisory Council minutes for January 29-30, 1981. The proposal included Dr. Seal's description of what each agency would contribute, with emphasis on the need for a "different kind of interagency work group." In truth, apart from meeting with the Public Health Service Interagency Group to Monitor Vaccine Development, Production and Usage, the only group that I "coordinated" was the MIDP staff previously noted.

Dr. Seal described the purpose and rationale of the program in the introduction:

> The purpose of a new vaccine development initiative is to develop within the HHS a clearly identified and recognized, coordinated approach to the further conquest of vaccine preventable diseases. New knowledge and technology emerging from basic research provide new opportunities to solve problems that have been largely insoluble with earlier technology and knowledge. The incentive for expanded efforts lies in recombinant DNA and hybridoma technologies and in the better understanding of the workings of the immune system. The new technologies permit radically different approaches to the problems of immunization. The goal of the initiative is to expedite the availability of needed vaccines, and its essence is the selection of a few candidate vaccines for intense effort with additional funding so as to bring these vaccines into use at least several years earlier than might otherwise be so…Efforts also will be made to improve pertussis vaccine by reducing reactogenicity.

To emphasize that progress had been made already in implementing the program, the submission to DHHS included the following:

> The Institute has held discussions with the Institute of Medicine (IOM) and is expecting a proposal from them as one step in implementing this initiative. The IOM

has been invited to undertake the review of potentially vaccine preventable diseases from the standpoint of socioeconomic and medical needs and to assess the cost benefits of vaccines for each of these diseases and the interest of industry in developing each vaccine and the prospective roles of government and the private sector. We expect these studies to get under way in early calendar year 1981 with the diseases listed herein given first priority. Eventually all vaccine preventable diseases will be reviewed in this manner including those where the exposure may only be under special circumstances (e.g., veterinarians, laboratory workers) or in the developing countries.

And speaking directly to the budget, the submission included the following regarding resources:

> The NIAID is proposing the creation of a special fund by FY 1984 that would represent an increase of over $25 million in the NIAID budget between 1981 and 1984. This would be reflected in a total of $25 million for the vaccine initiative under the contracts and agreements area of the FY 1983 budget submission and $30 million in FY 1974. There also would be an item of $12 million for other vaccine development, representing continuing of research and development at present levels of effort for vaccines not included in the initiative. Other participating agencies would also need to increase their efforts and will be requesting specifically identified funds as the projects to be included are identified. The initiative will also require an increase in staffing for the NIAID to manage the program.

Six positions were described. The proposal included three hastily assembled tables listing the status of current vaccine development efforts. Tables 1, 2, and 3 are attached so that the reader may judge the optimism with which staff approached this opportunity to assist investigators to turn 59 antigens into vaccines for 25 diseases.

As for resources, the $25 million plus requested was badly needed. When Dr. Krause arrived in 1975, the NIH budget was $2,108,886,000; the NIAID budget was $119,417,000. Dr. Krause felt that his institute's budget had fallen behind that of certain others, imposing a very restrictive payline, or score, on new research grants. Any requests for new contract proposals from industry would have to be backed up by new funds. Perhaps there was hope. By 1981, the NIH budget request increased by more than $1 billion to $3,569,405,000, and the NIAID budget request was for $232,077,000. But in 1981, $1.62 was required to purchase what $1 bought in 1975.

Since NIAID received no special appropriation of funds for its vaccine initiative, the program staff and contracts office had to apply talent and imagination to "accelerate" vaccine development. This included the wise use of seed money for contracts with industry, and seeking approval of the NIAID Advisory Council to adjust the scores (raise to pay) of meritorious vaccine-related grant proposals. Somehow, vaccine research and development intensified, and the institute's budget shared with all of NIH the admiration and generosity of Congress, particularly after the advent of AIDS.

A year after the proposed initiative for the Program for the Accelerated Development of Vaccines was endorsed by DHHS, it was assumed that the new secretary, Margaret Hechler, would continue to support the program. In the fall of 1981, just as the first cases of AIDS were recognized, the professional staff of MIDP met for 3 days to review the status of its vaccine development program. Each program officer reviewed the diseases and microbes in his or her portfolio, after which a consensus was reached as to those vaccines that should be assigned priority for accelerated development. Following review and discussion of more than 30 agents or groups of agents, excluding influenza, the staff updated three developmental listings: 1) Development completed, ready for expanded clinical trials; 2) encouraging progress made, further development needed; and 3) early development, basic studies in progress. Concurrently, the agents were placed in three categories for phased, sequential study: 1) Diseases for which safe, effective vaccines do not now exist, but that result in high morbidity, mortality, or socioeconomic costs in the U.S. population in general; 2) diseases of importance to special subsets of the U.S. population; and 3) diseases of importance to developing nations.

Next, the diseases were ranked according to priority of need in the United States and developing countries, and then ranked according to technical feasibility and the prospects for accelerated development using new and emerging technology. A consensus was reached as to how these rankings should be integrated. On this basis, MIDP staff assigned priority to 10 agents or agent pairs, 5 for use in the United States and 5 for use in developing countries, as follows:

United States	Developing Countries
1. H. influenzae	1. Malaria
2. Gonococcal	2. Typhoid/Escherichia coli
3. Parainfluenza/Respiratory Syncytial Virus (RSV)	3. Leprosy
4. Pertussis (improved)	4. Streptococcal, group A
5. Rotavirus	5. Shigella

As proposed, in the fall of 1982, the IOM of the National Academy of Sciences was asked to undertake a review of potential vaccine-preventable diseases from the standpoint of socioeconomic and medical needs and for an assessment of the

cost/benefit ratios of vaccines for each of these diseases to assist NIAID in setting priorities for development and to develop for NIAID a new model system for the decisionmaking process that can be applied to the setting of priorities in the future. AIDS was excluded because high priority had been assigned already to development of an HIV vaccine, and the secretary soon announced, with Dr. Robert Gallo at her side, that such a vaccine would be available in 2 years. IOM created a committee of 17 scientists under the chairmanship of Dr. Sam Katz, to be assisted by 6 consultants; a fine IOM staff under study director Dr. Roy Widdus; and liaison members from CDC, FDA, and the Army. The committee developed a method for ranking diseases of domestic importance based on a quantitative model in which vaccine candidates were ranked according to two principal characteristics: Expected health benefits (reduction of morbidity and mortality) and expected net savings of health resources. One vaccine automatically ranked higher on the priority list than another if it produced greater health benefits and greater savings. If a vaccine produced greater benefits but cost more (or produced a smaller savings), then a policy judgment was required to decide whether the additional benefits justified the extra expenditure. The method was applied to 14 diseases of importance in the United States and for which new or improved vaccines were judged technically feasible within the next decade (17).

The same IOM committees assisted by 18 consultants next considered diseases of importance in developing countries. The same method was applied to 29 vaccine candidates for 19 diseases of importance in such countries, where, as before, new or improved vaccines were judged technically feasible within the next decade. The five priority vaccines in each category are listed below with the dates when each study was completed rather than the publication date for comparison with the above MIDP listing of 1981 (18).

United States, 1984	Developing Countries, 1985
Hepatitis B (rDNa)	Malaria
RSV (attenuated/live)	Malaria (sporozoite)
H. influenzae type b (Hib)	Rotavirus (three candidates)
Influenza (attenuated/live)	Typhoid (Ty21a)
Varicella	Shigella

As noted previously, high priority had been assigned already by NIAID to AIDS and improved pertussis vaccines.

Before the two IOM reports were received, the first progress report on the Program for the Accelerated Development of Vaccines prepared by MIDP staff in November 1982 was submitted to the institute's Advisory Council in January 1983. It was Dr. John La Montagne, under whom MIDP became DMID, who named the 1992 annual report for me, and it has continued to flourish under his leadership and that of his successor Dr. Carole Heilman with the editorial guidance of a sequence of staff members: Dr. Gina Rabinovitch, Dr. Phil Baker, Dr. Bruce Gellin, and Dr. Mike Gerber. The current issue has been assembled and edited by our first professional writer, Sarah Landry, to whom I am most grateful.

Because of the thoughtful, sometimes tedious, work of MIDP staff, the annual report became increasingly popular and was distributed well beyond the Advisory Council. Before my retirement in 1987, Dr. Joseph L. Melnick, then Editor of Progress in Medical Virology, asked me to describe the Program for the Accelerated Development of Vaccines as it applied to new viral vaccines. I did so (Progress in Medical Virology, Vol. 35, pp. 1-20, Krager, Basel 1988) in the first publication about the program other than the IOM publications (19). The report remains its own best proponent.

How is it that I am able to write this piece 14 years after I retired at age 70 shortly after Dr. Anthony Fauci succeeded Dr. Krause as Director of NIAID? Dr. Fauci found an emeritus spot for me as a volunteer and housed me along with DMID staff as it more than doubled in size and moved from one satellite building to another. I also kept up with science by serving on an IOM committee created at the request of Dr. Kenneth Bart to review the program of its Board of Science and Technology for International Development for the study of respiratory infections in developing countries.

Dr. Bart next asked me to make a presentation at a symposium he was organizing on vaccines that would not become available in the next decade. The resulting publication reviewed the stages of vaccine development and reproduced tables from each of the two IOM reports that listed vaccines predicted to be available within a decade (20). These are reproduced as Tables 4 and 5. After reviewing impediments to development, I provided a table of diseases for which vaccines are not likely to be available in the next decade. This is reproduced as Table 6. I then served as a part-time consultant to the newly created National Vaccine Program Office (NVPO), first under the directorship of Dr. Anthony Robbins and then Dr. Bart. NVPO staff members at this time included Dr. Roy Widdus, now at WHO in Geneva; Dr. Richard Walker, now at FDA; and Dr. Feng Ying C. Lin, now with the National Institute of Child Health and Human Development (NICHD). USAID was still accepting proposals for vaccine research and needed an unbiased review process. Dr. Bart created the Consultative Group for Vaccine Development (CGVD) with me as the chairman. One of the members was Dr. Gerald Keusch who succeeded me as chairman and is now Director of the Fogarty International Center. Meetings of the CGVD served as a lively forum for discussion of global vaccines until USAID decided to use its funds for other purposes.

I continue as an observer of vaccine-related activities and will complete this summary of the first 20 years of efforts to accelerate vaccine development before considering the accomplishments of the program. As noted, NIAID periodically seeks advice and guidance from consultants. Two such groups were called on before the millennium.

On March 26, 1993, Dr. Fauci convened a blue ribbon panel to assist in assessing long-term goals for vaccine research and to recommend priorities for the area of anticipated resources for fiscal year 1993 and fiscal year 1994. The panel categorized six research objectives, each to be implemented by three to five initiatives, all focused primarily on research to accomplish three priorities:

1. Develop children's vaccines
2. Improve vaccine safety
3. Develop vaccines for emerging infectious diseases

One year later, Dr. Philip R. Lee, then Assistant Secretary for Health and Director of the National Vaccine Program, issued the "U.S. National Vaccine Plan—1994: Disease Prevention Through Vaccine Development and Immunization" (21). It included a summary of the report of the blue ribbon panel as Appendix 6, and a list of licensed vaccines currently distributed in the United States that contained two new vaccines licensed since the NIAID program began in 1981: Hib conjugate and typhoid vaccine live oral Ty21a.

In these same years, IOM and its assembled experts continued to be of great help to the Federal Government by providing objective reviews of adverse events associated with pertussis and rubella vaccines (22), childhood vaccines (23), and a new analysis of the relationship between diphtheria and tetanus toxoids and whole-cell pertussis (DTP) vaccine and nervous system dysfunction (24). A recent report rejected measles vaccines as a cause of autism (25).

In 1995, NIAID commissioned IOM to conduct a followup on the two reports issued 10 years earlier. This report (26) was to consider only vaccines directed against conditions of domestic health importance that could be developed within 20 years, so it began by listing the status of domestic candidate vaccines prioritized in 1985 (Table 4) and predicted to be completed within 10 years. Those licensed included Hib glycoconjugates mentioned above, plus hepatitis B recombinant, hepatitis A, varicella, and acellular pertussis. It was noted that a live-attenuated rotavirus vaccine had been licensed, but sale of this vaccine has been suspended in the United States. Also noted was the fact that a cold-adapted, live-attenuated vaccine for influenza viruses A and B was in phase III trials. These trials have now demonstrated safety and effectiveness in children and adults, and an application for licensure is pending. Of the candidate vaccines for international use listed in Table 5, only typhoid Ty21a and conjugated pneumococcal polysaccharide have been licensed in the United States. One other domestic disease whose infectious agent was discovered in 1981—Lyme disease and Borrelia burgdorferi—can now be added to the licensed vaccines list.

Thus, it is now possible to list in Table 7 the new vaccines (excluding combinations) that have been licensed since the Program for the Accelerated Development of Vaccines was initiated by NIAID 20 years ago.

In total, 12 new vaccines for 10 diseases have been licensed in the last 20 years. One of them, Japanese B encephalitis, is produced in Japan; we claim no credit for it. Another, Hib polysaccharide, has been replaced by the Hib conjugate with dramatic results. The pneumococcal conjugate, based on the Hib technology pioneered by Dr. John Robbins of NICHD, is a more potent immunogen in children and has been effective in preventing otitis media. As for typhoid, trials that compare the two vaccines, or a combination of the two, are needed. It must be acknowledged that Ty21a was produced by the Swiss Serum and Vaccine Institute and tested by Dr. Myron Levine with the support of the Department of Defense. The Vi polysaccharide also was developed at the initiative of Dr. Robbins and is produced by Pasteur Merieux Serum et Vaccine. They have replaced the much more reactogenic whole-cell typhoid vaccine that has been in use since it was made compulsory for the Army and Navy in 1911. And, of course, acellular pertussis antigens have been successfully combined with diphtheria and tetanus toxoids to produce a less reactogenic DTP vaccine. Of the two hepatitis vaccines, recombinant B has been successfully integrated into the childhood schedule while the A vaccine, now mostly limited to world travelers, deserves more widespread use. Use of varicella vaccine is now routine for children and is being evaluated for the prevention of herpes zoster (shingles) in older adults. Finally, Lyme disease vaccines are of note because of the time—8 years—from discovery of the organism by a NIAID scientist to licensure. A fear of the disease in endemic areas that were predominantly well off provided a market. In terms of "acceleration" of the 10 vaccines, I believe NIAID is entitled to claim a major role in the development of at least four: Pneumococcal, Hib, pertussis, and varicella. It certainly can claim the soon-to-be-licensed live-attenuated trivalent influenza vaccine as its own. My personal reflections on the history of some of these vaccines will be reviewed in relevant chapters of this report.

cancer and autoimmune diseases. As before, HIV vaccines were excluded, and this time the new committee, under Dr. Kathleen Stratton as Study Director, elected not to use the computer program of the prior committee, but developed a quantitative model that used as its primary measure a cost-effectiveness ratio of quality of life year (QALY) gained. Vaccines were ranked within four different categories from most favorable to less favorable based on cost of QALY saved. I have elected to reproduce only the highest category here:

Category I   Most Favorable   Saves Money and QALYs

- Cytomegalovirus vaccine administered to 12-year-olds

- Influenza virus vaccine administered to the general population (once per person every 5 years or one-fifth of the population per year)

- Insulin-dependent diabetes mellitus therapeutic vaccine

- Multiple sclerosis therapeutic vaccine

- Rheumatoid arthritis therapeutic vaccine

- Group B streptococcus vaccine to be administered to women during pregnancy and to high-risk adults

- S. pneumoniae vaccine to be given to infants and to 65-year-olds

Those interested in vaccine research, development, and marketing will find it useful to examine the other three categories of the IOM report. A candidate vaccine—B. burgdorferi—in Category IV (less favorable) has been marketed already. An understanding of the role of NIAID initiatives and support described in the chapters of the Jordan Report also should be helpful.

SUMMARY

What remains to be said about a program that began with great expectations and little funding? The program did not live up to Dr. Seal's expectations, to mine, or to those of consultants assembled by IOM. "Acceleration" is a relative term when applied to vaccine development, and expectations were unrealistic. It is hard to develop a vaccine, get it licensed, and move it to the market—consider AIDS, for example. Vaccine development requires patience and persistence on the part of the investigator and continuing support from the funding agencies. As is evident from this history, it requires close collaboration among NIAID, FDA, and industry. Vaccine is international in scope. Acellular pertussis vaccines were successfully tested in Italy and Sweden. Two vaccines to which NIAID contributed much, acellular pertussis and varicella, were pioneered by Japanese scientists. Vaccine development requires communication; neither Dr. Glasso nor I knew that acellular pertussis vaccine was being administered already to Japanese children when we prepared Table 3. The United States-Japan Cooperative Medical Sciences Program did not create panels on acute respiratory infections until several years after I retired. We could be criticized for waiting 2 years before seeking a contractor to produce such a vaccine for the United States.

Fortunately, there is no shortage of talk about vaccines. This, if not licensure, accelerated in the last 20 years. During this time, two private agencies—the National Foundation for Infectious Diseases and the Sabin Vaccine Institute—emerged as champions of vaccine research, development, and use. The International Society for Vaccines was created, faltered, and was revived. There are now many national and international conferences and congresses for the review of promising vaccines. At one such meeting, I heard Dr. Stanley Plotkin deliver the paper that he kindly agreed to include in this edition of the Jordan Report. I am most grateful to him and to the other authors for their thoughtful contributions. While staff members were assembling this report and soliciting these contributions to reflect recent advances in vaccinology and immunology, Dr. Gordon Ada, a long-time friend and contemporary, published the summary that I did not write (27).

Finally, I am happy to report that vaccinology—a term I first heard used by Jonas Salk and one that, I am told, was considered but rejected for the title of the journal Vaccine—is so flourishing that it requires a 7-pound book (28) to record its progress. The Bill & Melinda Gates Foundation has contributed large sums to target the development of AIDS, malaria, and tuberculosis vaccines. Because of AIDS, NIH has a new Vaccine Research Center. The budget has been expanded greatly.

Unfortunately, the infrastructure for vaccine production has not experienced the increased attention that has been given to vaccine development. There were 18 vaccine manufacturers in the United States in 1979; there are only 4 major ones today. Tetanus toxoid, one of the earliest effective vaccines, is in short supply because it is now made by only one company (Aventis Pasteur). Once again, influenza vaccine must be rationed in the fall. In recent years, scientists and administrators have not heeded the lessons of the past; history is now repeating itself because the adenovirus vaccine that once prevented the epidemics of acute respiratory disease peculiar to military recruits is no longer manufactured. Vaccines are the most powerful tools of preventive medicine. Once developed, ways must be found to assure their production and delivery to all U.S. citizens at appropriate ages.

In conclusion, I express my gratitude for the privilege of being taught by and working with outstanding scientists and professional associates. On behalf of DMID/NIAID and the entire vaccine community, I express admiration and thanks for the fine contributions made by Dr. Roy Widdus, Dr. Kathleen Stratton,

and the staff of IOM, and by the members of the many consultant groups assembled by them in fulfillment of NIAID contracts, a process that continues.

END NOTE

Dr. John R. Seal retired on September 30, 1981, shortly after the proposed initiative drafted by him had been accepted by DHHS. He served in the Navy with distinction as a medical officer in World War II and joined NIAID in 1965. His 16 years of service to NIAID consisted of 10 years as Scientific Director and 6 years as Deputy Director. He died in August 1984 and is buried in Arlington National Cemetery. With the concurrence

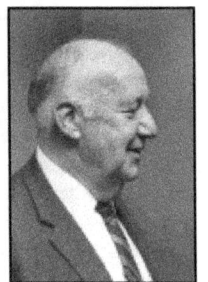

Dr. John R. Seal

of Dr. Carole Heilman, Dr. John La Montagne, and Dr. Anthony Fauci, this issue of the Jordan Report is dedicated to the memory of Dr. John R. Seal.

**Table 1: Development Completed
Ready for Expanded Clinical Trials**

Influenza A and B
    Attenuated (Cold-adapted and ts)
    Licensed, Inactivated

Hepatitis B
    Purified HB_SAg, Inactivated

Varicella
    Attenuated

Rocky Mountain spotted fever
    Inactivated, whole cell

Haemophilus influenzae type b
    Polysaccharide mixed with whole pertussis cells

Note: Tables 1, 2, and 3 are from 1980 proposal to DHHS

References

1 Dingle, J. H., & Fothergill, L. D. (1938). A fatal disease of pigeons caused by the virus of the eastern variety of equine encephalomyelitis. Science, 88, 549-550.

2 Commission on Acute Respiratory Diseases. (1947). Experimental transmission of minor respiratory illness to human volunteers by filter-passing agents. II. Immunity on reinoculation with agents from two types of minor respiratory illness and from primary atypical pneumonia. Journal of Clinical Investigation, 26, 974-982.

Table 4: Vaccines for Domestic Use Predicted by the Institute of Medicine to be Available Within a Decade

Pathogen	Type of Vaccine	Years to Licensure
Bordetella pertussis	Acellular	3-5
Coccidioiodes immitis	Killed spherule	6-7
Cytomegalovirus	Attenuated live	3
	rDNA glycoprotein	7-10
Haemophilus influenzae type b	Conjugated polysaccharide	3
Hepatitis A virus	Attenuated live	4
	Subunit	5
Hepatitis B virus	rDNA	1-2
Herpes simplex viruses 1 and 2	rDNA glycoprotein	5
	Attenuated live	8
Varicella virus	Attenuated live	2
Influenza viruses A and B	Purified hemagglutinating and neutralizing antibodies	4
	Attenuated live	6
Neisseria gonorrhoeae	Unspecified	10
Parainfluenza viruses	Trivalent, subunit	5
Respiratory syncytial virus	rDNA glycoprotein	5
	Attenuated live	5
Rotavirus	Attenuated live bovine	2-3
	Attenuated live human or reassortant	2-4
Streptococcus, group B	Conjugated polysaccharide	7

8 Jordan, W. S., Jr., Pillemer, L., & Dingle, J. H. (1951). The mechanism of hemolysis in cold hemoglobinuria. I. The role of complement and its components in the Doneth-Landesteiner reaction. Journal of Clinical Investigation, 30, 11-21.

9 Dingle, J. H., Badger, G. F., & Jordan, W. S., Jr. (1964). Illness in the home. Cleveland, OH: Press of Western Reserve University.

10 Ginsberg, H. S., Badger, G. F., Dingle, J. H., Jordan, W. S., Jr., & Katz, S. (1955). Etiologic relationship of the RI-67 agent to acute respiratory disease (ARD). Journal of Clinical Investigation, 34, 820-831.

11 Jordan, W. S., Jr., Badger, G. F., & Dingle, J. H. (1958). A study of illness in a group of Cleveland families. XV. The acquisition of adenovirus antibodies in the first five years of life; implications for the use of adenovirus vaccine. New England Journal of Medicine, 258, 1041-1044.

12 Jordan, W. S., Jr., Stevens, D., Katz, S., & Dingle, J. H. (1956). A study of illness in a group of Cleveland families. IX. Recognition of family epidemics of poliomyelitis and pleurodynia during search for respiratory disease viruses. New England Journal of Medicine, 254, 687-691.

13 Chanock, R. M. (1956). Association of a new type of cytopathic myxovirus with infantile croup. Journal of Experimental Medicine, 104, 555-576.

Table 5: Vaccines for International Use Predicted by the
Institute of Medicine to be Available Within a Decade

Pathogen	Vaccine	Years to Licensure
Dengue virus	Attenuated live vector virus	10
Escherichia coli (enterotoxigenic)	Purified antigens Attenuated, engineered	10 10
Japanese encephalitis virus	Cell culture-grown, inactivated	6-8
Mycobacterium leprae	Armadillo-derived 8-10	
Neisseria meningitidis	Conjugated polysaccharides for groups A, C, Y, and W135	4-6
Plasmodium species	P. falciparum synthetic or rDNA sporozoite antigen; P. falciparum, P. vivax, P. ovale, P. malariae	5-8 8-10
Rabies virus	Vero cell-grown, inactivated rDNA glycoprotein Live vector virus with glycoprotein gene	3 3 3
Salmonella typhi	Ty21a mutant Auxotrophic mutant	1 5-8
Shigella species	Plasmid-mediated determinants	10
Streptococcus A	Synthetic M protein	6-8
Streptococcus pneumoniae	Conjugated polysaccharides	5
Vibrio cholerae	Genetically defined live mutant Inactivated antigens	5-7 3-5
Yellow fever virus	Cell culture-grown, attenuated	2-4

14 Jordan, W. S., Jr., Gordan, I., & Dorrance, W. R. (1953). A study of illness in a group of Cleveland families. VII. Transmission of nonbacterial gastroenteritis; evidence for two different etiologic agents. Journal of Experimental Medicine, 98, 461-475.

15 Denny, F. W., Wannamaker, L. W., Brink, W. R., Rammelkamp, C. H., Jr., & Custer, E. A. (1950). Prevention of rheumatic fever. Treatment of the preceding streptococcic infection. Journal of the American Medical Association, 143, 151-153.

16 Gwaltney, J. M., Jr., Handley, J. O., Simon, G., & Jordan, W. S., Jr. (1966). Rhinovirus infections in an industrial population. I. The occurrence of illness. New England Journal of Medicine, 275, 1261-1268.

17 Institute of Medicine. (1985). New vaccines development: Establishing priorities, Vol. 1. Diseases of importance in the United States. Washington, DC: National Academy Press.

18 Institute of Medicine. (1985). New vaccines development: Establishing priorities, Vol. 2. Diseases of importance in developing countries. Washington, DC: National Academy Press.

19 Jordan, W. S., Jr. (1988). Program for the accelerated development of new viral vaccines. Progress in Medical Virology, 35, 1-20.

20 Jordan, W. S., Jr. (1989). Impediments to the development of additional vaccines: vaccines against important diseases which will not be available in the next decade. Rev. Inf. Dis., 11(3), 55603-55612.

21 Department of Health and Human Services/Public Health Service/National Vaccine Program Office. (1994). The U.S. National Vaccine Plan—1994: Disease prevention through vaccine development and immunization.

**Table 6: Examples of Diseases for Which
Vaccines Are Not Likely To Be Available in the Next Decade**

I. Ocular infections
  A. Conjunctivitis
    1. Adenoviruses
    2. Echovirus 70
  B. Blindness
    1. *Chlamydia trachomatis*
    2. *Onchocerca volvulus*
II. Acute respiratory infections
  A. Upper
    1. Coronaviruses
    2. Coxsackieviruses
    3. Rhinoviruses
  B. Lower
    1. *Klebsiella pneumoniae*
    2. *Legionella species*
    3. *Mycoplasma pneumoniae*
III. Gastrointestinal infections
  A. Diarrhea, viral
    Norwalk agent
  B. Diarrhea, bacterial
    Salmonella, nontyphoid
  C. Diarrhea, parasitic
    1. *Entamoeba histolytica*
    2. *Giardia lamblia*
IV. Liver infections
  A. Hepatitis, non-A, non-B
    1. Epidemic type
    2. Posttransfusion type
  B. Schistosomiasis
    1. *Schistosoma mansoni*
    2. *Schistosoma japonicum*

V. Genitourinary tract infections
  A. Sexually transmitted
    1. *Treponema pallidum*
    2. *Chlamydia trachomatis*
    3. *Haemophilus ducreyi*
  B. Other
    Schistosoma haematobium
VI. Nervous system infections
  A. Meningitis, viral
    1. Coxsackieviruses
    2. Echoviruses
  B. Encephalitis
    1. Arboviruses
    2. African trypanosomiasis
      a. *Trypanosoma brucei gambiense*
      b. *Trypanosoma brucei rhodesiense*
VII. Cutaneous infections
  A. Treponema pertenue
  B. Leishmaniasis
    1. *Leishmania tropica*
    2. *Leishmania major*
    3. *Leishmania braziliensis*
    4. *Leishmania mexicana*
VIII. Systemic infections
  A. Leishmaniasis, visceral
    1. *Leishmania donovani*
    2. *Leishmania infantum*
    3. *Leishmania chagasi*
  B. Filiariasis
    1. *Wuchereria bancrofti*
    2. *Brugia malayi*
    3. *Brugia timori*
  C. Epstein-Barr virus

22 Institute of Medicine. (1991). Adverse effects of pertussis and rubella vaccines. Washington, DC: National Academy Press.

23 Institute of Medicine. (1994). Adverse events associated with childhood vaccines: Evidence bearing on causality. Washington, DC: National Academy Press.

24 Institute of Medicine. (1994). DPT vaccine and chronic nervous system dysfunction: A new analysis. Washington, DC: National Academy Press.

25 Institute of Medicine. (2001). Immunization safety review: Measles-mumps-rubella vaccine and autism. Washington, DC: National Academy Press.

26 Institute of Medicine. (2000). Vaccines for the 21st century: A tool for decision making. Washington, DC: National Academy Press.

27 Ada, G. (2001). Vaccines and vaccination. New England Journal of Medicine, 345, 1042-1053.

28 Levine, M. W., Woodrow, G. C., Kaper, J. B., & Cobon, G. S. (Eds.). New generation vaccines (2nd ed.). New York: Marcel Decker.

**Table 7: New Vaccines Licensed
in the United States Since 1981**

Vaccine	Year

Haemophilus influenzae
    a. Hib polysaccharide
    b. Hib conjugate
	1985
	1987

Hepatitis B, recombinant	1986

Typhoid
    a. Live oral Ty21a
    b. Vi polysaccharide
	1989
	1994

Japanese B encephalitis	1992
Hepatitis A, inactivated	1995
Varicella, attenuated	1995
Pertussis, acellular	1996
Rotavirus, live, oral *	1998
Lyme disease, recombinant OspA**	1998
Streptococcus pneumoniae, 7 valent conjugate	2000

License revoked, 2000
** No longer produced*

Note: Hope that live intranasal influenza can be added

Author's Biography

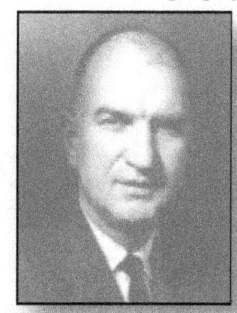

William Jordan, M.D.

Dr. Jordan has had a distinguished career in preventive medicine as a physician, teacher, and researcher in infectious diseases. He devoted his professional life to advancing research on infectious diseases and gave impetus to national and global disease prevention strategies by promoting research into vaccine development.

While at the Department of Preventive Medicine at Western Reserve University, Dr. Jordan played a pivotal role in the landmark Cleveland Family Study, the outcome of which was summarized in the book *Illness in the Home*. He later chaired the Department of Preventive Medicine at the University of Virginia, and the university established the William S. Jordan, Jr. Professorship of Medicine in Epidemiology.

From 1976 to 1987, Dr. Jordan served as Director of the Microbiology and Infectious Diseases Program (now the Division of Microbiology and Infectious Diseases) at the National Institute of Allergy and Infectious Diseases (NIAID) of the National Institutes of Health (NIH). A key part of his mission at NIAID, where he remains active today on a voluntary basis, was stimulating vaccine research. He launched NIAID's Program for the Accelerated Development of Vaccines in 1981 and created an annual report to review progress in vaccine research—now known as *The Jordan Report*.

The Ten Most Important Discoveries in Vaccinology During the Last Two Decades

The Ten Most Important Discoveries in Vaccinology During the Last Two Decades

Stanley A. Plotkin, M.D.

In science, it is particularly difficult to give ratings, as discoveries usually build on related discoveries, and it takes time before the importance of a discovery becomes evident. Nevertheless, it is often useful to look backward as well as forward, as history is a great teacher. This list is based on personal opinion, so there will be disagreement. Also, the names of individual researchers are not included.

ACELLULAR PERTUSSIS VACCINES

The idea of extracting protective antigens from pertussis organisms goes back to the 1960s. Workers in the United States and in Japan succeeded in isolating purified pertussis toxin and filamentous hemagglutinin in the early 1980s. However, acellular vaccines only came into their own in the 1990s.

The success of the acellular vaccines has had several beneficial byproducts. First, substitution of acellular for whole cell vaccines in most developed countries has eliminated the constant irritation of a vaccine that was highly reactogenic, even if permanent sequelae from the vaccine were exceedingly rare. For example, hypotonic hyporesponsive episodes were frightening, causing dissatisfaction with the vaccine despite the absence of sequelae. Second, the results of testing showed that purified antigens could protect vaccinees as well as suspensions of Bordetella bacteria, or more accurately that one could reconstitute protection using defined proteins. Vaccines containing from one to five antigens showed protection compared to placebo, but these data raised a heated controversy, fueled by commercial interests, as to the vaccines' relative importance. It is true that only the five-component vaccine, which contained all the known protective factors, was statistically proven to match the protection afforded by a good whole cell vaccine, but nevertheless, all acellular vaccines were efficacious. Third, the success of acellular vaccines provided a platform for pediatric combination vaccines based on purified pertussis proteins, rather than a mixture of pertussis bacteria.

COMBINATION VACCINES

The second important recent discovery was how to combine pediatric vaccines. It may seem strange to name combinations as a recent discovery, since Ramon combined diphtheria and tetanus toxoids in the 1920s, and diphtheria and tetanus toxoids and whole-cell pertussis (DTP) is itself a combination vaccine. However, more inclusive combinations are a major advance in vaccinology, removing the impediment of multiple injections and making room for newer valences in the pediatric schedule.

Recently, two companies have licensed vaccines containing diphtheria, tetanus, pertussis, Haemophilus influenzae type b (Hib), inactivated poliovirus (IPV), and hepatitis B in Europe. Despite the problem of interference between acellular pertussis and Hib vaccines, these combinations are apparently successful. Another combination, used in Canada, shows no interference problem. It is hoped that all of these combinations will be licensed in the United States.

Combination vaccines have facilitated the resurrection of IPV. The predictable occurrence of vaccine-associated paralytic poliomyelitis (VAPP) cases after oral poliovirus (OPV) vaccine has become a problem, even in developing countries. VAPP can be avoided by using IPV. The inclusion of purified, concentrated IPV in pediatric combination vaccines reduces the costs of vaccine purchase and administration to a significant degree.

VARICELLA VACCINE

Varicella vaccine took 20 years to develop, and finally achieved wide use in the mid 1990s. The licensure of varicella vaccine is significant in two respects. First, it offers control of the last major exanthem of childhood, which although usually self-limited, contributes significantly to life-threatening streptococcal sepsis, encephalitis, and pneumonia. Second, it is the first vaccine licensed for a human herpes group virus, offering prevention or moderation of primary disease and perhaps prevention of reactivated infection in the form of zoster, the virus responsible for shingles.

LIVE INFLUENZA VACCINE

Once again, this is a vaccine with deep roots in history. The idea of using attenuated mutant viruses given intranasally has been around for some time and actually was used in the former Soviet Union and in Japan. However, prior data concerning effectiveness were of poor quality and unconvincing. More recently, the strains developed by cold-adaptation and reassortment have been subjected to more thorough tests, with excellent results.

Trials in children have shown high efficacy, and trials in adults have shown a synergistic effect of live vaccine on immunogenicity of killed virus. The potential of the live vaccine is enormous. Universal vaccination of infants might control the reservoir of influenza in school children, thus offering protection to young siblings and elderly grandparents. If they too receive live vaccine, the grandparents themselves could profit from an augmentation in the efficacy of killed vaccine, which is not always high when the epidemic strain differs from that in the vaccine.

If live vaccine can be produced in sufficient quantity, it offers the best hope of aborting a pandemic caused by a new strain of influenza. Seed strains containing hemagglutinin genes from all 15 types should be prepared and stocked.

ROTAVIRUS VACCINE

It may be surprising to choose what may appear to be a vaccine failure as one of the ten most important recent discoveries in vaccinology. Nevertheless, there are two contradictory reasons for including rotavirus vaccine. First, despite the complication of intussusception, which caused withdrawal of the rotavirus vaccine based on the rhesus monkey strain, the fact is that this oral vaccine was shown to be highly effective against this serious, dehydrating disease. The protection afforded is on the same order as that after repeated natural infection, so it can be anticipated that any replicating rotavirus vaccine will also be protective. Thus, the second generation rotavirus vaccines now in clinical trial based on bovine or human strains are also likely to be efficacious. If that is true, and if they induce no or rare intussusception, the prospects for licensure in developed and developing countries are good. Second, the rotavirus vaccine marks the first occasion since the Cutter incident that a vaccine has been put on the market and then withdrawn because of an adverse reaction. This suggests that perhaps there should be an interval after licensure for data collection before a recommendation is made for universal use of a vaccine in children.

PROTEIN-CONJUGATED BACTERIAL POLYSCCHARIDES

The roots of this discovery go back to pre-World War II, but the exploitation of the immunologic effect of conjugating bacterial polysaccharides with proteins has happened only recently. The 1980s saw the application of this technology to Hib vaccine, with the first conjugate being licensed for infants in 1990. A reminder is not needed of the spectacular success of Hib vaccine, which promises to eradicate the disease and perhaps also the organism.

It appears that spectacular success will also attend the pneumococcal conjugate vaccine. Invasive disease with bacteremia caused by serotypes in the vaccine is likely to be prevented almost completely. Localized disease such as meningitis and pericarditis should also disappear.

Moreover, the vaccine trial revealed high efficacy against pneumonia with consolidation on x-ray, suggesting that pneumococcal pneumonia is more common in childhood than suspected. Application of the vaccine to the developing world could thus have great consequences on mortality, while application to the developed world could reduce the problem of

antibiotic-resistant pneumococci. However, the effect of vaccination on the epidemiology of pneumococcal serotypes and the possibility of replacement by nonvaccine serotypes will have to be watched carefully.

Protein-conjugated meningococcal polysaccharides are still in early stages, but the results with Group C conjugate in the United Kingdom already suggest that a large part of meningococcal meningitis and fulminant disease can be prevented.

GENETIC ENGINEERING

No doubt historians will look back at genetic engineering as one of the greatest discoveries of the 20th century. For vaccinologists, this discovery means that if one isolates the gene coding for a protective protein antigen, that gene can be inserted into cells of bacterial, yeast, or animal origin, which then produce the protein in large quantity. The most important result of this discovery thus far is the recombinant yeast that produces hepatitis B surface antigen, but the same technique has yielded antigens for Lyme disease, pertussis, and cholera vaccines produced in bacteria.

ATTENUATED VECTORS

In the 1980s, researchers determined that certain naturally or artificially attenuated organisms could carry genetic information from pathogens, and that during replication in an animal, they could transcribe, translate, and present that information to the immune system of the host. Thus, the field of vectorology was born. Soon virtually any organism, bacteria, virus, or parasite was suggested as a vector. Among the bacteria, the most popular vectors are Bacillus de Calmette-Guerin (BCG) and attenuated salmonella, whereas among the viruses, attention has been focused on poxviruses, adenoviruses, and alphaviruses, although other agents, such as Herpes simplex, adeno-associated viruses, and even retroviruses, have their advocates.

The study of vectors has evoked the concept of prime-boost. This is because although the vectored antigens have by themselves seldom given a sufficient B-cell response, the serial inoculation of vectors followed by proteins or plasmid DNA vaccines has elicited, respectively, strong B- and T-cell responses.

Poxviruses and alphavirus replicons will serve as illustrations. The poxviruses include vaccinia mutants, such as MVA and NYVAC, as well as naturally attenuated animal poxviruses. Recombinants are prepared from recombination events occurring in cells jointly infected with virus and transfected with the gene of interest. Canarypox is an example of a virus that replicates only abortively in humans. With respect to antibody production, the ability of poxvirus vectors to prime for antibody responses has been demonstrated by canarypox-HIV envelope recombinants, while the ability of poxviruses to stimulate strong cellular immunity has been demonstrated by canarypox-CMV. Alphaviruses as vectors depend on the ability to insert foreign genes in the genome, which are reflected in pseudovirions produced during abortive replication. The genome of the alphaviruses contains nonstructural genes necessary for replication and the structural genes. If the structural genes are replaced by foreign genes, replication of pseudoparticles can be induced by helper constructs containing the structural genes but disabled from making viral RNA. The structural proteins will assemble themselves together with the foreign proteins.

TRANSGENIC PLANTS AND PLANT VIRUSES

The use of orally administered fruits or vegetables containing vaccine antigens might also be considered an example of vectoring. However, the idea of delivering vaccines in the food chain is sufficiently different to give it a place of its own. There are two approaches to making vaccines in plants: Plants transgenic for genes coding for vaccine proteins, or chimeric plant viruses containing the same genes. Clinical trials have shown responses to a variety of antigens produced in plants, including *Escherichia coli* labile toxin, hepatitis B surface antigens, and rabies glycoprotein.

Developments in this field continue to be promising and already have begun to change ideas about the immunology of the gastrointestinal tract. If it can be discovered how to stimulate immunity to the antigens of pathogens without breaking tolerance against food antigens, plant or plant virus recombinants may become effective vaccine strategies.

This will require considerable immunologic effort, but my great hope for the new century is that immunologists will make more contributions to vaccinology. We know little about the mechanisms of antigenic dominance, adjuvants, interference, priming, and many other aspects of immune stimulation that could be used.

NAKED DNA

Naked DNA is the slang term for foreign genetic information inserted into a bacterial plasmid that is expressed on injection into the muscle or skin of the host. Antigen is produced in the muscle cell, but the antigen must be processed in bone marrow cells to achieve an immune response. In animals, superb responses have been generated after intramuscular and gene gun injection, but results in humans have thus far been somewhat disappointing when DNA is used alone.

Whether a DNA vaccine will be licensed depends on the answers to several questions:

1. Will intradermal or transcutaneous administration of DNA result in good antibody responses in humans?

2. Will an adjuvant be found to reduce the amount of DNA needed to obtain responses?

3. Will prime-boost combinations of DNA with other forms of vaccination give a complete immune response, that is, strong cellular responses and antibodies when needed?

The answers to these questions are likely to come earliest from studies of HIV and malaria vaccines.

Even if DNA never achieves the status of a vaccine for a particular infection, it already has had tremendous heuristic value as a tool for identifying protective antigens. As more and more pathogens are sequenced, their genes can be identified and tested for protection in animal models. This will simplify the selection of protective antigens that might have escaped attention otherwise. This strategy has already proven useful for the development of experimental vaccines against Group B meningococci and *Chlamydia pneumoniae*.

THE NEXT 10 YEARS

After looking backward, some predictions about the next decade include:

1. A new rotavirus vaccine will be licensed.

2. A meningococcal B vaccine based on mixtures of outer membrane proteins will be licensed.

3. Influenza will be controlled by the use of killed and live vaccines.

4. An HIV vaccine will show partial efficacy, but efforts to use it will be slowed by social factors.

5. Oral vaccines against enterotoxigenic *E. coli* and Shigella will be available for travelers.

6. Female adolescents will be immunized against some types of papillomavirus, cytomegalovirus, and Herpes simplex type 2.

7. A prophylactic vaccine will be used for those at high genetic risk of at least one chronic disease.

8. The varicella vaccine will be given to adults to modify the severity of herpes zoster.

9. High-risk patients with chronic diseases will be immunized against some nosocomial pathogens, like staphylococci and Pseudomonas.

10. Acellular pertussis vaccine will be recommended for newborn infants and adolescents.

Sources

Belshe, R. B., Gruber, W. C., Mendelman, P. M., et al. (2000). Efficacy of vaccination with live attenuated cold-adapted, trivalent, intranasal virus vaccine against a variant (A/Sydney) not contained in the vaccine. *Journal of Pediatrics, 136,* 168-175.

Black, S., Shinefield, H., Fireman, B., et al. (2000). Efficacy, safety and immunogenicity of heptavalent pneumococcal conjugate vaccine in children. Northern California Kaiser Permanente Vaccine Study Group. *Pediatric Infectious Disease Journal, 19,* 19/87-195.

Excler, J. L., & Plotkin, S. A. (1997). The prime-boost concept applied to HIV preventive vaccines. *AIDS, 11(A),* S127-S137, 1997.

Leitner, W. W., Ying, H., & Restifvo, N. P. (2000). DNA and RNA-based vaccines: Principles, progress and prospects. *Vaccine, 18,* 765-777.

Tacket, C. O., Mason, H. S., Losonsky, G., et al. (1998). Immunogenicity in humans of a recombinant bacterial antigen delivered in a transgenic potato. *Nature Medicine, 4,* 607.

Tubulekas, I., Berglund, P., Fleeton, M., et al. (1997). Alphavirus expression and their use as recombinant vaccines: A minireview. *Gene, 190,* 191-195.

Author's Biography

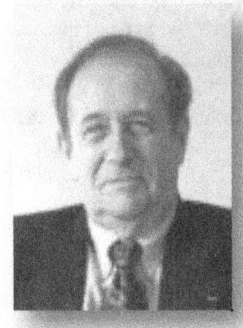

Stanley A. Plotkin, M.D.

Currently Medical and Scientific Advisor to Aventis Pasteur, Dr. Plotkin is the inventor of the rubella vaccine that is now the only one in use in the United States and most of the world. He has worked on other vaccines, including polio, rabies, varicella, acquired immunodeficiency syndrome (AIDS), and cytomegalovirus. While with the Centers for Disease Control and Prevention (CDC), he investigated in 1957 the last known outbreak of inhalation anthrax in the United States, prior to 2001, and helped demonstrate the efficacy of the current anthrax vaccine.

Dr. Plotkin has served as Chairman of the Infectious Diseases Committee and the AIDS Task Force of the American Academy of Pediatrics. He was liaison member of the Advisory Committee on Immunization Practices and Chairman of the Microbiology and Infectious Diseases Research Committee of the National Institutes of Health and holds the title of "Founding Father" of the Pediatric Infectious Diseases Society.

Dr. Plotkin has received the Bruce Medal in Preventive Medicine from the American College of Physicians, the Distinguished Physician Award from the Pediatric Infectious Diseases Society, and the French Legion of Honor Medal.

More than 500 articles are listed on Dr. Plotkin's bibliography, and he has edited several books, including *Vaccines*.

Vaccines and the Vaccine Enterprise: Historic and Contemporary View of a Scientific Initiative of Complex Dimensions

Vaccines and the Vaccine Enterprise: Historic and Contemporary View of a Scientific Initiative of Complex Dimensions

Maurice R. Hilleman, Ph.D., D.Sc.

INTRODUCTION

The modern era biologics enterprise began about 1950 and was built upon knowledge, concept, and technology developed during the previous century and a half. Progress during the entire two centuries of vaccine evolvement came in intermittent spurts that reflected mainly technologic advances, which created new feasibilities for vaccines. The present report is based mainly on the author's knowledge, experiences, and viewpoint gained during nearly six decades of engagement in academia, government, and industry. The focus is on history, technologic advance, and policy matters. (1-5)

BEGINNINGS

The foundations for prevention of diseases by vaccines were laid in the concepts and beliefs of ancient peoples (1, 3) who noted that certain clinically definable diseases were contagious, and that, for some, a first experience imparted immunity against a second exposure. Such observations must have led to the ancient Chinese practice of variolation in which artificial inoculation of pus taken from a patient with smallpox led usually to a modified disease and imparted immunity against subsequent natural exposure. This practice was introduced into England in the early 1700s by Lady Mary Wortley Montagu (2).

A folklore developed during the late 1700s that was based on the observation that mild disease following infection with cowpox of cattle prevented smallpox of man. This led to the practice, by some, of purposeful human inoculation (vaccination) of cowpox pus. The practices of variolation and vaccination led to the first scientific studies of the phenomenon by Edward Jenner in England in 1796 (6). The science of vaccinology was created based on the proofs of principle that were provided by Jenner for smallpox. Manufacture and use of smallpox vaccine spread throughout the world.

NEW APPLICATION OF SCIENCE

The 17th, 18th, and 19th centuries' science (1) was extremely important to vaccine progress since it consisted of a period of transition in which democratic principles gradually replaced the theistic and political structures of the time. During the 17th and 18th centuries, Galileo developed methods for scientific investigation, Hooke discovered cells, and Leeuwenhoek discovered microbes. A trial and error approach in pursuit of logical concepts was followed. Belief in spontaneous generation of life was attacked and the germ theory for disease was substituted. The 19th century to 1875 was marked by realism and materialism,

which replaced the idealism and humanitarianism of the past. Schleiden and Schwann established a cellular basis for living organisms, and studies of altered structure and function of abnormal cells provided the basis for the science of histopathology.

The most important upheaval came with Darwin's theories of evolution and the origin of species. Institutionalized beliefs were replaced by the demand for knowledge that is supported by evidence.

ENLIGHTENED EMPIRICISM 1875-1930

The final quarter of the 19th century was a time of breakthrough discoveries in science and medicine that created whole new fields, including microbiology and applied immunology. The principal architects (1, 3) for the new science were Louis Pasteur, Robert Koch, Emil von Behring, and Paul Ehrlich. Pasteur put an end to the recurring theory of spontaneous generation and conceived of disease as similar to putrefaction and fermentation. This came as a sequel to his discovery of microbial contamination and the spoilage of wine and beer. Following on Koch's technologies for microbial purification and cultivation, Koch and Pasteur proceeded to discover a number of human microbial pathogens and to prepare vaccines against them. Emil von Behring was the discoverer of antibodies who proceeded to develop the field of passive immunotherapy. Ehrlich developed the means for quantifying antibodies and demonstrated differential staining of microbes and tissues with aniline dyes. From this came his concept for specific receptor/ligand binding and his development of the world's first therapeutic drug, salvarsan against syphilis.

The great advances made by these four pioneers and those who followed led to production of vaccines by laboratories around the world. Vaccines and therapeutics created a need for something better than local and haphazard standardization and control. The end of World War I was followed by the formation of the League of Nations and creation of the Permanent Commission on Biological Standardization (7), which developed systems and methods to assure safety and potency of biological preparations.

PREMODERN ERA: TRANSITION, WAR, AND RECOVERY

The period between 1930 and 1950 (1, 3, 4), which included World War II, was a time of transition to the modern era.

Goodpasture's discovery (8) of microbial propagation in embryonated hens' eggs provided an important technologic advance that would lead to new vaccines, including influenza. Use of the new technology of tissue culture propagation of viruses led to Theiler's 17D yellow fever vaccine (9), the first viral vaccine following Pasteur's antirabies immunogen.

The entry of the United States into World War II in the European and Pacific theaters created a great need for new vaccines. A number of pharmaceutical companies with biologics capability became the source for vaccines that needed to be developed and manufactured under military procurement on a cost-plus basis (1, 3, 4). Especially important were the vaccines against epidemic typhus, Japanese B encephalitis, and viral influenza, as well as a six-valent polysaccharide vaccine against pneumococcal disease, which was developed and produced in the laboratories of E. R. Squibb and Sons. The influenza and typhus vaccines were made possible by the breakthrough technology of propagation in embryonated hens' eggs.

During World War II, and continuing through the Korean and Vietnam wars, the principal center for infectious diseases research for all the military services was at the Walter Reed Army Institute of Research located in the Walter Reed Army Medical Center in Washington, DC (1, 3, 4, 10). The Walter Reed laboratories focused heavily on basic and applied research on viral and bacterial diseases. From the program in the Department of Respiratory Diseases (3, 4) came the discovery of the phenomenon and the dynamics of what is now called drift and shift in the antigenic specificity of influenza virus (11), which determines epidemic and pandemic disease occurrence. The first detection and identification of the 1957 pandemic influenza virus was a product of that effort (3, 4, 12). This early alert allowed production of 40 million doses of vaccine before subsidence of the pandemic. The adenoviruses (3, 4, 13) were codiscovered at Walter Reed and at the U.S. National Institutes of Health (NIH). A killed vaccine was developed at Walter Reed and was proven highly effective in field studies at Fort Dix, New Jersey (14). The efforts of the Department of Microbiology at Walter Reed in studies with meningococcal bacterial polysaccharides led to subunit vaccines that came to dominate the modern era of bacterial vaccinology (see below). The advances in viral vaccinology relied on the new technology for cell culture (see below), and the meningococcal vaccine was a continuation of the early work on pneumococcal polysaccharide vaccines pioneered at Squibb during World War II.

MODERN ERA VACCINES

The year 1950 has been chosen as the beginning of the modern era (1, 3, 4) of vaccines since it marks the time of the breakthrough technology of Enders' cell culture propagation of viruses (15) that led to the development of poliovirus and a large number of other vaccines. Several of the large pharmaceutical companies participated in poliovaccine development, made possible by the efforts of the National Foundation for Infantile Paralysis to fund and create a vaccine against poliomyelitis (16).

During the 1960s, the NIH funded contract research with several U.S. pharmaceutical manufacturers to develop new vaccines under an academically directed mission called the Vaccine Development Board. For reasons undisclosed, the initiative developed nothing of significance and was eventually discontinued.

During early 1957, Dr. Vannevar Bush (1, 3, 4), then President of the Carnegie Foundation and Chairman of Merck Sharp and Dohme, conceived the potential importance of viruses to science and medicine. He mandated (1, 3, 4, 10) that a major new virus laboratory for basic and applied research be established within the Merck research complex that would be among the world leaders. Such an essentially freestanding laboratory was built and it was accorded novelty by the granting of strong central authority to the director in return for assumption of total responsibility and accountability. Decisionmaking was rapid and effective. The venture embraced all the basic sciences and disciplines plus engineering development, data analysis, and government liaison. In addition, the responsibility for planning and implementation of clinical research was vested in the department and was carried out principally by partnering (1, 3, 4, 10) with the Children's Hospital of Philadelphia and the Louisiana State University International Center for Medical Research and Training in San Jose, Costa Rica. These research and development operations, working under the single roof concept (17), were highly efficient and effective and led to the pioneering development and licensure of nearly all the new vaccines of the modern era following poliovaccine. The lessons learned may be instructive to future vaccine research endeavors since fragmentation of effort may be inefficient and nonproductive. Important developments included the individual measles, mumps, and rubella vaccines and the combined measles-mumps-rubella (MMR) vaccine (18), plus the plasma derived (19, 20) and recombinant yeast (20) hepatitis B vaccines and killed hepatitis A vaccine (20, 21).

The sum and substance of vaccine developments during the nearly 6 decades of research are listed in Table 1. These vaccines represented pioneering basic research from beginning to end without concern for later developments by others. Nearly all the vaccines encountered hurdles that required major new technologic discoveries to make the vaccines possible. Such hurdles are recorded in detail elsewhere (1, 3, 4), but cogent examples are listed in Table 2.

It is a reality that the period from the mid 1980s to the end of the century was a time of relative quiescence for vaccines (1, 3, 4), marked only by completion of licensure of varicella, conjugated *Haemophilus influenzae*, and hepatitis A vaccines, which had been pioneered before 1985, but entered into the final stages of development later in the century. Vaccines against Lyme disease and against rotaviruses are licensed new products of recent date, but neither has achieved widespread use at present. The current inventory of vaccines licensed in the United States is against about 25 disease entities shown in Table 3.

THE 21ST CENTURY — TRANSITION TO AN UNCERTAIN FUTURE

Science, and with it vaccinology, faces a wave of transition (1) rooted in the late 20th century and is now in need of successes that will assure its favored status at a time of change in national policies and worldwide imperatives. (1)

PUBLIC POLICY

Gibbons, in his recent treatise (22), brings a reminder and a new vision to the contract between science and society in which society itself (the people) makes choices, empowers, and holds accountable in its relationships to government, higher education, and industry. It can impose sanctions if its expectations are not met. The previous contract, which demanded only the creation and imparting of useful knowledge, now has new expectations that include transparency and public participation. The instruments for control lie with congressional legislation, Federal appropriations, and policy affairs.

The great success of the Office of Scientific Research and Development under the direction of Dr. Bush during World War II (1, 23) clearly established the merit of Government support of civilian research to provide technologies and solutions to military problems. After the war and working under a mandate from President Roosevelt, Dr. Bush wrote his 1945 treatise: "Science: The Endless Frontier" (24). The plan became public policy in the late 1940s for continuing public support for basic research discovery, primarily in academia. A basic tenet of Dr. Bush's plan (1, 24) held that science carried out in universities should have a sharp demarcation between what is academic research and what is needed by industry to begin research and development to create useful products.

The era of Dr. Bush's policy came to an end in the mid 1990s at a time of public dissatisfaction with science, and when budgets for science were deeply slashed, with consideration given to ending public support for science (1, 25, 26). This changed quickly, however, with the appearance of a more robust economy. The Ehlers report to Congress (27) in 1998 represented the start of a defined new public policy that has not yet been formalized. The Ehlers report, in contrast to Dr. Bush's policy, called for a new model in which there would be continuum between basic academic research and industrial development, bringing commercial possibilities to the point of feasibility, which would justify commercial commitment of risk capital in pursuit of useful products. In Gibbons' view (22), Government is to be held responsible for filling the gap of required knowledge between basic research and initiation of commercial research and development.

In fulfilling its mission to advise Government, the U.S. National Academy of Sciences has been commissioned to conduct investigations and to provide guidelines for the governmental agencies and for legislative considerations by Congress. Among its reports were proposals to bring about improved mechanisms for review and awarding of grants for scientific research (28, 29), for improving science education (30) at the precollege level (K-12), and for public education. The Committee on Science, Engineering, and Public Policy (31) was established whereby the academy issues an annual assessment for accountability and an evaluation of the federally supported programs in research and technology. (1, 4)

CHANGING WORLD INITIATIVES

The World Health Organization (WHO), an agency of the United Nations, came into being about 1950 and undertook a mission to bring protection against infectious diseases to the underdeveloped nations of the world. Early activity was centered on procurement and distribution of low-cost vaccines through its United Nations International Children's Emergency Fund (UNICEF) operation. In the mid 1970s, the Expanded Program for Immunization (EPI) (1, 32) was created by the WHO to bring six needed vaccines to all of the world's children. In 1990, UNICEF assembled a small group of knowledgeable scientists to create a blueprint for developing simplified vaccines of low cost and ease of administration for the poor and underdeveloped nations. A report was issued under the title of the Declaration of New York (32). The vaccines would provide broad coverage with fewest doses while providing long-term immunity. The declaration was adopted by the International World Summit for Vaccines and by the World Health Assembly in the same year. Following this, the EPI was discontinued and was replaced by the Children's Vaccine Initiative (CVI) under several United Nations' agencies and the Rockefeller Foundation, which were proactive in vaccine development and in vaccination (32). Following a decade of useful programs, the CVI was dissolved and replaced by the Global Alliance for Vaccines and Immunization (GAVI) (33) under the WHO, the World Bank, and UNICEF to provide vaccines, financial resources, country coordination, and research and development activities.

What seemed severe restriction through lack of funding was greatly relieved by donations from the Bill and Melinda Gates Foundation and other private organizations and by contributions from governments (33). One GAVI initiative provides for payment for vaccines by poor nations at prices based on their gross national product per individual. Present principal focus is on vaccines against three diseases: Tuberculosis, malaria, and AIDS (see reference 1).

FUTURE OF VACCINOLOGY

The year 2001 finds the NIH well funded and with further intended increases in annual appropriations until 2003. The NIH provides enthusiastic support for development of new vaccines not only against infectious diseases, but also those for treating cancer, autoimmune diseases, and the amyloidoses, including Alzheimer's disease and the infectious prion diseases (e.g., Creutzfeldt-Jakob), which arise from misfolding of proteins in the body (34) to render them insoluble.

TRANSITION TO SIMPLIFICATION

At the close of the last century, the vaccine research establishment found itself with an amazing array of technologies for preparing vaccine antigens and of facilitators that would enhance the immune system in providing protection against disease. These technologies included recombinant expression systems; recombinant vectors, including plasmid DNA; and delivery systems that elicit humoral and cellular immune responses. The new sciences of genomics, proteomics, and informational technologies, together with rapid throughput assays for identifying appropriate antigens, will likely be a bonanza for new vaccine development (1, 34).

Though whole live and killed organisms and complex protein and polysaccharide vaccines continue to be pursued, subunit vaccines now receive much attention (34). The limitations imposed by the shortened length of genetic insertion into vectors and expression systems decrease the complexity of antigens (the number of epitopes) that can be included.

It has been a long-term objective of reductionists (34) to forget whole organisms and full-length proteins while in pursuit of simple peptide vaccines that consist of little more than a restricted assemblage of epitopes, even without need for added adjuvants and immune modulators. This objective, while attractive, may be very difficult to accomplish since such a vaccine would need to identify and incorporate appropriate B-cell, cytotoxic T-cell, and T-helper determinants. B-cell determinants are usually conformational and need to be displayed in native folded pattern. Cytotoxic T cells and T-helper 1 and 2 cells recognize linear arrays of amino acids of specific sequence. They require, in addition, that the available fragmented epitopes be of sufficient diversity in charge distribution pattern to be able to find adequate anchorage points in the grooves of different major histocompatibility complex (MHC) molecules, which are of polymorphic (allelic) diversity in the human population. Added to this is the need to assure adequate memory cell responses. Delivery of epitopes that are expressed endogenously by recombinant vectors may have a greater chance to find suitable compatibility for MHC presentation than if given exogenously.

It may be noted that the acid test for a successful vaccine is licensure and use. To date, only two recombinant expressed subunit vaccines exist, hepatitis B and Lyme disease, even though the technology was proven 15 years ago. No recombinant vector vaccine has been licensed to date.

When pursuing vaccines in the 21st century, researchers may need to exercise selective choices amid the huge redundancy of technologies (35). It may be said finally that the mandate of the Declaration of New York (32) will serve as a useful guideline for the vaccines of developed as well as underdeveloped nations, especially with respect to possible future vaccine delivery by oral, transcutaneous, or mucosal application.

Table 1: More Than Five Decades of Vaccine and Globulin Development and Dates of Licensure

Viral Vaccines	
Killed	
Japanese B encephalitis*	1945
Pandemic A2 influenza**	1957
Adenovirus**	1958
Purified poliovirus	1960
Purified influenza	1969, 70
Adjuvanted influenza	1973
Hepatitis B	
Plasma derived	1981
Recombinant expression	1986
Hepatitis A	1996
Live	
Measles	
Edmonston B, plus IgG	1963
More attenuated	1968
Mumps	1967
Rubella	1969
Combined vaccines	
Measles – smallpox	1967, 70
Mumps – rubella	1970
Measles – rubella	1971
Measles – mumps	1973
Measles-mumps-rubella	
(MMR) 1971	
Varicella	1995
Marek's disease***	1971, 75
Bacterial Vaccines	
Bacterial Subunit	
Meningococcus A	1974
Meningococcus C	1975
Combined Meningococcus	
A, C	1975
A, C, Y, W-135	1982
Pneumococcus	
14 types	1977
23 types	1983
Haemophilus influenzae	
Conjugate	1989
Immune globulins	
Hepatitis B	1978
Hepatitis A	1979

*Squibb ** Walter Reed *** Virus cancer of chickens
Remaining are Merck

Table 2: Examples of Technologic Breakthroughs Essential to Development of Modern Era Vaccines

- Cell culture technology and poliovaccine precedents

- Elimination of avian leukemia virus from chicken flocks and from measles virus vaccine

- Initial attenuation of measles vaccine virulence through coadministration of measles immune globulin

- Further attenuation of measles virus to eliminate need for immune globulin

- Discovery of propagability and attenuation of rubella virus in duck cell culture

- Achievement of potency and safety of combined live virus vaccines

- Development of safe and effective combined live vaccines

- Discovery of hepatitis A virus and its propagability in cell culture

- Evaluation of principles for a safe and effective hepatitis B vaccine derived from human carrier plasma; later evolution of recombinant expressed vaccine

- Discovery and development of means for removal of oncogenic monkey polyomavirus from vaccines

Table 3: Vaccines Against Bacterial and Viral Disease Agents Licensed in the United States (Abbreviated Generic List)

Bacterial
Diphtheria
Tetanus
Pertussis (acellular)
Botulinum toxin A
Lyme disease (OspA)
Plague
Pneumococcus (and conjugate)*
Meningococcus (and conjugate)*
Haemophilus influenzae (and conjugate)
Tuberculosis [Bacillus de Calmette-Guerin (BCG)]
Typhoid fever (live)
Typhoid fever Vi
Cholera
Anthrax

Viral
Poliovirus (live and killed)
Measles
Mumps
Rubella
Varicella
Yellow fever
Adenovirus
Hepatitis A
Hepatitis B
Influenza
Rabies
Rotavirus (withdrawn)

* Recent licensure. Based on the *Jordan Report 2000*.

References

1 Hilleman, M. R. (in press). Overview of vaccinology in historic and future perspective: The whence and whither of a dynamic science with complex dimensions. In H. Ertl (Ed.), *DNA vaccines.* Georgetown, TX: Landes Bioscience.

2 Plotkin, S. L., & Plotkin, S. A. (1999). A short history of vaccination. In S. L. Plotkin & W. A. Orenstein (Eds.), *Vaccines* (3rd ed., pp. 1-27). Philadelphia: W. B. Saunders.

3 Hilleman, M. R. (2000). Vaccines in historic evolution and perspective: A narrative of vaccine discoveries. *Vaccine, 18,* 1436-1447.

4 Hilleman, M. R. (1999). Personal historical chronicle of six decades of basic and applied research in virology, immunology, and vaccinology. *Immunological Reviews, 170,* 7-27.

5 Castiglioni, A. (1958). *A history of medicine* (2nd ed.). New York: Alfred A. Knopf.

6 Jenner, E. (1798). *An inquiry into the causes and effects of the variolae vaccinae.* London: Low.

7 Hilleman, M. R. (1999). International biological standardization in historic and contemporary perspective. In F. Brown, E. Griffiths, F. Horaud, & G. C. Schild (Eds.), A celebration of 50 years of progress in biological standardization and control at WHO [Special issue]. *Developments in Biological Standardization, 100,* 19-30.

8 Woodruff, A. M., & Goodpasture, E. W. (1931). The susceptibility of the chorioallantoic membrane of chick embryos to
infection with the fowl-pox virus. *American Journal of Pathology, 7,* 209-222.

9 Theiler, M., & Smith, H. H. (1937). The use of yellow fever virus
modified by in vitro cultivation for human immunization. *Journal
of Experimental Medicine, 65,* 787-800.

10 Galambos, L., & Sewell, J. C. (1995). *Networks of innovation.*
New York: Cambridge University Press.

11 Hilleman, M. R., Mason, R. P., & Buescher, E. L. (1950).
Antigenic pattern of strains of influenza A and B. *Proceedings of
the Society for Experimental Biology and Medicine, 75,* 829-
835.

12 Meyer, H. M., Jr., et al. (1957). New antigenic variant in Far
East influenza epidemic. *Proceedings of the Society of Experimental Biology and Medicine, 95,* 609-616.

13 Hilleman, M. R., & Werner, J. H. (1954). Recovery of new
agent from patients with acute respiratory illness. *Proceedings
of the Society of Experimental Biology and Medicine, 85,* 183-
188.

14 Hilleman, M. R., et al. (1956). Prevention of acute respiratory
illness in recruits by adenovirus (RI-APC-ARD) vaccine.
*Proceedings of the Society of Experimental Biology and
Medicine, 92,* 377-383.

15 Enders, J. F., Weller, T. H., & Robbins, F. C. (1949). Cultivation
of the Lansing strain of poliomyelitis virus in cultures of various
embryonic tissues. *Science, 109,* 85-87.

16 Robbins, F. C. (1988). Polio—historical. In S. A. Plotkin & E.
A. Mortimer, Jr. (Eds.), *Vaccines* (pp. 98-114). Philadelphia: W. B.
Saunders.

17 Hilleman, M. R. (1999). The business of science and the
science of business in the quest for an AIDS vaccine. *Vaccine,
17,* 1211-1222.

18 Buynak, E. B., et al. (1969). Combined live measles, mumps,
and rubella virus vaccines. *Journal of the American Medical
Association, 207,* 2259-2262.

19 Hilleman, M. R. (1979). Plasma-derived hepatitis B vaccine—a
breakthrough in preventive medicine. In R. W. Ellis (Ed.),
Hepatitis B vaccines in clinical practice (pp. 17-39). New York:
Marcel Dekker.

20 Hilleman, M. R. (1996). Three decades of hepatitis
vaccinology in historic perspective. A paradigm of successful
pursuits. In S. A. Plotkin, B. Fantini (Eds.), *Vaccinia, vaccination, vaccinology: Jenner, Pasteur and their successors* (pp.
199-209). New York: Elsevier.

21 Hilleman, M. R. (1993). Hepatitis and hepatitis A vaccine: A
glimpse of history. *Journal of Hepatology, 18,* S5-S10.

22 Gibbons, M. (1999). Science's new social contract with
society. *Nature, 402* (Suppl.), C81-C84.

23 Zachary, G. P. (1997). *Endless frontier. Vannevar Bush,
engineer of the American century.* New York: Free Press.

24 Bush, V. (Reprinted 1990). *Science: The endless frontier. A
report to the President on a program for post-war scientific
research, July 1945.* Washington, DC: National Science
Foundation.

25 Press, F. (1992, April 27). *Science and technology policy for a
new era, Presidential address.* Washington, DC: National
Academy of Sciences.

26. U.S. National Academy of Sciences Committee on Criteria for
Federal Support of Research and Development. (1995). *Allocat-
ing Federal funds for science and technology.* Washington, DC:
National Academy Press.

27 *Ehlers report. A report to Congress by the House Committee
in Science. Unlocking our future toward a new national
science policy.* (1998, September 24).

28 Alberts, B. M., et al. (1999). Proposed changes for NIH's
Center for Scientific Review. *Science, 285,* 666-667.

29 Dove, A. (1999). NIH proceeds with overhaul of grant system.
Nature, 5, 1219.

30 President's Committee of Advisors on Science and Technology, Panel on Educational Technology. (1997, March). *Report to
the President on the use of technology to strengthen K-12
education in the United States.* Executive Office of the President
of the United States.

31 U.S. National Academy of Sciences Committee on Science,
Engineering, and Public Policy. (1998). *Observations on the
President's fiscal year 1999 Federal science and technology
budget.* Washington, DC: National Academy Press.

32 Basch, P. F. (1994). *Vaccines and world health. Science,
policy and practice* (pp. 181-199). New York: Oxford University
Press.

33 Nossal, G. J. V. (2000). The global alliance for vaccines and
immunization—A millennial challenge. *Nature Immunology,
1,* 5-8.

34 Hilleman, M. R. (2001). *Overview of the needs and realities for developing new and improved vaccines during the twenty-first century.* Manuscript submitted for publication.

35 Hilleman, M. R. (1998). A simplified vaccinologists' vaccinology and the pursuit of a vaccine against AIDS. *Vaccine, 16,* 778-793.

Author's Biography

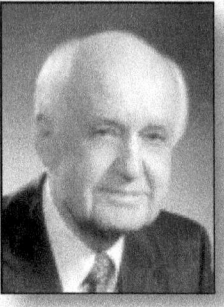

Maurice R. Hilleman, Ph.D., D.Sc.

Dr. Hilleman is Director of the Merck Institute for Vaccinology at Merck & Co., Inc., where he previously held the position of Director and Senior Vice President for the Division of Virus and Cell Biology Research. His 58-year career has been spent in academia, Government, and industry. Dr. Hilleman has served extensively as consultant and advisor to public and private organizations worldwide, particularly relating to policy, education, and disease intervention through vaccines.

He has been recognized for the quality, diversity, and numbers of his basic research discoveries in viruses, vaccines, immunology, and cancer and for his pioneering concepts and achievements in applied research that netted 32 new vaccines.

Dr. Hilleman is author or coauthor of 500 scientific publications. He is an elected member of the U.S. National Academy of Sciences, Institute of Medicine of the Academy, American Philosophical Society, and American Academy of Arts and Sciences.

Dr. Hilleman's most distinctive honors include the Lasker Medical Research Award, National Medal of Science given by President Reagan, Robert Koch Gold Medal (Germany), Maxwell Finland Award, Decoration for Distinguished Service in Scientific Discoveries given by the U.S. Secretary of Defense, and numerous prizes and lifetime achievement awards.

Vaccine Technologies

Vaccine Technologies

Margaret A. Liu, M.D.; Jeffrey B. Ulmer, Ph.D.; and Derek O'Hagan, Ph.D.

INTRODUCTION

Despite the successful development of many vaccines, it has not been feasible in many cases to simply use the same approaches to make new vaccines. This has been due to various factors, biological and social. Three main reasons drive the development of new vaccine technologies:

1. New technologies are needed to generate stronger and broader immunity not effectively induced by earlier types of vaccines.

2. As regulatory and safety standards have increased, the requirements for safety and manufacturing processes have increased, thereby rendering certain older vaccines (such as whole-cell pertussis or Japanese encephalitis vaccine made in mouse brain) less acceptable.

3. To make vaccination more acceptable from the patient's perspective and more feasible globally, new technologies are needed to reduce the use of needles or to facilitate delivery of vaccines to places lacking skilled professionals and proper equipment.

As an example of the need to generate broader immunity, consider the influenza vaccine. The current influenza vaccine must be remade each year because changes in circulating strains render the antibody-inducing inactivated viral vaccine potentially ineffective against the new strains. Mismatches of the circulating strains with the anticipated ones used for the vaccine, or the emergence of unexpected new strains midseason result in disease even in vaccinated individuals. In contrast to the highly changeable exterior hemagglutinin and neuraminidase proteins against which the antibody response of the inactivated vaccine are directed, the internal nucleoprotein and matrix protein are much more highly conserved among strains and even between viral subtypes. If a vaccine could be made that generated a response against conserved parts of the virus [such as a cytotoxic T lymphocyte (CTL) response], one could potentially have a vaccine that would protect against multiple strains within or between subtypes.

Human immunodeficiency virus (HIV) provides another example of the rationale for new technologies. Attenuated or inactivated versions of HIV are considered by many as too risky to use as a vaccine. Unlike other viruses for which vaccines have been effectively made using weakened or inactivated versions, HIV integrates into the infected person's genome leading to permanent infection, and is, as yet, incurable and eventually fatal.

Thus, if a vaccine strain, even though weakened, were to cause disease in an immunocompromised individual or were to revert to virulence, or if an inactivated vaccine were to contain traces of live virus, the vaccine could cause infection and disease. While this rarely happens for certain of the existing vaccines, such as polio, the resulting disease is not chronic, nor so frequently fatal. Even for diseases that are not as lethal as HIV, rare but adverse outcomes have become less accepted. So, for example, after clinical occurrences of intestinal intussusception were observed following immunization with the then newly licensed rotavirus vaccine (with an excess risk of about 1:10,000), the vaccine was withdrawn in 1999.

Ironically, the research and development of new means of vaccine delivery has been necessitated by the success of vaccines. Currently, infants receive multiple immunizations for an increasing number of diseases: Measles, mumps, rubella, diphtheria, tetanus, pertussis, polio, hepatitis B, hemophilus influenzae B, varicella, pneumococcus, and often hepatitis A. This increasing number of injections has fueled the drive to develop combination vaccines and alternative delivery systems designed to reduce the number of injections and to maintain or increase the potency of responses against each component.

VACCINE ADJUVANTS AND DELIVERY SYSTEMS

One approach to improve the performance of vaccines involves the use of a diverse range of vaccine delivery systems. Generally, the terms adjuvants and delivery systems have been used interchangeably in relation to vaccines, although in certain situations a clear distinction can be made. Immunological adjuvants were originally described as substances used in combination with a specific antigen that produced a more robust immune response than the antigen alone. This broad definition encompasses a very wide range of materials, including a number of particulate delivery systems (e.g., emulsions, liposomes, iscoms, and microparticles), whose principal mode of action is to deliver antigens into the key cells and/or sites that are responsible for the induction of immune responses. In contrast, certain entities act directly on cells of the immune system to increase or modulate immune responses against coadministered antigens.

Adjuvants

Adjuvants are potent and, in many cases, necessary components of effective vaccines. Conventional and experimental adjuvants are reviewed in detail by Vogel and Edelman. The power of experimental adjuvants, such as MPL, quil A, and iscoms, is well documented in animal models, yet none are approved for human use. This is due, in part, to potential side effects, but also to a poor understanding of their mechanism of action and to the only recent insights into signaling of the innate immune system. It has long been known that exposure to pathogens (or stress) results in a rapid production (in minutes) of proinflammatory cytokines (e.g., tumor necrosis factor-a), thereby providing a first line of defense prior to the onset of the adaptive immune response. This is manifest through the action of antiviral and antibacterial cytokines, recruitment and activation of macrophages to kill intracellular pathogens, and facilitation of antigen presentation resulting in the initiation of antigen-specific immune responses. Recently, much has been learned about the specific receptors involved in the recognition of pathogen-associated molecular patterns (PAMPs) and the ensuing signal transduction cascade, leading to the upregulation of cytokine expression. Indeed, it has been shown that specific PAMPs signal through specific Toll-like receptors (TLRs) present on the surface of immune cells (see Table 1). Moreover, recent data have implicated this pathway in directing the activation of the type of adaptive immune response [i.e., T helper (Th) 1 versus Th2 type of helper T cell response]. One such PAMP, immunostimulatory CpG-containing DNA derived from invertebrates, has generated much excitement. CpG signals through TLR9, induces a potent immunostimulatory response on cells *in vitro*, and has strong adjuvant effects on protein-based vaccines in animal models. Preliminary data from human clinical trials show promise.

These data provide evidence for a direct link between the innate and adaptive immune responses, and that the use of adjuvants can facilitate and potentiate this link. Furthermore, the growing understanding of the innate immune system now provides the basis for rational and high-throughput adjuvant discovery. On the one hand, based on knowledge of the specific ligands (PAMPs) and receptors (TLRs) involved in immune signal transduction, it may be possible to rationally design adjuvant-active compounds. On the other hand, the existence of cell-based assays and reasonable *in vitro* correlates of *in vivo* adjuvant activity (i.e., cytokine production) offers the possibility of screening large numbers of compounds without regard to their structure. These complementary approaches should yield novel and potent compounds that increase the effectiveness of vaccines. Although immunological adjuvants have persistently defied easy classifications, they are often readily identifiable as components of bacteria and viruses, which are recognized as danger signals by receptors on innate immune cells. Nevertheless, delivery systems are often used to direct the adjuvants to key cells to enhance their potency. Hence, for an optimal adjuvant effect, it is becoming increasingly common to use delivery systems to deliver antigen and adjuvants into the same immunocompetent cells.

Following the discovery of some very potent adjuvants in recent years, there has been concern that these agents might activate

immunity to such an extent that autoimmune conditions might be triggered. This is a reasonable concern for adjuvants that mimic components of pathogenic micro-organisms and provide potent proinflammatory signals. However, the timing and localization of the proinflammatory stimuli may prove to be important. In this context, limiting the systemic distribution of adjuvants and focusing their effects specifically on the key immune cells is likely to be beneficial. Hence, an important contribution of particulate delivery systems may be to limit the toxicity of new-generation adjuvants by limiting their distribution in vivo. Additional practical issues that are important for the development of adjuvants and delivery systems include biodegradability, stability, ease of manufacture, cost, and applicability to a wide range of vaccines. Ideally, for ease of administration and enhanced patient compliance, the adjuvant should allow the vaccine to be administered by a mucosal route, preferably orally.

Delivery Systems

Although the precise mechanisms of action of most adjuvants still remain only partially understood, if the geographical concept of immune reactivity is accepted, in which antigens that do not reach the local lymph nodes do not induce responses, it becomes easier to propose mechanistic interpretations of the important effects of adjuvants, which work primarily as delivery systems. Delivery systems may function to improve antigen access to lymph nodes in a number of ways: Increase cellular infiltration into the injection site so that more cells are present to take up antigen, directly promote the uptake of antigen into antigen presenting cells (APCs) through activating phagocytosis, or directly deliver antigen to the local lymph node by exiting from the injection site and moving into the lymphatics. The most important APCs involved in antigen capture are thought to be dendritic cells (DCs), which have the unique ability to present antigen to naive T cells in lymph nodes. Immunization with a number of delivery systems, including emulsions, microparticles, liposomes, and iscoms, has been shown to result in recruitment of significant numbers of APCs into the injection site, which are then able to take up the delivery system, along with associated antigens and adjuvants, prior to trafficking to the local lymph nodes. Particulate adjuvants (e.g., emulsions, microparticles, iscoms, liposomes, virosomes, and virus-like particles) have comparable dimensions to the pathogens that the immune system evolved to combat. Therefore, these particulates are normally taken up efficiently by phagocytic cells of the innate immune system and function mainly to deliver associated antigen into these cells. Adjuvants may also be included in particulate delivery systems to further enhance the level of response or to focus the response through a desired pathway (e.g., Th1 or Th2).

In 1997, a squalene oil in water microemulsion (MF59) was introduced into the market in Italy as an adjuvant for influenza vaccine (FluadÔ). MF59 has been shown to be safe and well tolerated in a number of clinical trials involving a wide range of experimental vaccines. Liposomal vaccines, based on phospho-lipids and viral membrane proteins from influenza virus (virosomes), also have been on the market in Europe for several years and have shown improved potency over traditional influenza vaccines. Iscoms, which comprise the saponin adjuvant Quil A, incorporated into lipid particles of cholesterol, phospholipids, and viral membrane antigens have been evaluated extensively in preclinical and clinical studies. Although iscoms are considered the optimal approach for the induction of CTL responses using protein antigens in preclinical models, their potency and tolerability remains to be further established in human subjects. In recent years, microparticles constructed from biodegradable polymers have shown considerable promise as antigen delivery systems, particularly for DNA vaccines. Microparticles also offer unique opportunities for the development of single-dose vaccines due to the controlled release of entrapped antigens. However, progress has been slow in this area, largely due to the problems of instability of entrapped antigens and due to inefficiencies of microencapsulation for many antigens.

Antigen Delivery Systems for Mucosal Immunization

Although most vaccines have been traditionally administered by intramuscular or subcutaneous immunization, mucosal administration of vaccines offers a number of important advantages, including easier administration, reduced adverse effects, and the potential for frequent boosting. In addition, local immunization induces mucosal immunity at the sites where many pathogens initially establish infection of hosts. Oral immunization would be particularly advantageous in isolated communities where access to healthcare professionals is difficult. Moreover, mucosal immunization would avoid the potential problem of infection due to the reuse of needles. Several orally administered vaccines, which are based on live-attenuated organisms, including polio, *Vibrio cholerae*, and *Salmonella typhi*, are commercially available. In addition, a wide range of approaches is currently being evaluated for mucosal delivery of vaccines, including many approaches involving nonliving adjuvants and delivery systems.

The most attractive route for mucosal immunization is oral due to the ease and acceptability of administration through this route. However, due to the presence of low acidity in the stomach, an extensive range of digestive enzymes in the intestine, and a protective coating of mucus that limits access to the mucosal epithelium, oral immunization has proven extremely difficult with nonliving antigens. However, novel delivery systems and adjuvants may be used to significantly enhance responses following oral immunization.

Encapsulation of antigens into particulate delivery systems, including liposomes, microparticles, and iscoms, has been extensively evaluated for mucosal delivery of vaccines. How-ever, all of these approaches share some serious limitations. Uptake of the delivery system into the mucosal-associated lymphoid tissue is often very inefficient, resulting in most of the formulation not reaching its intended site of action. This problem is most apparent following oral delivery, necessitating high doses for oral immunization, but is also a problem following intranasal immunization. In addition, many of the particulate delivery systems used do not have sufficient stability to withstand the challenging environment in the gut, including low pH, gastric enzymes, bile salts, etc. Nevertheless, polymeric microparticles can be specifically designed to survive the low pH of the stomach and to release the entrapped antigen within the vicinity of the local lymphoid tissue. Hence, so-called enteric-coated formulations have some attributes of a desirable formulation for oral delivery. The use of enteric-coated formulations can also overcome the problem of limited uptake of particulates into lymphoid tissue since these formulations are not designed for uptake, rather the antigen is released locally for direct uptake. However, most protein and DNA-based vaccines are unlikely to be sufficiently immunogenic to induce potent immune responses even in this situation, and additional formulation components may prove necessary to protect the antigens against enzymatic degradation or to promote uptake. More potent responses may be expected if the antigen can bind directly to the epithelium and carry its own inbuilt adjuvant potential (e.g., secreted bacterial toxins, particularly mutated enterotoxins). Overall, the significant challenges to the development of effective oral vaccines using nonreplicating delivery systems should not be underestimated, and success in smaller animal models using high doses of antigen should not be overinterpreted. As an alternative approach, intranasal immunization offers many advantages, since this route does not expose antigens to the range of secreted enzymes and low pH of the gut and offers easy self-administration with a variety of commercially available devices. Moreover, on many occasions, potent immune responses have been induced in a number of different species following intranasal immunization with particulate delivery systems using doses significantly lower than those used for oral immunization.

Vaccine Delivery Devices

In its broadest sense, the concept of vaccine delivery systems can be expanded to include a diverse range of devices and physical delivery systems that are designed to improve the potency of vaccines or to allow immunization using novel, noninvasive routes. Approaches that have been evaluated in the clinic with encouraging data include the gene-gun approach, which propels gold beads coated with DNA into the epidermis; devices designed to fire powdered vaccines into the skin through the use of helium gas; and vaccine patches, which are topically applied to the skin to induce immunization. Of these approaches, topical immunization is the one that engenders the most excitement since it offers the opportunity to avoid needles while using technology that is already well established for drug delivery. Nevertheless, this approach faces very significant challenges for routine acceptance, particularly as a primary immunization regimen. When this approach was first described, there was a great deal of skepticism about whether or not the data would prove reproducible, largely because the observations were so surprising and contrary to what had been observed previously. However, as this approach has advanced into initial clinical trials, it has become more broadly accepted by the vaccine community. The challenges facing this approach should not be underestimated since, so far, relatively low immune responses have been induced with high doses of potent immunogens. Nevertheless, the technology is still in its early stages of development, and improvements are likely to result in significant increases in potency, perhaps resulting in the ability of this approach to be used as an effective booster vaccine in well-primed individuals.

Gene-Based Vaccines

As the understanding of the cellular and molecular processes involved in the generation of different arms of the immune system increased during the last two decades, new approaches to selectively generate immunity have been attempted. The ability to make recombinant proteins expanded the means to target a single antigen for a vaccine beyond the simple purification of particular proteins or polysaccharides from the pathogen itself. One area of significant effort has been the development of vaccines designed to specifically generate CTL, as well as specific types of helper T cell responses.

CTLs have long been considered to be important in the host's immune response against infections by viruses, intracellular bacteria, and parasites, as well as against cancer. Within the last 20 years or so, it became clear that an antigen generally is needed to be present in the cytoplasm of an APC in order for epitopes derived from it to be able to associate with major histocompatibility complex (MHC) class I molecules to then elicit a CTL response. Conversely, if a protein is exogenous to a cell, it usually is not taken up into this MHC class I processing pathway, and hence does not generally result in the induction of CTL, but rather results in the production of Th cells. This knowledge has helped guide efforts to design vaccines that will generate CTL. For example, efforts have been made to introduce peptides derived from antigens directly onto the MHC class I molecules or to deliver the genes encoding the antigens into the cells in order for the cells to then produce the proteins endogenously in the cytoplasm. Many different delivery systems are thus under development that deliver the genes encoding various antigens, rather than simply delivering the protein antigens themselves.

Infection by live viruses will result in their proteins being made intracellularly as they replicate, often leading to induction of CTL. However, because of concerns about the safety of certain live viruses even if attenuated (*vide supra*, HIV), efforts have

been made to use nonpathogenic organisms to deliver genes encoding heterologous antigens (i.e., encoding protein antigens from a different organism). For example, modified vaccinia or adenoviruses have been altered to carry the genes for various pathogens such as HIV, generally coding for one or a few antigens. An intact replicative HIV could not be made, but simply specific antigens to induce a response that would be potentially protective. Bacteria also have been modified to either encode a heterologous gene [e.g., Bacillus de Calmette-Guerin (BCG)] or to deliver a plasmid encoding a protein antigen. For the latter, attenuated versions of mucosal pathogens such as Shigella or Salmonella offer the possibility of orally delivered vaccines. Such vector systems have the potential limitation of inducing an immune response against themselves, possibly limiting their repeat use for either boosters or other vaccines. Similarly, previous exposure, such as to adenovirus, may mean that many people already have an immune response that may limit the effectiveness of the vaccine.

Thus, another approach has been the use of DNA vaccines, simple plasmids of DNA encoding the desired antigen. The plasmids have the advantages of being simpler to manipulate and manufacture than viral or bacterial vectors and of not having the potential risk of causing disease by reversion or otherwise. In addition, DNA vaccines do not have the same limitation of antivector immunity as do heterologous vector systems. However, DNA vaccines do have the ability to induce the innate immune response that is separate from the encoded protein. The DNA vaccines consist of bacterial (plasmid) DNA and contain sequences that are recognized by mammalian immune systems as being foreign (CpG motifs), which results in the activation of innate immunity. Thus, this is a property that is intrinsic to the gene sequences that make up the DNA vaccine quite separate from the antigen encoded by the vaccine. To date, early clinical trials of DNA vaccines have shown limited potency; hence, a number of second generation DNA vaccines are in development using various delivery systems and devices. In addition, a new approach to immunization, called mixed modality vaccination or prime-boost, is being evaluated. It involves an initial vaccination that uses one type of vaccine, then boosting is done with a different type of vaccine. For example, promising preclinical results have been obtained by immunizing first with DNA then boosting with a vaccinia or adenovirus vector encoding the same antigen, or with a recombinant protein version of the same antigen that the DNA vaccine encoded.

SUMMARY

During the past 20 years, the technologies applied to vaccine development have radically changed from using the pathogen itself to harnessing the developments of a variety of scientific disciplines to use new forms of antigens (such as the gene encoding an antigen), new adjuvants besides alum, and new delivery systems. As a result, numerous vaccines are in development with the goal of inducing new types of or specific forms of immunity, using new routes of delivery, providing increased safety if necessary, increasing stability, and lowering cost. While much remains to be accomplished before some of these technologies become realities, the pace of new vaccine development over the past 20 years has been remarkable.

Suggested Reading

Amara, R. R., et al. (2001). Control of a mucosal challenge and prevention of AIDS by a multiprotein DNA/MVA vaccine. *Science, 292*(5514), 69-74.

Barouch, D. H., et al. (2000). Control of viremia and prevention of clinical AIDS in rhesus monkeys by cytokine-augmented DNA vaccination. *Science, 290*(5491), 486-492.

Barr, I. G, Sjolander, A., & Cox, J. C. (1998). ISCOMs and other saponin based adjuvants. *Advanced Drug Delivery Reviews, 32,* 247-271.

Bendelac, A., & Medzhitov, R. (2002). Adjuvants of immunity: Harnessing innate immunity to promote adaptive immunity. *Journal of Experimental Medicine, 195*(5), F19-F23.

Calarota, S. A., et al. (2001). Gene combination raises broad human immunodeficiency virus-specific cytotoxicity. *Human Gene Therapy, 12*(13), 1623-1637.

Dubensky, T. W., Jr., Liu, M. A., & Ulmer, J. B. (2000). Delivery systems for gene-based vaccines. *Molecular Medicine 6*(9), 723-732.

Edelman, R. (1997). Adjuvants for the future. In M. M. Levine, G. C. Woodrow, J. B. Kaper, & G. S. Cobon (Eds.), *New generation vaccines* (pp. 173-192). New York: Marcel Dekker, Inc.

Krieg, A. M., & Davis, H. L. (2001). Enhancing vaccines with immune stimulatory CpG DNA. *Current Opinion in Molecular Therapeutics, 3*(1), 15-24.

Le, T. P., et al. (2000). Safety, tolerability and humoral immune responses after intramuscular administration of a malaria DNA vaccine to healthy adult volunteers. *Vaccine, 18*(18), 1893-1901.

Levine, M. M., & Dougan, G. (1998). Optimism over vaccines administered via mucosal surfaces. *Lancet, 351,* 1375-1376.

Medina, E., & Guzman, C. A. (2001). Use of live bacterial vaccine vectors for antigen delivery: Potential and limitations. *Vaccine, 19*(13-14), 1573-1580.

Michalek, S. M., O'Hagan, D. T., Gould-Fogerite, S., et al. (1999). Antigen delivery systems: Nonliving microparticles, liposomes, cochleates, and ISCOMS. In P. L. Ogra, J. Mestecky, M. E. Lamm, W. Strober, J. Bienenstrock, & J. R. McGhee (Eds.), *Mucosal immunology* (2nd ed., pp. 759-778). San Diego: Academic Press.

O'Hagan, D., Singh, M., Ugozzoli, M., et al. (2001). Induction of potent immune responses by cationic microparticles with adsorbed HIV DNA vaccines. *Journal of Virology, 75*(19), 9037-9043.

O'Hagan, D. T., MacKichan, M. L., & Singh, M. (2001). Recent developments in adjuvants for vaccines against infectious diseases. *Biomolecular Engineering, 18*(3), 69-85.

Roy, M. J., et al. (2000). Induction of antigen-specific CD8+ T cells, T helper cells, and protective levels of antibody in humans by particle-mediated administration of a hepatitis B virus DNA vaccine. *Vaccine, 19*(7-8), 764-778.

Ulmer, J. B., et al. (1993). Heterologous protection against influenza by injection of DNA encoding a viral protein. *Science, 259*(5102), 1745-1749.

Vogel, F. R., & Powell, M. F. (1995). A compendium of vaccine adjuvants and excipients. In M. F. Powell & M. J. Newman (Eds.), *Vaccine design: The subunit and adjuvant approach* (pp. 141-228). New York: Plenum Press.

Widera, G., et al. (2000). Increased DNA vaccine delivery and immunogenicity by electroporation in vivo. *Journal of Immunology, 164*(9), 4635-4640.

Table 1: Receptor-Mediated Signaling of the Innate Immune System

Pathogen-Associated Molecular Pattern (PAMP)	Toll-Like Receptor (TLR)
Lipopeptides, proteoglycan, yeast cell wall	TLR2
dsRNA	TLR3
Lipopolysaccharide (LPS), heat shock protein (HSP), respiratory syncytial virus (RSV)	TLR4
Bacterial flagellin	TLR5
Zymosan	TLR6
Imiquimod	TLR7
CpG	TLR9

Certain ligands from pathogens (PAMPs) are thought to stimulate the innate immune system through receptor-mediated signal transduction leading to the upregulation of cytokine production.

Author's Biography

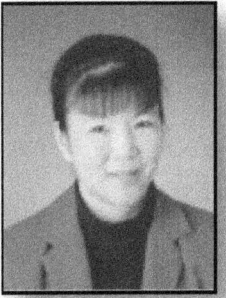

Margaret A. Liu, M.D.

Dr. Liu is Vice Chairman of Transgene and Consultant for the Bill & Melinda Gates Foundation. She also is a member of the National Institute of Allergy and Infectious Diseases (NIAID) Council, the chairman of the Scientific Advisory Group of the International Vaccine Institute in Seoul, a member of the Board of Directors of the American Society of Gene Therapy, and a member of the Science Advisory Board of the Elizabeth Glaser Pediatric AIDS Foundation. Dr. Liu was elected a member of the American Society for Clinical Investigation and a fellow of the Molecular Medicine Society.

For her pioneering work in the area of DNA vaccines, Dr. Liu has received the Rose Lectureship at Columbia University College of Physicians and Surgeons (1993); the Inaugural Saul Krugman Memorial Lecture at New York University (1996); the M. R. Hilleman Lecture at Children's Hospital of Pennsylvania (1997); the Walter F. Enz Memorial Lecture Series at the University of Kansas (1999); and the Oon International Fellowship in Preventive Medicine at Cambridge University, England (2000). In addition, she has spoken in the Karolinska Research Lecture Series at the request of the Nobel committee (2001).

Author's Biography

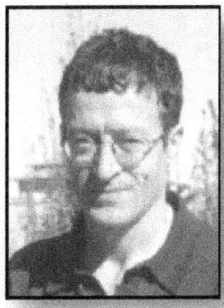

Derek O'Hagan, Ph.D.

Since 1995, Dr. O'Hagan has worked at Chiron Corporation in Emeryville, CA. He is Director of Vaccine Adjuvants and Delivery Systems, a position he has held since 2000.

Dr. O'Hagan has made a number of pioneering contributions in the use of systemic and mucosal delivery systems for a wide range of vaccines, including proteins, peptides, DNA, and protein polysaccharide conjugate vaccines.

Dr. O'Hagan was awarded the Conference Science Medal of the Royal Pharmaceutical Society of Great Britain in 1997 and the Young Investigator Research Achievement Award of the Controlled Release Society in 1999. He is a member of the Board of Scientific Advisors of the Controlled Release Society.

Dr. O'Hagan is on the editorial boards of *Vaccine*, *Pharmaceutical Research*, and *Critical Reviews*[6] *in Therapeutic Drug Carrier Systems*. He has published more than 80 papers, 15 reviews, 12 book chapters, and 2 books. In addition, he has filed more than 25 patents.

Author's Biography

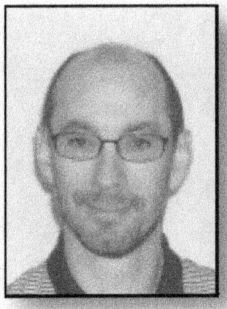

Jeffrey B. Ulmer, Ph.D.

After completing his postdoctoral training in the laboratory of Nobel laureate Dr. George Palade at Yale University School of Medicine, Dr. Ulmer spent 8 years at Merck Research Laboratories where he conducted seminal work on DNA vaccines. Since 1998, Dr. Ulmer has been at Chiron Corporation where he is Senior Director of Vaccines Research and is responsible for protein, DNA, and adjuvant technologies for vaccines.

Dr. Ulmer is on the editorial board of *Expert Opinion on Biological Therapy* and has published more than 100 scientific papers in the fields of biochemistry, cell biology, immunology, and vaccines.

Progress in Immunologic Adjuvant Development: 1982-2002

Progress in Immunologic Adjuvant Development: 1982-2002

Frederick R. Vogel, Ph.D., and Carl R. Alving, Ph.D.

Immunologic adjuvants are any agents that act to enhance, accelerate, modify, or prolong specific immune responses to vaccine antigens. Gel-type adjuvants, first described in the 1920s (1), commonly are prepared from aluminum salts (alum) and remain the only adjuvants in U.S.-licensed vaccine formulations. Adjuvants designed to augment or replace aluminum salts have been undergoing significant preclinical development and clinical evaluation in the past two decades. Many of these new adjuvants have been shown to be more effective than gel-type adjuvants in enhancing antibody and cell-mediated immune responses. These adjuvants can be used to improve the performance of new and existing vaccines by enhancing the immunogenicity of weaker immunogens, such as highly purified or recombinant antigens, or by reducing the amount of antigen or the frequency of booster immunizations needed to provide protective immunity. Some types of novel adjuvants also permit mucosal administration of vaccines by the oral and nasal routes and even transcutaneous delivery.

CLASSIFICATION OF ADJUVANTS

During the past 20 years, numerous natural and synthetic compounds have been evaluated and tested as immunologic adjuvants. Adjuvants have been classified using a variety of classification schemes. Table 1 shows a classification of adjuvants based on physical and chemical properties.

A compendium of vaccine adjuvants and excipients published in 1995 cataloged many of the immunologic adjuvants under development and testing at that time (2). A second edition of this publication is maintained on the NIAID Web site (www.niaid.nih.gov/aidsvaccine/pdf/compendium.pdf). This edition is designed to be a living document into which new adjuvants, results, and contact information can be added.

REFINING THE UNDERSTANDING OF ADJUVANT MECHANISMS

Understanding of the human immune system has advanced significantly during the past 20 years. Adjuvant researchers are applying much of this new knowledge to understanding the mechanisms of adjuvant action. Adjuvants function through three basic mechanisms: 1) Effects on antigen delivery and presentation, 2) induction of immunomodulatory cytokines, and 3) effects on antigen presenting cells (APCs).

Adjuvant Effects on Antigen Delivery and Presentation

The original mechanism of action attributed to adjuvants was the "depot effect" in which gel-type adjuvants or emulsion-based adjuvants (e.g., Freund's adjuvant) associate with antigen and effectively increase its biological and immunologic "half-life" at the site of injection. Although this mechanism does play a role, during the past 20 years this explanation of adjuvant activity has proven too simplistic by itself and has been refined to include the improved delivery of antigen to APCs and to the secondary lymphoid organs. The immunogenicity of synthetic peptides and other soluble antigens that otherwise would be rapidly cleared from the injection site without sufficient delivery to the draining lymph nodes can be improved using gel-type or emulsion-based adjuvants. Particulate adjuvants, such as some liposomes and microspheres, also can protect antigens from proteolytic destruction in the stomach, allowing the antigen to pass into the intestines intact for presentation to the gut-associated lymphoid system. Particulate adjuvants can also target antigen to APCs (macrophages and dendritic cells). Adjuvants such as the cholera toxin B (CT-B) subunit also can deliver antigen to macrophage cells of the gut to induce mucosal immune responses (25) and permit transcutaneous antigen delivery (26).

Adjuvants also function through enhancement of antigen presentation. After phagocytosis by macrophages of exogenous particulate antigen formulations consisting of synthetic beads with surface-conjugated antigen, or liposomes containing encapsulated antigen and lipid A, the antigen is released into the cytoplasm where it is treated as an endogenous antigen. The antigen is then processed through the major histocompatibility complex (MHC) class I presentation pathway, and this can lead to induction of cytotoxic T lymphocytes (27, 28). Ingestion of liposomal lipid A by macrophages can also enhance MHC class II presentation of liposome-encapsulated antigen by macrophages (29).

Induction of Immunomodulatory Cytokines by Adjuvants

Adjuvants also can induce the production of various cytokines and chemokines, which then direct helper lymphocyte subsets or APCs to modulate immune responses. Several cytokines have been used as experimental vaccine adjuvants, including interleukin (IL)-2 and interferon gamma (IFNg). Certain cytokine mixtures, including granulocyte-macrophage colony-stimulating factor (GM-CSF), tumor necrosis factor-alpha (TNF-a), and IL-12 emulsified with incomplete Freund's adjuvant, can serve to steer the immune response in a desired direction (30). The T helper (Th) 1 versus Th2 paradigm, although continually undergoing evolution and refinement, gave adjuvant researchers a reference point to classify the activity of various immunologic adjuvants that act primarily through the induction of immunomodulatory cytokines (31). In mice, adjuvants that enhance Th1-like responses, evidenced by delayed-type hypersensitivity (DTH) reactions, also elicit immunoglobulin (Ig) G2a antibody subclass responses. Adjuvants such as CT, *Escherichia coli* heat-labile toxin (LT), and alum can shift the immune response toward Th2-like responses, predominantly enhancing antibody production, including IgA or IgE. IgE-mediated allergies are associated with

Th2 responses to allergens. The ability of adjuvants to preferentially induce Th1 over Th2 responses or even to "correct" immune responses that have naturally proceeded to the Th2 pathway is a common goal for the development of prophylactic vaccine or for therapeutic vaccines designed to combat allergies.

IL-12 is a recently characterized cytokine that may play a pivotal role in the adjuvant activities of several microbial adjuvants. The adjuvant activity of IL-12 has been demonstrated in a leishmania vaccine in mice. Immunization of BALB/c mice with *Leishmania major* antigens and IL-12 induced Leishmania-specific CD4[+] Th1 cells and conferred protection against infection against *L. major*. Immunization of control animals with antigen alone elicited Th2 responses that were not protective (32).

Table 1: Types of Immunologic Adjuvants

Type of Adjuvant	General Examples	Specific Examples/References
1. Gel-type	Aluminum hydroxide/phosphate ("alum adjuvants") Calcium phosphate	(3) (4)
2. Microbial	Muramyl dipeptide (MDP) Bacterial exotoxins Endotoxin-based adjuvants Bacterial DNA	(5) Cholera toxin (CT), Escherichia coli heat-labile toxin (LT) (6) Monophosphoryl lipid (MPL) A (7) CpG oligonucleotides (8)
3. Particulate	Biodegradable polymer microspheres Immunostimulatory complexes (ISCOMs) Liposomes	(9) (10) (11)
4. Oil-emulsion and surfactant-based adjuvants	Freund's incomplete adjuvant Microfluidized emulsions Saponins	(12)MF59 (13)SAF (14, 15) QS-21 (16)
5. Synthetic	Muramyl peptide derivatives Nonionic block copolymers Polyphosphazene (PCPP) Synthetic polynucleotides	Murabutide (17) Threonyl-MDP (18) L121 (15) (19) Poly A:U, Poly I:C (20)
6. Cytokines	Interleukin (IL)-2, IL-12, granulocyte-macrophage colony-stimulating factor (GM-CSF), interferon gamma (IFNg)	(21, 22)
7. Genetic	Cytokine genes or genes encoding costimulatory molecules delivered as plasmid DNA	IL-12, IL-2, IFNg, CD40L (23, 24)

Adjuvant Effects on APCs

During the past two decades, adjuvant researchers have begun to study the effect of adjuvants on APCs, and in particular the dendritic cell. Dupuis and his coinvestigators demonstrated that fluorescein-labeled gD2 antigen from type 2 herpes simplex virus contained in the emulsion-based adjuvant MF59 was internalized by dendritic cells after intramuscular injection in mice (33). The maturation of dendritic cells bearing antigen is required for optimal presentation of antigen and induction of immune responses through stimulation of T cells (34). Adjuvants that induce dendritic cell maturation enhance immune responses through T-cell activation. Ahonen, et al., demonstrated that a synthetic adjuvant R-848 that previously was shown to induce IL-12 and IFNa secretion induces the maturation of human monocyte-derived dendritic cells. Maturation of dendritic cells was demonstrated through the induction of cell surface expression of CD83 and increased cell surface expression of CD80, CD86, CD40, and human leukocyte antigen (HLA)-DR. R-848 also induced cytokine and chemokine secretion from dendritic cells. R-848 was shown to enhance dendritic cell antigen presenting functions, as measured by increased T-cell proliferation and T-cell cytokine secretion in allogeneic and autologous T-cell systems (35). Understanding the ability of adjuvants to increase antigen uptake and maturation of dendritic cells is critical to the rational design of vaccine adjuvants.

CHANGING TARGETS OF VACCINES

Vaccine targets, requirements, and expectations also have been expanding. This includes therapeutic vaccine targets, including allergy, autoimmunity, and cancer, as well as new preventative vaccines. During this time period, there also has been a marked increase in the number of required and recommended childhood immunizations, with varicella, pneumococcal conjugate, and *Haemophilus influenzae* type b (Hib) conjugate vaccines added to the vaccination series. During the same time, multicomponent acellular pertussis vaccines began to replace whole-cell pertussis vaccine, and an injectable inactivated poliovirus (IPV) vaccine began to replace the live-attenuated oral poliovirus (OPV) vaccine. Therefore, the development of vaccines formulated in combinations is being pursued as a common goal in the vaccine industry to reduce the number of injections required to accomplish the required childhood immunizations. A combination vaccine is defined by the Food and Drug Administration (FDA) as "two or more live organisms, inactivated organisms, or purified antigens combined either by manufacture or mixed immediately before administration (36)." Among the first combination vaccines were diphtheria and tetanus toxoids and whole-cell pertussis (DTP), and trivalent polio vaccines. The desire to develop combination vaccines often requires the reduction of the concentration of antigens that are normally given as single immunizations. The use of adjuvants to provide the dose-sparing effect required for these formulations may be key to the success or failure of this approach.

The past 20 years has seen significant advances in basic immunology, much of which can be applied to the study of adjuvants and their proposed mechanisms of action. Vaccine science is steadily moving away from the empirical approaches by which it was characterized in the past to more rational strategies of vaccine design in terms of dose, route of administration, and presentation. Vaccines that can be administered by means other than percutaneous injection are also under development; oral and transcutaneous immunization are already in preclinical and clinical evaluation.

IMPROVEMENTS IN ADJUVANT SAFETY TESTING

The benefits of incorporating adjuvants into vaccine formulations to enhance immunogenicity must be weighed against the risk of these agents inducing adverse reactions. Local adverse reactions include inflammation at the injection site or, rarely, the induction of granulomas or sterile abscesses. Systemic reactions to adjuvants observed in laboratory animals include malaise, fever, adjuvant arthritis, and anterior chamber uveitis, although retrospective analyses of previous human cohorts, including a large group of soldiers administered an influenza vaccine containing IFA, suggest that such models may not always accurately reflect expected toxicity in humans (37). Such reactions may be due to synergy between biologically active antigens, such as bacterial exotoxins or endotoxins, and the adjuvant. These combinations might promote, through the induction of inflammatory cytokines, reactions that would not be seen with more inert antigens combined with the same adjuvant. Therefore, even though separate and extensive preclinical toxicity studies may have been performed on the adjuvant and the vaccine antigens to be incorporated into a candidate vaccine formulation, a final safety evaluation of the vaccine slated for phase I clinical testing should be conducted. This evaluation should be conducted in a small animal species in which the antigen has been found to be immunogenic and that can be reproducibly immunized via the same route anticipated for use in humans. The dose and frequency of immunization also should meet or exceed those anticipated for use in the clinical trial. Such a test, conducted in rabbits, was designed through a collaborative effort among the Center for Biologics Evaluation and Research, FDA, and NIAID and continues to be evaluated with vaccine formulations containing novel adjuvants (38).

FUTURE ADJUVANT RESEARCH AND DEVELOPMENT

Optimization of the immunogenicity of modern single and combination vaccines constructed of subunit antigens will require the use of a larger array of immunologic adjuvants than the aluminum compounds in today's licensed vaccines. The selection of adjuvants for use in vaccine formulations is important in optimizing vaccine efficacy, improving vaccine compliance, and reducing cost. They should be chosen for use with a particular antigen based on the route of administration and the immune responses desired. Standardized methods currently under development for the evaluation of adjuvant safety should be implemented for testing human candidate vaccines formulated with novel adjuvants. The methods and models adopted for use in the safety evaluation of adjuvanted vaccines must be appropriate for the formulation and the route of administration.

References

1 Glenny, A., Pope, C., Waddington, H., & Wallace, U. (1926). The antigenic value of toxoid precipitated by potassium alum. *Journal of Pathology and Bacteriology, 29,* 31-40.

2 Vogel, F. R., & Powell, M. F. (1995). A compendium of vaccine adjuvants and excipients. In M. F. Powell & M. J. Newman (Eds.), *Vaccine design: The subunit and adjuvant approach* (pp. 141-248). New York: Plenum Press.

3 Aggerbeck, H., & Heron, I. (1995). Adjuvanticity of aluminium hydroxide and calcium phosphate in diphtheria-tetanus vaccines—I. *Vaccine, 13,* 1360-1365.

4 Relyveld, E. H. (1986). Preparation and use of calcium phosphate adsorbed vaccines. *Developments in Biological Standardization, 65,* 131-136.

5 Chedid, L., Audibert, F., & Jolivet, M. (1986). Role of muramyl peptides for the enhancement of synthetic vaccines. *Developments in Biological Standardization, 63,* 133-140.

6 Freytag, L. C., & Clements, J. D. (1999). Bacterial toxins as mucosal adjuvants. *Current Topics in Microbiology and Immunology, 236,* 215-236.

7 Ulrich, J. T., & Myers, K. R. (1995). Monophosphoryl lipid A as an adjuvant. Past experiences and new directions. *Pharmaceutical Biotechnology, 6,* 495-524.

8 Corral, R. S., & Petray, P. B. (2000). CpG DNA as a Th1-promoting adjuvant in immunization against *Trypanosoma cruzi. Vaccine, 19,* 234-242.

9 Gupta, R. K., Chang, A. C., & Siber, G. R. (1998). Biodegradable polymer microspheres as vaccine adjuvants and delivery systems. *Developments in Biological Standardization, 92,* 63-78.

10 Morein, B., & Bengtsson, K. L. (1999). Immunomodulation by iscoms, immune stimulating complexes. *Methods, 19,* 94-102.

11 Wassef, N. M., Alving, C. R., & Richards, R. L. (1994). Liposomes as carriers for vaccines. *Immunomethods, 4,* 217-222.

12 Jensen, F. C., Savary, J. R., Diveley, J. P., & Chang, J. C. (1998). Adjuvant activity of incomplete Freund's adjuvant. *Advanced Drug Delivery Reviews, 32,* 173-186.

13 Ott, G., Barchfeld, G. L., Chernoff, D., Radhakrishnan, R., van Hoogevest, P., & van Nest, G. (1995). MF59. Design and evaluation of a safe and potent adjuvant for human vaccines. *Pharmaceutical Biotechnology, 6,* 277-296.

14 Allison, A. C., & Byars, N. E. (1992). Syntex adjuvant formulation. *Research in Immunology, 143,* 519-525.

15 Allison, A. C. (1999). Squalene and squalane emulsions as adjuvants. *Methods, 19,* 87-93.

16 Kensil, C. R. (1996). Saponins as vaccine adjuvants. *Critical Reviews in Therapeutic Drug Carrier Systems, 13,* 1-55.

17 Lederer, E. (1986). New developments in the field of synthetic muramyl peptides, especially as adjuvants for synthetic vaccines. *Drugs Under Experimental and Clinical Research, 12,* 429-440.

18 Allison, A. C. (1997). Immunological adjuvants and their modes of action. *Archivum Immunologiae et Therapiae Experimentalis (Warszawa), 45,* 141-147.

19 Payne, L. G., Jenkins, S. A., Andrianov, A., & Roberts, B. E. (1995). Water-soluble phosphazene polymers for parenteral and mucosal vaccine delivery. *Pharmaceutical Biotechnology, 6,* 473-493.

20 Johnson, A. G. (1994). Molecular adjuvants and immunomodulators: New approaches to immunization. *Clinical Microbiology Reviews, 7,* 277-289.

21 Banyer, J. L., Hamilton, N. H., Ramshaw, I. A., & Ramsay, A. J. (2000). Cytokines in innate and adaptive immunity. *Reviews in Immunogenetics, 2,* 359-373.

22 Nohria, A., & Rubin, R. H. (1994). Cytokines as potential vaccine adjuvants. *Biotherapy, 7,* 261-269.

23 Kim, J. J., Yang, J., Manson, K. H., & Weiner, D. B. (2001). Modulation of antigen-specific cellular immune responses to DNA vaccination in rhesus macaques through the use of IL-2, IFN-gamma, or IL-4 gene adjuvants. *Vaccine, 19,* 2496-2505.

24 Iwasaki, A., Stiernholm, B. J., Chan, A. K., Berinstein, N. L., & Barber, B. H. (1997). Enhanced CTL responses mediated by plasmid DNA immunogens encoding costimulatory molecules and cytokines. *Journal of Immunology, 158,* 4591-4601.

25 Holmgren, J., Lycke, N., & Czerkinsky, C. (1993). Cholera toxin and cholera B subunit as oral-mucosal adjuvant and antigen vector systems. *Vaccine, 11,* 1179-1184.

26 Scharton-Kersten, T., Yu, J., Vassell, R., O'Hagan, D., Alving, C. R., & Glenn, G. M. (2000). Transcutaneous immunization with bacterial ADP-ribosylating exotoxins, subunits, and unrelated adjuvants. *Infection and Immunity, 68,* 5306-5313.

27 Rock, K. L. (1996). A new foreign policy: MHC class I molecules monitor the outside world. *Immunology Today, 17,* 131-137.

28 Rao, M., & Alving, C. R. (2000). Delivery of lipids and liposomal proteins to the cytoplasm and Golgi of antigen-presenting cells. *Advanced Drug Delivery Reviews, 41,* 171-188.

29 Verma, J. N., Rao, M., Amselem, S., et al. (1992). Adjuvant effects of liposomes containing lipid A: Enhancement of liposomal antigen presentation and recruitment of macrophages. *Infection and Immunity, 60,* 2438-2444.

30 Ahlers, J. D., Dunlop, N., Alling, D. W., Nara, P. L., & Berzofsky, J. A. (1997). Cytokine-in-adjuvant steering of the immune response phenotype to HIV-1 vaccine constructs: Granulocyte-macrophage colony-stimulating factor and TNF-alpha synergize with IL-12 to enhance induction of cytotoxic T lymphocytes. *Journal of Immunology, 158,* 3947-3958.

31 Moingeon, P., Haensler, J., & Lindberg, A. (2001). Towards the rational design of Th1 adjuvants. *Vaccine, 19,* 4363-4372.

32 Scott, P., & Trinchieri, G. IL-12 as an adjuvant for cell-mediated immunity. (1997). *Seminars in Immunology, 9,* 285-291.

33 Dupuis, M., Murphy, T. J., Higgins, D., et al. (1998). Dendritic cells internalize vaccine adjuvant after intramuscular injection. *Cellular Immunology, 186,* 18-27.

34 Banchereau, J., & Steinman, R. M. (1998). Dendritic cells and the control of immunity. *Nature, 392,* 245-252.

35 Ahonen, C. L., Gibson, S. J., Smith, R. M., et al. (1999). Dendritic cell maturation and subsequent enhanced T-cell stimulation induced with the novel synthetic immune response modifier R-848. *Cellular Immunology, 197,* 62-72.

36 Falk, L. A., & Ball, L. K. (2001). Current status and future trends in vaccine regulation — USA. *Vaccine, 19,* 1567-1572.

37 Page, W. F., Norman, J. E., & Benenson, A. S. (1993). Long-term follow-up of army recruits immunized with Freund's incomplete adjuvanted vaccine. *Vaccine Research, 2,* 141-149.

38 Goldenthal, K. L., Cavagnaro, J. A., Alving, C. R., & Vogel, F. R. (1993). Safety evaluation of vaccine adjuvants. National Cooperative Vaccine Development Working Group. *AIDS Research and Human Retroviruses, 9,* S45-S49.

Author's Biography

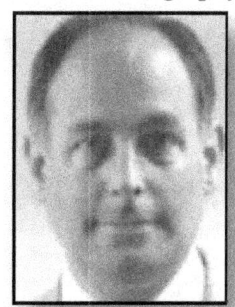

Frederick R. Vogel, Ph.D.

Dr. Vogel is Project Leader at Aventis Pasteur and is based in Marcy L'Etoile, France. From 1999 to 2002, he was Formulation Platform Leader, Product Development, at Aventis Pasteur in Swiftwater, PA.

Prior to joining Aventis Pasteur, Dr. Vogel served as Program Officer in the Division of AIDS, National Institute of Allergy and Infection Diseases (NIAID), in Bethesda, MD. His previous pharmaceutical experience was with Lederle-Praxis Biological, Pearl River, NY, where he was Senior Research Scientist.

Dr. Vogel's primary scientific interest is the study of adjuvants and delivery systems for vaccines. He is a member of the American Society for Microbiology.

Author's Biography

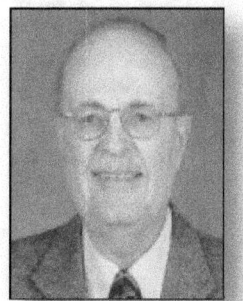

Carl R. Alving, Ph.D.

Dr. Alving has been Research Investigator at Walter Reed Army Institute of Research since 1970 and Chief of the Department of Membrane Biochemistry since 1978. He is also Adjunct Professor of Microbiology and Immunology at Uniformed Services University of the Health Sciences.

He developed the first highly successful application of liposomes as drug carriers—for treatment of leishmaniasis. Dr. Alving is the co-inventor of needle-free transcutaneous immunization, a technology being commercially developed for immunization by skin patch. He has been author or coauthor on more than 200 scientific publications on vaccine adjuvants, lipid biochemistry and immunology, and liposomes as drug carriers and carriers of vaccines, and he sits on numerous editorial boards. Dr. Alving holds 20 issued U.S. patents.

Dr. Alving is a member of the American Association of Immunologists, American Society for Biochemistry and Molecular Biology, and American Society for Microbiology; a founding member of the International Endotoxin Society and International Liposome Society; and a fellow of the American Association for the Advancement of Science. He was the third recipient of the Alec Bangham Award for lifetime contributions to liposome research and was elected Chair of the Fifth Gordon Research Conference on Drug Carriers in Biology and Medicine.

Changes in the Regulations for Vaccine Research and Development

Changes in the Regulations for Vaccine Research and Development

Norman W. Baylor, Ph.D., and Loris D. McVittie, Ph.D.

INTRODUCTION

Over the past 20 years, there have been many new vaccines licensed for use in the United States (Table 1). Although there are general requirements (e.g., good manufacturing practices, labeling, licensing procedures, conduct of clinical trials) codified in the Federal regulations for all biological products, there are no specific minimum standards codified in the regulations for the manufacture and clinical evaluation of any of the vaccines listed in Table 1. The Food and Drug Administration (FDA) is constantly challenged to develop standards for assessing the safety and efficacy of new vaccines under development. Instead of incorporating new standards into the regulations, the license application itself contains all of the standards for each specific new vaccine. The FDA also publishes guidance and other regulatory documents on specific topics to assist manufacturers and clinical investigators in developing new products. Some of these will be discussed in more detail below.

Regulatory History

The regulation of biologics, vaccines in particular, has developed historically around safety concerns. It has been nearly a century since Congress enacted the 1902 Biologics Control Act. This was the first U.S. legislation that regulated the sale and interstate traffic of viruses, serums, toxins, and analogous products. These provisions were revised and codified in Section 351 of the Public Health Service Act (PHS Act) of 1944. This congressional mandate established a regulatory program whereby manufacturers of biological products must be licensed to distribute these products and must provide adequate demonstration that they are pure, potent, and safe for their intended purposes.

The regulation of biologics can be divided into two phases: Premarketing, which consists of the investigational and licensing phase, and postmarketing, which involves surveillance of the product performance after licensure. The PHS Act allows only licensed products to be shipped from one State to another. With the passage of the Kefauver-Harris amendments to the Food, Drug, and Cosmetic Act (FD&C Act) in 1962, the FDA obtained the legal authority to regulate clinical research in the United States when an experimental (investigational) product moves across State or international borders.

The authority to revoke or deny a license on the basis that the product is ineffective or misbranded is not explicit in Section 351 of the PHS Act. However, all biological products, including vaccines, are defined to be drugs. Thus, the FD&C Act also pertains to biological products. Applicable provisions of the FD&C Act containing explicit authority to control the effectiveness and misbranding of all drugs were redelegated in 1972 for use to control the effectiveness and misbranding of biological products.

On July 1, 1972, the Division of Biologics Standards of the National Institute of Allergy and Infectious Diseases, which was charged with administering and enforcing Section 351 of the PHS Act, was transferred by the Secretary of Health, Education and Welfare to the FDA and became the Bureau of Biologics (BoB). This resulted in the transfer of the regulations pertaining to biologics from Part 73 of Chapter I of Title 42 of the *Code of Federal Regulations* (*CFR*) to Chapter I of Title 21 of the *CFR* (1). In 1982, the BoB was renamed the Office of Biologics Research and Review (OBRR) and combined with the Office of Drugs Research and Review to form the Center for Drugs and Biologics. In 1987, the OBRR was renamed the Center for Biologics Evaluation and Research (CBER).

Legal Authority

A single set of basic regulatory criteria applies to vaccines, regardless of the technology used to produce a vaccine. The legal authority for the regulation of vaccines resides in Section 351 of the PHS Act as well as specific sections of the FD&C Act. These statutes are implemented through regulations codified in the *CFR*. The *CFR* contains current regulations of all U.S. Federal agencies. There are 50 titles, and the FDA regulations are found in Title 21. The regulations that specifically apply to vaccines and other biologics are located in 21 *CFR* 600 through 680. Vaccine manufacturers must also comply with current good manufacturing practices written in 21 *CFR* 210 and 211. The *CFR* regulations cover the methods, facilities, and controls to be used for the manufacture, processing, packing, and holding of drugs and biologics to assure that such products meet the requirements of the FD&C Act as to safety and have the identity, strength, quality, and purity characteristics that they are purported to possess. These regulations detail the minimum requirements for the preparation of drug products for administration to humans or animals. Other specific regulations that apply to vaccines and biologics are 21 *CFR* Part 50—protection of human subjects, Part 56—institutional review boards, Part 58—good laboratory practices, Part 201—labeling, and Part 312—investigational new drug applications.

CHANGES TO THE REGULATIONS

The Prescription Drug User Fee Act of 1992 (PDUFA I) enabled the FDA to accelerate its drug and biological evaluation process. This legislation resulted in a commitment by the FDA to perform complete reviews, not necessarily approvals, of regulatory submissions for new or currently marketed products and provide feedback to manufacturers (applicants) within specified timeframes.

The Clinton administration's reinventing Government initiative ordered all Federal agencies to review their regulations and eliminate or revise those that were outdated. As a result of this initiative, the FDA issued a notice of proposed rulemaking in the *Federal Register* of October 13, 1995, for the removal of a number of outdated or unnecessary regulations in 21 *CFR* 100 to 801 (2). The FDA issued a final rule in August 1996 to remove certain biologics regulations that were considered obsolete or no longer necessary to achieve public health goals (3). Among these regulations were the additional standards for bacterial products (including bacterial vaccines), 21 *CFR* 620, and additional standards for viral vaccines, 21 *CFR* 640. Although not all bacterial and viral vaccines were actually covered in the additional standards as written in the regulations, the elimination of the regulations that did exist allowed for a more flexible approach in the development of product specifications without having to adhere to codified standards that quickly become obsolete.

The passage of the FDA Modernization Act of 1997 (FDAMA) focused on reforming the regulation of drugs and biologicals as well as food and cosmetics. The FDAMA reauthorized the PDUFA I and extended it through September 30, 2002. In the past 5 years, the PDUFA II program has further compressed the timeframes by which regulatory submissions are to be reviewed.

The codified initiatives under the FDAMA included measures to modernize the regulation of biological products by bringing them in harmony with the regulations for drugs. This included eliminating the need for establishment license applications. Prior to the FDAMA, a product license application and an establishment license application (ELA) were required to be submitted for review by the FDA. Section 123 of the FDAMA amended Section 351 of the PHS Act to require that a single biologics license be in effect for all biological products in interstate commerce. On October 20, 1999, the final rule "Biological Products Regulated Under Section 351 of the Public Health Service Act; Implementation of the Biologics License; Elimination of the Establishment License and Product License" was published (4). This final rule addressed procedures for handling Biologics License Applications (BLAs) and issuance of biologics licenses for all products subject to licensure under the PHS Act, and amended the licensing regulations in 21 *CFR* 601 to reflect the changes to the licensing requirement of Section 351.

In July 1997, the FDA amended the biologics regulations for reporting changes to an approved application (5). These regulations describe the nature and extent of information that must be submitted to the CBER by manufacturers of licensed products to support changes in product manufacture, testing, or clinical use. The FDA proposed that for reporting purposes, changes to a licensed product be divided into three categories based on the potential of change described to substantially, moderately, or minimally affect product safety, purity, potency, or effectiveness in an adverse way. The "changes to be reported" regulations are found in 21 *CFR* 601.12.

REGULATORY DOCUMENTS

The FDA also publishes guidance documents that do not have the force of law, but provide useful recommendations in specific developing areas of science. Guidance documents can clarify certain sections of the *CFR* or provide expanded discussions of current scientific and regulatory expectations regarding product development. The use of such documents to provide guidance, rather than regulations to enumerate requirements, allows the agency to be more timely, flexible, and responsive to rapidly evolving scientific fields. With the enactment of the PDUFA and FDAMA; significant advances in many areas of immunology, microbiology, virology, and related sciences; and participation of the United States in efforts of the International Conference on Harmonization (ICH) (a joint project between the regulatory authorities of Europe, Japan, and the United States and pharmaceutical industry experts) all leading to an increasingly complex regulatory environment, the number of guidance-containing documents has grown dramatically. Many of these documents are relevant to vaccine development. The following section provides a brief discussion of those documents most often referenced by FDA reviewers in their assessment of regulatory submissions.

The "Points to Consider in the Characterization of Cell Lines Used to Produce Biologicals" (1993) describes basic concepts in cell banking and characterization, including testing for tumorigenicity and adventitious agents. In the years since this document was developed, concerns regarding the possible presence of adventitious agents (which may have arisen from contaminated raw materials or been introduced during the manufacturing process) and the ability to detect these agents have increased. The CBER is currently working to revise and update guidance in this area, which affects cell banks and viral seeds. The ICH also has published "Guidance on Quality of Biotechnological/ Biological Products: Derivation and Characterization of Cell Substrates Used for Production of Biotechnological/Biological Products" (Q5D, 1998), which is generally applicable to many vaccine products not made in primary cell lines.

Additional guidance regarding adventitious viral clearance (i.e., virus removal or inactivation) may be found in "Points to Consider in the Manufacture and Testing of Monoclonal Antibody Products for Human Use" (1997) and in the ICH document "Viral Safety Evaluation of Biotechnology Products Derived From Cell Lines of Human or Animal Origin" (Q5A, 1995). Although the ICH document excludes most vaccines from the scope of its coverage, the concepts discussed are considered generally relevant for many traditional vaccine approaches.

The emphasis by the FDA and ICH on cell and viral issues underscores the importance of thorough, well-documented, scientifically sound testing and characterization from the earliest stages of product development. As always, it is incumbent upon product manufacturers to keep abreast of agency recommendations and requirements to ensure satisfactory product quality and safety and to avoid regulatory hurdles caused by poor decisionmaking and recordkeeping during the development process.

As an example of the need for appropriate product quality control from the onset of product development, consider the concern that has arisen regarding the potential presence of causative agents of transmissible spongiform encephalopathies in products exposed to animal-derived raw materials at any stage of development and manufacture. This concern, albeit remote and theoretical at this time, has prompted not only rigorous prospective qualification of bovine materials, such as serum used for cell culture, but also retrospective searches for documentation of materials used in cell bank and viral seed preparations. Throughout the 1990s, the FDA and CBER sent a series of "Dear Manufacturer" letters cautioning against the use of undocumented or inappropriately sourced bovine materials. Although agency policy is evolving, there has been and continues to be a clear expectation that only appropriate material should be used during all stages of product manufacture. Current information regarding regulatory expectations and scientific concerns may be found on the CBER Web site (http://www.fda.gov/cber).

In addition to the guidance provided in the documents listed above, the CBER's Office of Vaccines Research and Review (OVRR) has sent several letters to sponsors of investigational new drugs (INDs) covering new considerations for testing for adventitious retroviruses [letter of Dec. 14, 1998 (www.fda.gov/cber/ltr/viral121498 htm)] and for characterization of products derived from the Vero cell continuous line [letter of Mar. 12, 2001 (www.fda.gov/cber/ltr/vero031301 htm)]. The use of such letters to convey concerns or make recommendations regarding emerging technologies or scientific issues facilitates the establishment of clearer communication between the agency and sponsors in these complex policy areas.

Another rapidly expanding area of interest is the development of DNA vaccines. The nature of these products dictates that specific preclinical studies be carried out to address issues of integration, biodistribution, and persistence of the vaccine construct in subjects. The "Points to Consider on Plasmid DNA Vaccines for Preventive Infectious Disease Indications" (1996) provides extensive discussion and recommendations regarding these and other relevant issues.

Of great utility for the developers of all new vaccines is the "Guidance for Industry for the Evaluation of Combination Vaccines for Preventable Diseases: Production, Testing and Clinical Studies" (1997). This document provides a concise discussion of many generally applicable principles of vaccine development with regard to performance and documentation of manufacturing and quality control testing, as well as elements of clinical trial design and conduct. Combination vaccines, which are those intended to prevent multiple diseases or a single disease caused by different strains or serotypes of the same organism, have been interpreted to fall under the purview of 21 CFR 610.17, which dictates that licensed products may not be combined with other licensed or unlicensed products unless a license is obtained for the combination. Moreover, according to 21 CFR 601.25(d)(4), each component of the combination must contribute to the claimed effects of the combination and must not interfere with each other's performance. The combination vaccines guidance document discusses special challenges presented in demonstrating the safety and effectiveness of these products, such as the compatibility of active components and potential for immunological interference.

With the implementation of the new BLA to obtain marketing approval, guidance was developed in the "Content and Format of Chemistry, Manufacturing and Controls [CMC] Information and Establishment Description Information for a Vaccine or Related Product" (1999). This document provides a detailed outline of the CMC and establishment sections of the BLA. The CMC section requires descriptions of the method of manufacture, batch records, in-process controls, and product consistency and stability; the guidance document discusses these and other points in detail to assist manufacturers preparing a license application. Similarly, the establishment section, which takes the place of the formerly separate ELA, should contain information regarding specific facility systems (e.g., water and ventilation) and contamination and cleaning issues. It should be noted that many facilities issues will also be addressed during the prelicensure inspection that will be conducted by various agency experts.

Recently, the "Guidance for Industry on Considerations for Reproductive Toxicity Studies for Preventive Vaccines for Infectious Disease Indications" (2000) was developed because of the potential for preventive vaccines to be used in females of childbearing potential as well as pregnant women. While preclinical studies addressing this issue are now expected to be completed during the prelicensure stage of product development, this document also discusses the establishment of pregnancy registries for products in commercial use.

While not specific for vaccines, many other documents published by the ICH are useful in assessing vaccine quality, with regard to manufacturing issues and clinical performance. Documents on stability, assay validation, specifications, preclinical testing, clinical data collection and organization, as well as other topics are available on the CBER Web site (http://www.fda.gov/cber) and may provide helpful guidance to developers of various vaccine products.

Guidance is also available on the many administrative procedures and policies that have arisen from the PDUFA and FDAMA. For example, different types of meetings with the agency are described in "Guidance for Industry on Formal Meetings With Sponsors and Applicants for PDUFA Products" (2000). This document describes the procedures to be followed in requesting a meeting, which were devised to help ensure that meetings can be held in a timely manner with relevant staff in attendance. Additional guidance on the CMC content of meeting packages to be submitted by manufacturers of IND products is available in the document entitled "IND Meetings for Human Drugs and Biologics—Chemistry, Manufacturing, and Controls Information" (2001). Critical guidance for potential license applicants is found in the Refusal to File Guidance, which describes criteria by which a license application may be considered to be so incomplete as to be unreviewable.

FUNCTION OF THE OFFICE OF VACCINES RESEARCH AND REVIEW

The CBER's OVRR is responsible for regulating vaccines and related products produced by manufacturers licensed in the United States. The OVRR is one of six offices established in January 1993 during the reorganization of the CBER. This office is comprised of two laboratory-based divisions (Division of Bacterial, Parasitic and Allergenic Products and Division of Viral Products) as well as a nonlaboratory-based division [Division of Vaccines and Related Products Applications (DVRPA)] comprised of nonlaboratory-based scientists and physicians.

DVRPA has the responsibility for the initial receipt and administrative processing of biological INDs and BLAs for vaccines and related products submitted by the regulated industry. This division has the responsibility along with the laboratory-based research divisions for the review of viral, bacterial, rickettsial, and parasitic vaccines, toxins, toxoids, diagnostic substances for dermal tests, venoms, and allergenic extracts. The review process in the OVRR begins with an initial review by multidisciplinary review teams consisting of microbiologists, virologists, immunologists, toxicologists, statisticians, physicians, and consumer safety officers for scientific content and compliance with the regulations. Reviewers are selected on the basis of their expertise with the type of product, its method of manufacture, and clinical indication.

Approval of a new vaccine application or supplement (applications are submitted for new products, whereas supplements to those applications must be submitted when significant manufacturing, facility, or equipment changes are made to the product, or a new indication is sought) involves the satisfactory review of all manufacturing and clinical data, a review of protocols for manufacturing and testing, the results of confirmatory testing within the OVRR, and a prelicensing inspection by product experts in the OVRR and good manufacturing practice

experts from the CBER's Division of Manufacturing and Product Quality. In addition, the preapproval process usually involves a review and discussion of applications by the OVRR's Vaccines and Related Biological Products Advisory Committee prior to approval.

SUMMARY

There are hundreds of vaccines in clinical trials throughout the world. Many of these investigational vaccines contain novel adjuvants, some are DNA vaccines, and others are recombinant subunit vaccines. The FDA has the difficult charge of regulating these vaccines to assure they are safe and efficacious. It continues to face new challenges, dealing with such safety concerns as the use of novel cell substrates and the evaluation of these cell substrates for known and unknown adventitious agents. The FDA's regulations and guidance documents will continue to evolve in response to new technologies.

Table 1: Vaccines Licensed in the United States Between 1981 and 2001

Date	Vaccine
1981-1990	Meningococcal A, C, Y, W-135 vaccines
	Hepatitis B vaccine
	Pneumococcal polyvalent 23 vaccine
	Haemophilus influenzae type b (Hib) polysaccharide vaccine
	Hib conjugate vaccine
	Typhoid live oral Ty21A vaccine
1991-2001	Diphtheria and tetanus toxoids and acellular pertussis (DTaP) vaccine
	Japanese encephalitis vaccine
	Diphtheria and tetanus toxoids and whole-cell pertussis (DTP)-Hib conjugate combination vaccine
	DTaP-Hib conjugate combination vaccine
	Hepatitis A vaccine
	Typhoid polysaccharide vaccine
	Varicella vaccine
	Hib conjugate-hepatitis B combination vaccine
	Rotavirus vaccine
	Lyme vaccine
	Pneumococcal conjugate vaccine

References

1 *Federal Register*, Volume 37, Number 154, p. 12865.

2 *Federal Register*, Volume 60, Number 198, p. 53480.

3 *Federal Register*, Volume 61, Number 149, p. 40153.

4 *Federal Register*, Volume 64, Number 202, p. 56441.

5 *Federal Register*, Volume 62, Number 142, p. 39890.

Guidance Documents

"Points to Consider in the Characterization of Cell Lines Used to Produce Biologicals" (1993)

"Guidance on Quality of Biotechnological/Biological Products: Derivation and

Characterization of Cell Substrates Used for Production of Biotechnological/Biological Products" (Q5D, 1998)

"Points to Consider in the Manufacture and Testing of Monoclonal Antibody Products for Human Use" (1997)

"Viral Safety Evaluation of Biotechnology Products Derived From Cell Lines of Human or Animal Origin" (Q5A, 1995)

"Points to Consider on Plasmid DNA Vaccines for Preventive Infectious Disease Indications" (1996)

"Guidance for Industry for the Evaluation of Combination Vaccines for Preventable Diseases: Production, Testing and Clinical Studies" (1997)

"Content and Format of Chemistry, Manufacturing and Controls Information and Establishment Description Information for a Vaccine or Related Product" (1999)

"Guidance for Industry on Considerations for Reproductive Toxicity Studies for Preventive Vaccines for Infectious Disease Indications" (2000)

"Guidance for Industry on Formal Meetings With Sponsors and Applicants for PDUFA Products" (2000)

"IND Meetings for Human Drugs and Biologics—Chemistry, Manufacturing, and Controls Information" (2001)

Author's Biography

Dr. Baylor is Associate Director for Regulatory Policy in the Office of Vaccines Research and Review, Center for Biologics Evaluation and Research (CBER), Food and Drug Administration (FDA). After his postdoctoral training, Dr. Baylor joined Program Resources Incorporated as a Senior Research Scientist at the National Cancer Institute-Frederick Cancer Research Facility (NCI-FCRF). His research at NCI-FCRF included the study of transcriptional regulation of human T-cell leukemia virus (HTLV-I). Dr. Baylor joined the Office of Vaccines Research and Review, CBER, FDA, as a scientific reviewer in 1991. He served as Acting Deputy Director of the Division of Vaccines and Related Applications, as well as Acting Deputy Director of the Office of Vaccines Research and Review. Dr. Baylor has been in his current position since 1994, and also serves as FDA's liaison to the Advisory Commission for Childhood Vaccines.

Author's Biography

Dr. McVittie is Chief of the Viral Vaccines Branch, Division of Vaccines and Related Products Applications, Office of Vaccines Research and Review, Center for Biologics Evaluation and Research (CBER), Food and Drug Administration (FDA). She joined CBER in 1990 as a scientific reviewer in the Division of Biological Investigational New Drugs. Dr. McVittie also has served recently as Acting Deputy Director of the Division of Viral Products, Office of Vaccines Research and Review, CBER.

Vaccine Efficacy
and Safety Evaluation

Vaccine Efficacy and Safety Evaluation

Mary A. Foulkes, Ph.D., and Susan S. Ellenberg, Ph.D.

Benefit-to-risk considerations are needed to support informed public health policy decisions and personal choices regarding vaccinations. Such considerations require that the efficacy and the safety profile be evaluated thoroughly for any given vaccine. From this perspective, we discuss the continuing process of vaccine development and evaluation through to widespread public use.

VACCINE DEVELOPMENT

Vaccine efficacy has long been defined as the reduction in the infection rate attributable to the vaccine (1, 2). It is sometimes estimated as prevention of disease after deliberate exposure in challenge studies, or by induction of immunogenicity when a specific immune response measured serologically has been shown to be adequate to prevent infection. Efficacy, whether measured directly as prevention of the targeted disease or indirectly by measuring immune response, is generally evaluated in prospective, randomized controlled trials. Double-blind trials with placebo controls are often necessary to minimize bias in patient recruitment and assignment and in evaluation of outcomes.

Initial testing of new vaccines involves measuring immune responses in phase I and II trials. Immunogenicity is a measure of the ability of the vaccine to elicit the desired or intended immunologic response. Antibody titers provide a measure of an individual subject's direct response to the vaccine, and in principle, should indicate whether that subject is likely to be protected from the disease in question. Additionally, safety assessments, primarily evaluation of local and systemic reactions, are very important in establishing a rationale for future development. Often, multiple doses are evaluated to arrive at an optimal dose for further investigation. Similarly, multiple routes of delivery can be evaluated (e.g., injection; tablet; inhalation; or edible products such as potatoes, bananas, or tomatoes). This information can provide an initial, relatively imprecise measure of risk/benefit ratio.

Phase III trials to assess efficacy are conducted after early phase trials establish preliminary evidence of the vaccine's safety and immunogenicity. The appropriate size of phase III vaccine trials depends upon a variety of factors, including the primary outcome measure, the disease rate in the absence of vaccination, the minimum effect size of interest, and the acceptable error rates (a and b). Sample sizes needed to study efficacy based on levels of immune response are usually much smaller than those needed to evaluate prevention of clinical disease, and vaccines to prevent common diseases can be evaluated in smaller trials than

vaccines to prevent rare diseases. For example, the efficacy of varicella vaccine was clearly established in a clinical trial that included less than 1,000 subjects; on the other hand, the World Health Organization Vaccine Trial Registry includes numerous phase III efficacy trials of cholera, *Haemophilus influenzae* type B (Hib) meningitis, and pneumococcal vaccines enrolling tens of thousands of subjects. The first randomized vaccine trial, the Francis field trial of the Salk polio vaccine, required nearly half a million children in order to reliably assess the vaccine's efficacy (3).

If the focus of a vaccine trial includes not only efficacy but also safety with respect to a specific adverse event, additional factors to consider in determining sample size would be the rate of that adverse event in the absence of vaccination, and the magnitude of the difference in the event rate between the vaccinated and nonvaccinated groups that one would wish to detect. Due to the association of intussusception with rhesus rotavirus vaccine (4), for example, trials of new rotavirus vaccine candidates will have to focus on the rate of intussusception as well as on the usual measures of vaccine efficacy. When the rate of a relatively rare adverse event determines the sample size, the trial may be considerably larger than trials designed with vaccine efficacy as the sole driving focus.

As with all new pharmaceutical products, evaluation of safety is a critical concern in all phases of vaccine development, from early phase I through phase IV (5, 6, 7). Active adverse event monitoring is very important throughout the process of experimental vaccine evaluation. Phase I trials are often designed as dose-finding studies, looking for immediate toxicity and unanticipated adverse events, measuring antibody titers, injection site reactions (erythema, induration, pain and tenderness), allergic reactions, and other short-term (hours to days) outcomes. These may even be conducted in an inpatient facility to permit close observation, reporting of signs and symptoms, and collection of sera and other specimens. Phase II trials, often placebo controlled, are designed to further establish safety. These trials capture the occurrence and magnitude of fever, irritability, injection site redness, swelling, and pain, as well as the longer term (weeks to months) response to vaccine. Safety events are scrutinized as isolated events and as consolidated events, e.g., any respiratory adverse event during the follow-up period. The eligibility for these trials becomes progressively less restrictive in each successive phase, approaching the target population of potential vaccinees. Phase III controlled trials, often double blind, are designed to directly estimate vaccine efficacy with health outcomes (requiring months of follow-up), such as infection, hospitalization, or absenteeism from school or employment, rather than exclusively immunologic end points, except in cases in which the immune response is considered to be a satisfactory surrogate for clinical protection. In addition to evaluating efficacy, phase III trials often address duration of protection.

Prelicensure studies typically provide adequate safety data on relatively common adverse events, but usually cannot provide estimates of the risk of more serious but rare adverse events. Experience with similar or earlier generation vaccines [e.g., oral poliovirus (OPV), whole-cell pertussis, or rhesus rotavirus vaccines] can suggest appropriate adverse events for focused attention in safety studies. Hypotheses related to vaccine safety often require larger and/or longer studies than have been conducted traditionally prior to licensure.

As more vaccines have been added to the pediatric immunization schedule, and as the incidence of serious infectious disease has declined, parent groups and the lay media have focused increasing attention on possible vaccine-associated adverse events. With memory of the infectious disease epidemics of the past fading, previously acceptable margins of uncertainty may be larger than can be tolerated. Expansion of the prelicensure safety information as discussed above may be inevitable.

Vaccine formulations often include additives: Adjuvants such as aluminum hydroxide, aluminum phosphate, and calcium phosphate; preservatives such as thimerosal; and thermal or alkaline stabilizers such as $MgCl_2$. The effects of these additives on the immune response and on adverse events need to be evaluated thoroughly during development and postlicensure. Recent concerns about exposing infants to mercury compounds have led to the discontinuation of vaccines manufactured with thimerosal, a mercury-containing preservative, for use in the United States (8). As the result of concerns about exposure to products that could potentially transmit bovine spongiform encephalopathy (BSE), stabilizers of bovine origin are no longer used. Investigational adjuvants, used to enhance immune response, also may raise safety concerns, particularly with therapeutic vaccines for which it may be difficult to distinguish between adverse events caused by the administered product and adverse events that are part of the disease process that is being treated (9). Severe local reactions [localized cystic reactions requiring surgical intervention (10)] and the subsequent perceived safety profile of incomplete Freund's adjuvant (IFA) have limited its use in recent years and have impacted the development of newer adjuvants. Other examples include the evaluation of a variety of adjuvants, including a liposome-based adjuvant in malaria vaccine (11), or multiple adjuvants with different physical and chemical properties in an experimental human immunodeficiency virus type 1 (HIV-1) vaccine (12).

Each new vaccine development poses unique challenges, but the development of HIV vaccines is particularly challenging. Since HIV is known to have a high rate of mutation of the HIV-1 envelope protein (13), there are subtle biological and geographic differences in variants of the virus that may be changing over time. To ensure impact on the rate of HIV transmission, public policy considerations must include not only vaccine efficacy, but also population-level benefits (direct and indirect effects), including behavioral changes, vaccine coverage rates, secondary transmission rates, mixing patterns, and other factors (14). Phase III trials of HIV candidate vaccines are ongoing. One of the limiting factors in moving trials forward is the lack of known correlates of protection that could simplify and speed the evaluation of candidate vaccines. Candidate vaccines might prevent infection, prevent or delay progression to clinical disease, or reduce HIV-1 transmission in humans. The choice of target for an HIV vaccine affects not only the vaccine design and development, but also the ultimate public health impact, given multiple clades with geographic-specific prevalence. Those factors specific to HIV vaccine trials that may increase the trial size, duration, and/or complexity include the need for rapid trial results, the gradual accumulation of maximum protection, accuracy levels of detection assays, and HIV exposure avoidance counseling (15). Trials may need increased sample size due to the potentially small effect size, which may be the result of competing behavioral interventions, excessive loss to follow-up, or a need for broader inclusion of various subpopulations.

POSTLICENSURE SURVEILLANCE

Since preventive vaccines are administered to millions of healthy individuals, they necessarily undergo extensive and continuous safety evaluation. Most safety monitoring of licensed vaccine is based on passive reporting systems, such as the Vaccine Adverse Events Reporting System (VAERS) in the United States (16) and the Yellow Card system used by the Medicines Control Agency in the United Kingdom (17). Passive systems have many known limitations, including underreporting of events, incomplete and often inaccurate information on the event itself and the medical history of the vaccinee, and the inability to distinguish coincidentally occurring serious events from those with a true causal association with the vaccine (18). Passive surveillance approaches offer hypothesis-generating but not hypothesis-testing capabilities.

Improved surveillance approaches are feasible with sophisticated computer systems linking routine clinical data with immunization records. Examples of such systems include the Canadian Immunization and Monitoring Programme Active (IMPACT) system (19), and the Vaccine Safety Datalink [VSD] (20) in which a number of health maintenance organizations (HMOs), such as Kaiser Permanente Northern California and Group Health Cooperative of Puget Sound, collaborate with the Centers for Disease Control and Prevention (CDC) on vaccine safety investigations. These systems have been instrumental in describing the safety profile of pneumococcal, varicella, hepatitis B, Hib, and other vaccines. They can provide postvaccination rates of local and systemic reactions, hospitalization, emergency room use, sudden infant death syndrome (SIDS), and other events. They also can provide the setting for randomized controlled trials, comparisons to historical (prevaccine) controls, case-control studies, or comparisons of observed safety profiles of different vaccines (21).

Once a vaccine is generally available, safety monitoring continues with respect to the production, distribution, storage, and delivery. Package inserts for licensed vaccines include recommendations for storage and handling. The widespread use of vaccines rapidly after licensure can exacerbate these safety considerations. The classic historical example is the Cutter incident. In the production of inactivated poliovirus (IPV) vaccine from Cutter Laboratories, not all of the wild poliovirus was inactivated in two of the vaccine lots, leading to 260 cases of paralytic polio clearly caused by the vaccine. This incident had the potential, fortunately unrealized due to the positive public reception to the vaccine, to seriously undermine the entire vaccination program (22). As a consequence of this devastating event, CDC established surveillance programs to continuously monitor vaccine adverse effects (23). Refinement of postlicensure safety assessments has continued, and oral vaccine has been superseded by inactivated vaccine. The Department of Health and Human Services Advisory Committee on Immunization Practices (ACIP) recommended in 1999 that IPV be used exclusively in the United States to eliminate the shedding of live vaccine virus and the risk of vaccine-associated poliomyelitis.

An instructive example of the rapidity with which postlicensure safety evaluation can provide important new information following the introduction of a new vaccine is the experience with the tetravalent rhesus-human reassortant rotavirus vaccine (RRV) approved by the Food and Drug Administration (FDA) in 1998 and then recommended for universal administration to infants (24). The initial placebo-controlled trials of RRV demonstrated the vaccine's efficacy in reducing the incidence and severity of rotavirus. Although several cases of intussusception had occurred among approximately 10,000 vaccinees, the observed rate did not appear to exceed the expected number based on estimated background rates in this age group; further, a case of intussusception also had been observed among the controls (25). Passive surveillance (VAERS) provided the initial indication of a safety concern; the reporting of 15 cases of intussusception following RRV during the first 10 months after licensure represented about half the number that might have been expected during that interval, based on the expected background rate and the estimated vaccine coverage (26). Given the unknown but likely substantial underreporting, these reports generated concern and prompted the rapid design and implementation of a large case-control study. Simultaneously, ACIP recommended the immediate suspension of the RRV immunization program. When the case-control study was completed, showing a strong causal association between the vaccine and

intussusception (27), the American Academy of Pediatrics Committee on Infectious Diseases withdrew its recommendation for rotavirus vaccination (28), and the manufacturer voluntarily recalled the product.

VACCINE ADVERSE EVENT SURVEILLANCE METHODS

Just as vaccine development and new routes of delivery are evolving, so are the methods for surveillance of adverse events. One surveillance method, used in the United Kingdom and Canada to monitor the adverse events associated with vaccines, is based on the linkage of vaccination records (dates and vaccine batch numbers) and hospital discharge diagnosis records. This method controls for confounding by indication without requiring information on noncases (29, 30). The proportion of cases vaccinated is compared to the proportion vaccinated in the population as a whole, without the detailed vaccination record data for the entire population. The advantage is that this method provides an estimate of relative incidence of the clinical event conditioned not only on the occurrence of the event (as with the usual case series), but also on the vaccination history (31). The risk associated with a specific dose of a multidose regimen, the duration and magnitude of any increased risk, as well as risks attributable to particular strains of vaccine could be compared by this approach. The potential associations between diphtheria and tetanus toxoids and whole-cell pertussis (DTP) vaccination and febrile convulsion and between measles-mumps-rubella (MMR) vaccination and idiopathic thrombocytopenia purpura (ITP) were investigated by this method. With increasing availability of administrative computerized records, and more combination vaccines delivering more antigens simultaneously, this approach provides an additional method for identifying adverse events without requiring vaccination data on the entire population.

The VSD permits a variety of study approaches, including case series, case-control studies, and cohort studies, with the additional strength of chart validation and prospectively recorded vaccination history (19, 20). In the VSD, vaccination records are linked to pharmacy prescriptions, demographic data, and medical outcome records at several HMOs. While not broadly representative of the U.S. population, opportunities exist with this approach to investigate diverse vaccination exposures and acutely emerging public health questions. As HMOs are added to the VSD, and the population becomes more representative, the VSD will provide even more valuable data.

Computer-intensive methods such as data mining are being used to explore and analyze very large datasets to identify potential associations between vaccines and adverse outcomes. Data mining methods are not dependent upon strong model assumptions as are, for example, discriminant analysis or multiple linear regression. Some data mining applications rely on existing analytic techniques such as logistic regression or recursive partitioning. The application of data mining techniques to VAERS, using empirical Bayesian estimation, has been described using the data on the rhesus rotavirus vaccine association with intussusception as an example (32). It remains to be seen how effective the routine application of data mining techniques to passive surveillance data will be in providing early signals of true vaccine safety issues.

COMBINATION VACCINES

Combination vaccines have been in use in the United States since the 1940s. They offer increased convenience and therefore the potential for increased vaccine coverage, particularly as the pediatric vaccination schedule continues to expand. The evaluation of combination vaccines administered in the same syringe is complex, but the impact of combination vaccines on clinical staff, parents, and infants is clear. Numerous investigators have demonstrated the savings attributable to combination vaccines in total staff time associated with vaccine preparation, injection, and administrative issues (shipping, handling, storage), as well as in reducing infant crying time and multiple visits (33, 34). Fewer injections also diminish missed vaccination visits, simplify the overall vaccination schedule, and facilitate broader vaccine coverage. Antigenic competition, decreased immunogenicity or increased reactogenicity, choice of control groups for comparison in prospective trials, standardized assessment of adverse reactions, and determination of serologic correlates of protection all complicate the evaluation of combination vaccines (35, 36). Standardized assessment of adverse events in trials comparing combination vaccine with separately administered components has been recommended for pre- and postlicensure studies (37). More safety data may be needed for some combination vaccines if the available safety data for the individual components are limited (38).

RISK COMMUNICATION

The continued success of immunization programs and infectious disease control depends to a great extent upon targeted, accurate, and timely communication with potential vaccinees and their parents. Given that public understanding of infectious disease and of the immune system can be limited and is sometimes erroneous, and that confusion of causality and temporal association occurs all too frequently, public education regarding the need for and the efficacy and safety of vaccines is vital to global public health. Recent examples of the concerns surrounding the use of the hepatitis B vaccine in France (39, 40, 41) and the MMR vaccine in the United Kingdom (42) demonstrate that public health programs must improve their capacities to communicate more clearly and effectively to the public about the benefits and risks of vaccination. Although investigation of these concerns showed little or no evidence of any adverse consequences of the vaccines in question, the extensive publicity that the concerns received had major negative effects

on immunization programs. Re-emergence of serious diseases following lowered levels of vaccine coverage has been seen in several countries (43) and may be on the horizon again if more effective means of communicating with the public about the importance and value of vaccination are not developed and implemented.

References

1 Greenwood, M., & Yule, U. G. (1915). The statistics of anti-typhoid and anti-cholera inoculation, and the interpretation of such statistics in general. *Proceedings of the Royal Society of Medicine, 8*(Part 2), 113-194.

2 Orenstein, W. A., Bernier, R. H., Dondero, T. J., et al. (1985). Field evaluation of vaccine efficacy. *Bulletin of the World Health Organization, 63,* 1055-1068.

3 Francis, T. F., Korns, R. F., Voight, R. B., et al. (1955). An evaluation of the 1954 poliomyelitis vaccine trials. Summary report. *American Journal of Public Health, 45*(5, Part 2).

4 Zanardi, L. R., Haber, P., Mootrey, G. T., Niu, M. T., et al. (2001). Intussusception among recipients of rotavirus vaccine: Reports to the Vaccine Adverse Event Reporting System. *Pediatrics, 107*(6), e97.

5 Tacket, C. O., Rennels, M. B., & Mattheis, M. J. (1997). Initial clinical evaluation of new vaccine candidates: Phase 1 and 2 clinical trials of safety, immunogenicity, and preliminary efficacy. In M. M. Levine, G. C. Woodrow, J. B. Kaper, & G. S. Cobon (Eds.), *New generation vaccines* (2nd ed., pp. 35-45). New York: Marcel Dekker.

6 Clemens, J. D., Naficy, A., & Rao, M. R. (1997). Long-term evaluation of vaccine protection: Methodological issues for phase 3 trials and phase 4 studies. In M. M. Levine, G. C. Woodrow, J. B. Kaper, & G. S. Cobon (Eds.), *New generation vaccines* (2nd ed., pp. 47-67). New York: Marcel Dekker.

7 Goldenthal, K. L., Kleppinger, C., & McVittie, L. D. (in preparation). The clinical evaluation of preventive vaccines. In *Biologics development: A regulatory overview* (3rd ed.). Parexel.

8 Notice to readers. Thimerosal in vaccines: A joint statement of the American Academy of Pediatrics and the Public Health Service. (1999). *Morbidity and Mortality Weekly Report, 48,* 563-565.

9 Goldenthal, K. L., Cavagnaro, J. A., Alving, C. R., & Vogel, F. R. (1993). Safety evaluation of vaccine adjuvants. *AIDS Research and Human Retroviruses, 9,* S47-S51.

10 Davenport, F. M. (1968). Seventeen years experience with mineral oil adjuvant influenza virus vaccines. *Annals of Allergy, 26,* 288-292.

11 Fries, L. F., Gordon, D. M., Richards, R. L., et al. (1992). Liposomal malaria vaccine in humans: A safe and potent adjuvant strategy. *Proceedings of the National Academy of Sciences, 89,* 358-362.

12 Powell, M. F., Eastman, D. L., Lim, A., et al. (1995). Effect of adjuvants on immunogenicity of MN recombinant glycoprotein 120 in guinea pigs. *AIDS Research and Human Retroviruses, 11,* 203-209.

13 Kuiken, C., et al. (1999). Human retroviruses and AIDS. In *Theoretical biology and biophysics* (pp. 1-789). Los Alamos, New Mexico: Los Alamos National Laboratory Press.

14 Halloran, M. E., Haber, M., Longini, I. M., Jr., & Struchiner, C. J. (1991). Direct and indirect effects in vaccine efficacy and effectiveness. *American Journal of Epidemiology, 133,* 323-331.

15 Dixon, D. O., Rida, W. N., Fast, P. E., & Hoth, D. F. (1993). HIV vaccine trials: Some design issues including sample size calculations. *Journal of Acquired Immune Deficiency Syndromes, 6,* 485-496.

16 Chen, R. T., Rastogi, S. C., Mullen, J. R., et al. (1994). The Vaccine Adverse Event Reporting System (VAERS). *Vaccine, 12,* 542-550.

17 Chen, R. T. (2000). Special methodological issues in pharmacoepidemiology studies of vaccine safety. In B. L. Strom (Ed.), *Pharmacoepidemiology* (pp. 707-732). Chichester: Wiley.

18 Ellenberg, S. S., & Braun, M. M. (in press). Monitoring the safety of vaccines: Assessing the risks. *Drug Safety.*

19 Morrs, R., Halperin, S., Dery, P., et al. (1993). IMPACT monitoring network: A better mousetrap. *Canadian Journal of Infectious Diseases, 4,* 194-195.

20 Chen, R. T., Glasser, J. W., Rhodes, P. H., et al. (1997). Vaccine Safety Datalink project: A new tool for improving vaccine safety monitoring in the United States. The Vaccine Safety Datalink Team. *Pediatrics, 99,* 765-773.

21 Niu, M. T., Rhodes, P., Salive, M., et al. (1998). Comparative safety of two recombinant hepatitis B vaccines in children: Data from the Vaccine Adverse Event Reporting System (VAERS) and Vaccine Safety Datalink (VSD). *Journal of Clinical Epidemiology, 51,* 503-510.

22 Nathanson, N., & Langmuir, A. D. (1995). The Cutter incident. Poliomyelitis following formaldehyde-inactivated poliovirus vaccination in the United States during the spring of 1955. II. Relationship of poliomyelitis to Cutter vaccine. 1963. *American Journal of Epidemiology, 142,* 109-140.

23 Robbins, F. C. (1988). Polio — Historical. In S. A. Plotkin & E. A. Mortimer (Eds.), *Vaccines* (pp. 98-114). Philadelphia: Saunders.

24 Centers for Disease Control and Prevention. (1999). Rotavirus vaccine for the prevention of rotavirus gastroenteritis among children: Recommendations of the Advisory Committee on Immunization Practices (ACIP). *Morbidity and Mortality Weekly Report, 48,* (RR-2) 1-23.

25 Rennels, M. B., Parashar, U. D., Holman, R. C., et al. (1998). Lack of an apparent association between intussusception and wild or vaccine rotavirus infection. *Pediatric Infectious Disease Journal, 17,* 924-925.

26 Centers for Disease Control and Prevention. (1999). Intussusception among recipients of rotavirus vaccine — United States, 1998-1999. *Morbidity and Mortality Weekly Report, 48,* 577-581.

27 Murphy, T. V., Cargiullo, P. M., Massoudi, M. S., et al. (2001). Intussusception among infants given an oral rotavirus vaccine. *New England Journal of Medicine, 344,* 564-572.

28 Centers for Disease Control and Prevention. (1999). Withdrawal of rotavirus vaccine recommendation. *Morbidity and Mortality Weekly Report, 48,* 1007.

29 Farrington, C. P. (1995). Relative incidence estimation from case series for vaccine safety evaluation. *Biometrics, 51,* 228-235.

30 Farrington, P., Pugh, S., Colville, A., et al. (1995). A new method for active surveillance of adverse events from diphtheria/tetanus/pertussis and measles/mumps/rubella vaccines. *Lancet, 345,* 568-569.

31 Farrington, C. P. (1995). Relative incidence estimation from case series for vaccine safety evaluation. *Biometrics, 51,* 228-235.

32 Niu, M. T., Erwin, D. E., & Braun, M. M. (2001). Data mining in the U.S. Vaccine Adverse Event Reporting System (VAERS): Early detection of intussusception and other events after rotavirus vaccination. *Vaccine, 19,* 4627-4634.

33 Pellissier, J. M., Coplan, P. M., Jackson, L. A., & May, J. E. (2000). The effect of additional shots on the vaccine administration process: Results of a time-motion study in 2 settings. *American Journal of Managed Care, 6,* 1038-1044.

34 Pinchichero, M. E. (2000). New combination vaccines. *Pediatric Clinics of North America, 47,* 407-426.

35 Decker, M. D., & Edwards, K. M. (2001). Combination vaccines. *Infectious Disease Clinics of North America, 15,* 234-240.

36 Midthun, K., Horne, A. D., & Goldenthal, K. G. (1998). Clinical safety evaluation of combination vaccines. In S. Plotkin, F. Brown, & F. Horaud (Eds.), Preclinical and clinical development of new vaccines. *Developments in Biological Standardization, 95,* 209-230.

37 Decker, M. D., & Edwards, K. M. (1995). Issues in design of clinical trials of combination vaccines. In J. C. Williams, K. L. Goldenthal, D. L. Burns, & B. P. Lewis (Eds.), *Combination vaccines and simultaneous administration* (pp. 234-240). New York Academy of Sciences.

38 Ellenberg, S. S. (2001). Evaluating the safety of combination vaccines. *Clinical Infectious Diseases, 33*(Suppl. 4), S319-S322.

39 Hepatitis B immunization — WHO position. (1998). *Weekly Epidemiological Record, 73,* 329.

40 Monteyne, P., & Andre, F. E. (2000). Is there a causal link between hepatitis B vaccination and multiple sclerosis? *Vaccine, 18,* 1994-2001.

41 Ascherio, A., Zhang, S. M., Hernan, M. A., et al. (2001). Hepatitis B vaccination and the risk of multiple sclerosis. *New England Journal of Medicine, 344,* 322-327.

42 Taylor, B., Miller, E., Farrington, C. P., Petropoulos, M., et al. (1999). Autism and measles mumps and rubella vaccine: No epidemiological evidence for a causal association. *Lancet, 353,* 2026-2029.

43 Gangarosa, E. J., Galazka, A. M., Wolfe, C. R., Phillips, L. M., Gangarosa, R. E., Miller, E., & Chen, R. T. (1998). Impact of anti-vaccine movements on pertussis control: The untold story. *Lancet, 351,* 356-361.

Author's Biography

Dr. Foulkes is Deputy Director of the Office of Biostatistics and Epidemiology, Center for Biologics Evaluation and Research, Food and Drug Administration. She has held a variety of positions in academia, private industry, and government. Dr. Foulkes served more than 14 years at the National Institutes of Health, including working in the Division of Acquired Immunodeficiency Syndrome of the National Institute of Allergy and Infectious Diseases (NIAID). She has participated in the design, conduct, interim monitoring, analysis, and reporting of numerous randomized, controlled clinical trials in cardiovascular disease, neurological disorders, oncology therapies, human immunodeficiency virus (HIV) prevention and therapy, and vaccine efficacy.

Author's Biography

Dr. Ellenberg is Director of the Office of Biostatistics and Epidemiology at the Center for Biologics Evaluation and Research at the Food and Drug Administration. She has published extensively in statistical and medical journals on topics such as surrogate end points; data monitoring committees; clinical trial designs; adverse event monitoring; and special issues in cancer, acquired immunodeficiency syndrome (AIDS), and vaccine trials. Dr. Ellenberg also has played a leading role in the development of international standards for clinical trials performed by the pharmaceutical industry. She is a fellow of the American Statistical Association and the American Association for the Advancement of Science and is an elected member of the International Statistical Institute

The Evolution of
Vaccine Risk
Communication
in the United States:
1982-2002

The Evolution of Vaccine Risk Communication in the United States: 1982-2002

Geoffrey Evans, M.D., and Ann Bostrom, Ph.D.

OVERVIEW

Over the past 20 years, vaccine risk communication has evolved from nearly nonexistent to becoming an integral part of immunization practice today. There are several reasons for this; some obvious, others less so. Advances in medicine and biotechnology have led to public debate over the imprecise nature of health risks. The task of informing the public about these risks is made difficult by limited understanding of what are often rare adverse effects. With immunization, the seeming disappearance of many infectious diseases has paradoxically created a heightened perception of vaccine risk and uncertainty. The challenge to effectively communicate vaccine risks and benefits has increased accordingly. With the Internet and its limitless opportunities for information (and misinformation) comes the need for even more effective techniques and strategies for effectively communicating vaccine risks and benefits. Building on insights from research on health and environmental risk perception, communication, and decision making, vaccine risk communicators are developing validated empirical approaches to the design and evaluation of risk communication, and a cadre of researchers and new institutional structures to assist in these efforts. This article reviews the changing vaccine benefit/risk paradigm; factors affecting vaccine risk communication; and the roles and influences of institutional development, government regulation, and the media. It concludes with a discussion of the current state of risk communication science and its relevance to future vaccine communication design and content. A timeline reflecting events over the past two decades is shown in Table 1, and a list of vaccine risk communication resources is provided in Table 2.

BACKGROUND

Concerns about vaccine risk originated in the late 1700s when smallpox vaccine was introduced, followed by similar controversy over rabies vaccination nearly 100 years later. As time passed, the life-saving benefits of vaccines spoke volumes, making acceptable the relatively infrequent, albeit serious, reactions associated with each vaccine. Polio eradication campaigns of the mid-20th century were proof of the need for, and public trust and faith in, vaccines. However, by the 1970s, unquestioned acceptance of vaccination was changing in Western Europe and Japan. With pertussis disease at low levels, attention began to focus on the adverse events (truly related or not) that sometimes follow immunization. Consumer movements questioning the safety and efficacy of whole-cell pertussis vaccine eventually led to diminished or discontinued use, and resurgence of epidemic disease.

America's wake-up call came in 1982 with the airing of the controversial Emmy-winning program "DTP: Vaccine Roulette." Showing images of severely impaired children and suggesting that serious reactions to diphtheria and tetanus toxoids and whole-cell pertussis (DTP) vaccine were as frequent as 1 in 700 infants, the show (and its derivatives) generated great concern among parents. Standard resources like the American Academy of Pediatrics (AAP) Committee on Infectious Diseases *Redbook* and Important Information Statements from the Centers for Disease Control and Prevention (CDC) were ill equipped to answer the program's allegations, inquiries having to do with Japan's use of a safer alternative (i.e., acellular pertussis vaccine), or State immunization laws. Other than the popular "parenting manuals," there was little information on vaccines for parents. Consumer support groups began appearing in part to fill this information gap. Perspectives on immunization were changing, and not just for the short term.

Sources

Centers for Disease Control and Prevention. (1978). *Important information statements on diphtheria, tetanus, and pertussis vaccines.*

Committee on Infectious Diseases. (1982). *Report of the Committee on Infectious Diseases.* American Academy of Pediatrics.

Freed, G. L., Katz, S. L., & Clark, S. J. (1996). Safety of vaccinations: Miss America, the media and public health. *Journal of the American Medical Association, 276, 1869-1872.*

Gangarosa, E. J., Galezka, A. M., Wolfe, C. R., et al. (1998). Impact of anti-vaccine movements on pertussis control: The untold story. *Lancet, 351, 356-361.*

Plotkin, S. L., & Plotkin, S. A. (1999). A short history of vaccination. In S. A. Plotkin & W. A. Orenstein (Eds.), *Vaccines* (3rd ed., pp. 1-12). Philadelphia: W. B. Saunders Co.

Thompson, L., & Nuell, D. (1982). *DTP: Vaccine roulette* [video recording]. Washington, DC: WRC-TV (NBC).

SHIFT IN VACCINE RISK-BENEFIT PERCEPTION

After the introduction of acellular pertussis vaccine in Japan, Europe, and more recently the United States, controversy over the use of DTP vaccine waned. Its genesis, however, is relevant for present-day vaccine safety concerns. The success of vaccination has produced generations of parents, and physicians, with little or no first-hand experience of vaccine-preventable disease. With benefits apparently assured, adverse events following immunization—particularly of unknown cause—attract increased attention from cautious parents. It is only natural to conclude that events closely following immunization are causally related, whether or not they are. Temporal association is especially compelling when alternative explanations are lacking and parents are told the condition is idiopathic. Those who turn to science for help or reassurance often find a disturbing lack of data. Even when there is scientific evidence, disagreement by experts over its meaning can confuse those looking for answers. Addressing all of this effectively requires an understanding of how individuals assess and make decisions about vaccine risks, including whom and what influences these decisions.

Sources

Evans, G., Bostrom, A., Johnston, R. B., Fisher, B. L., & Stoto, M. A. (Eds.). (1997). *Risk communication and vaccination: Workshop summary.* Washington, DC: National Academy Press.

Howson, C. P., Howe, C. J., & Fineberg, H. V. (Eds.). (1991). *Adverse effects of pertussis and rubella vaccines.* Institute of Medicine. Washington, DC: National Academy Press.

EXTERNAL FACTORS AFFECTING VACCINE RISK COMMUNICATION

Parental decisions about vaccination are influenced by external factors (i.e., medical, sociopolitical) as well as personal factors. The increasing popularity of alternative health options affects vaccine decisions. In one survey, parents cited homeopathy and its benefits of natural immunity as the most common reason for immunization refusal, although at least one group of homeopathic practitioners denies it is "anti-vaccination." Inconsistent viewpoints on immunization are also reflected in a survey of chiropractors that found a third agreeing with the statement that there is no scientific proof that immunization prevents disease.

Vaccine decisions involve ethical considerations as well. Because the decision not to vaccinate increases the risk to the community as well as the individual, the duty of society to protect healthy (and susceptible) children may conflict with the right of families to make health decisions for their children. The presence of State immunization laws for school (and daycare) entry has led to a polarized debate on individual rights and civil liberties. Few issues have raised as much controversy. In 1999, consumer efforts in 15 States led to draft legislation to either rescind mandates or provide exemptions based on philosophical grounds. Compulsory immunization also complicates risk communication since messages regarding mandated vaccination may be perceived differently from those about voluntary vaccination. Information needed for informed decisionmaking

takes on greater urgency when decisions are involuntary, causing consumers to question the adequacy of vaccine adverse event reporting and long-term studies of vaccine safety and efficacy. Moreover, immunization mandates are inconsistent with the voluntary decisionmaking, an inherent principle of informed consent.

Beyond individual autonomy and informed consent is trust, a key determinant in risk decisions. Health communication is only effective when its recipients view the source as credible and impartial, which in part explains why conflict of interest inquiries have become so common. If there is even a perception of a conflict of interest, messages can leave people suspicious or confused and lead some to turn to less authoritative sources. The trust placed in authority derives from the perception that the authority shares public values. One way of achieving this is to involve the public in policy formulation. Trust may be lost when decisions are made behind closed doors and unexpected harm results. Recent examples include the French Government's handling of possible human immunodeficiency virus (HIV) contamination of the blood supply, and the experience of bovine spongiform encephalopathy (BSE) contamination of meat in the United Kingdom, both of which resulted in deaths after the public was reassured about potential risk.

Dialogue and decisionmaking partnerships can bridge gaps and forge better understanding. Nothing is assured, however, by being informative or inclusive. As a 1989 hallmark National Research Council report points out, informing the public may not reduce conflict at all, but actually sharpen it. Yet, as was stated in an Institute of Medicine (IOM) workshop on risk communication, "[P]olitics is about decision making in the absence of complete information," which is nearly always the case with technological hazards. Only by understanding how people view certain risks and what is acceptable can efforts to promote behavioral outcomes be successful. Public discussions on smallpox vaccine policy that took place in 2002 are one example of participatory decisionmaking.

Sources

Altman, L. K. (2002, June 6). Preventive smallpox vaccinations urged for health workers. *New York Times.* http://www.nytimes.com/2002/06/07/health/07SMAL.html.

Colley, F., & Haas, M. (1994). Attitudes on immunization: A survey of American chiropractors. *Journal of Manipulative and Physiological Therapeutics, 17,* 584-590.

Evans, G., Bostrom, A., Johnston, R. B., Fisher, B. L., & Stoto, M. A. (Eds.). (1997). *Risk communication and vaccination: Workshop summary.* Washington, DC: National Academy Press.

Feudtner, C., & Marcuse, E. K. (2001). Ethics and immunization policy: Promoting dialogue to sustain consensus. *Pediatrics, 107(5),* 1158-1164.

Fisher, P. (1990). Enough nonsense on immunization. *British Medical Journal, 79*, 198-200.

National Research Council. (1989). *Improving risk communication.* Washington, DC: National Academy Press.

Simpson, N., Lenton, S., & Randall, R. (1995). Parental refusal to have children immunised: Extent and reasons. *British Medical Journal, 310,* 227.

PERSONAL FACTORS AFFECTING VACCINE RISK COMMUNICATION

No matter how well intentioned or well designed a risk message may be, individual risk perception and decisionmaking have to be taken into account if the communication is to be effective. Individuals tend to use heuristics, or shortcuts, in thinking about otherwise complex issues of risk. Among those related to immunization are bandwagoning, which is the tendency for parents to vaccinate if "everyone else is doing it" without fully evaluating the options themselves; altruism, when individuals are willing to accept personal risk if society as a whole will benefit (i.e., herd immunity); and less commonly, freeloading logic, which relies on high vaccination rates and herd immunity to protect an unvaccinated child. Vaccine decisions also can be influenced by cognitive biases. Omission bias, or the perception that actions are riskier than inactions, operates on the premise that vaccination, because it involves taking an action, is riskier than disease, even if the expected mortality and morbidity rates are lower with the vaccine.

Social and cognitive factors also influence consumers' and providers' vaccine risk perceptions and decisionmaking. Individuals perceive risk based on their experiences, attitudes, education, beliefs, values, and culture as well as the nature of the risk. Some risks are more acceptable to parents than others. For example, risks that are voluntary and controllable tend to be more acceptable than involuntary risks, an issue that comes into play with mandatory immunization. Risks may be perceived differently depending on how they are framed, as people tend to avoid sure losses, but prefer certain benefits to equivalent uncertain benefits. It follows that parents who view vaccines as risky may choose to vaccinate only when they perceive a high threat of disease. Others who view vaccines as generally safe may be more likely to vaccinate in response to messages emphasizing the benefits of immunization rather than the risks of disease.

While there is a fairly limited (but growing) body of empirical evidence on vaccine risk perceptions and the demand for risk communication, the available data show that parents generally want to have relevant and practical information on vaccine risks, including mention of rare, serious risks that may occur. They have basic questions—and sometimes serious concerns—about side effects, such as what to expect, when to expect it, how

severe it will be, what to do (if anything), and when to call the doctor.

Sources

Asch, D. A., Baron, J., Hershey, J. C., et al. (1994). Omission bias and pertussis vaccination. *Medical Decision Making, 14*, 118-123.

Ball, L. K., Evans, G., & Bostrom, A. (1998). Risky business: Challenges in vaccine risk communication. *Pediatrics, 101*(3), 453-458.

Davis, T. C., Fredrickson, D. D., Arnold, C. L., et al. (2001). Childhood vaccine risk/benefit communication in private practice office settings: A national survey. *Pediatrics, 107*(2).

Fischhoff, B., Bostrom, A., & Quadrel, M. J. (1993). Risk perception and communication. *Annual Review of Public Health, 14,* 183-203.

Fitzgerald, T. M., & Glotzer, D. E. (1995). Vaccine information pamphlets: More information than parents want? *Pediatrics, 95(3), 331-334.*

Gellen, B. G., Maibach, E. W., & Marcuse, E. K. (2000). Do parents understand immunizations? A national telephone survey. *Pediatrics, 106*(5), 1097-1102.

Slovic, P. (1987). Perceptions of risk. *Science, 236,* 280-285.

Tversky, A., & Kahneman, D. (1981). The framing of decisions and the psychology of choice. *Science, 211,* 453- 458.

THE ROLE OF CONSUMERS

Consumers, in an advocacy or watchdog role, have significantly influenced immunization policy. Working with the media and policymakers, consumer groups successfully pursued a number of safety initiatives in the early 1980s, including: 1) Expanded research on vaccine adverse events, 2) a national adverse event surveillance system, 3) dedicated parent information materials, and 4) a safer alternative to the whole-cell pertussis vaccine. Starting with enactment of the National Childhood Vaccine Injury Act of 1986 (NCVIA), each affected the form and content of vaccine risk communication, and all were in place by the mid-1990s. Changing from the live oral poliovirus (OPV) vaccine to the "safer" inactivated poliovirus (IPV) vaccine product was also related to efforts by a polio consumer group opposed to further use of OPV.

Against this backdrop of activism are repeated surveys showing that the vast majority of parents believe in immunization and follow State mandates and their physician's recommendations. Yet, concerns about vaccine safety have grown over time, increasing attention on vaccine risk communication.

The popularization of the Internet has brought the reality of mass communication to people's fingertips through using email, browsing the World Wide Web, participating in LISTSERV discussion groups, or posting to Web pages or Internet chat rooms or bulletin boards. Recent surveys show that two-thirds of Americans are now online, and of the 80 percent who use it for decisions on health, just more than half find the information credible. There is virtually no limit to the information (and misinformation) that is easily accessible to laypersons and professionals.

A first-time parent entering the word "vaccine" on a standard Internet search engine (e.g., Google, Yahoo, Excite) will find an overwhelming number of links to Web sites, many of which are hosted by consumer groups. The Web sites belonging to consumer groups or individuals provide a wide variety of information. A few offer links to peer-reviewed journals, government Web sites, and pro-vaccine institutions. These Web sites also may present anecdotal information and misconceptions about vaccines or vaccination. These range from the linkage of vaccines to specific idiopathic illnesses [e.g., sudden infant death syndrome (SIDS), diabetes], to the value of alternative medicine, the dangers of immunization-related immune overload, and allegations of collusion between government and industry with profit motives as the basis for decisions on immunization policy and the withholding of vaccine safety information. Adding to the potential confusion is the lack of consistency across such Web sites, which leaves readers who do not have access to scientific method and peer review with no clear means of vaccine benefit-risk assessment or validation.

In the mid-nineties, public health officials became concerned about their relative absence on the increasingly active Internet, where the available vaccine information was dominated by consumer groups. Concerted efforts to maintain a balance contributed to increased and improved government and private vaccine-related Web sites. The Web sites of Federal health agencies and allied nongovernmental organizations usually contain peer-reviewed information on current safety issues, policy statements, vaccine use recommendations, and links to complementary Web sites. Their readers are generally left with the impression that the benefits of vaccination outweigh the risks.

Sources

Blizard, R. T., & Volkert, J. J. (2001, August 3). *Americans supportive of childhood vaccinations.* Gallup News Service.

Blizzard, R. T., & Volkert, J. J. (2001, August 3). *Gallup poll.* Gallup News Service.

Centers for Disease Control and Prevention. (1999, June 17). *Advisory Committee on Immunization Practices meeting.*

Centers for Disease Control and Prevention. (2001). National, state, and urban area vaccination coverage levels among children aged 19-35 months—United States, 2000. *Morbidity and Mortality Weekly Report, 50*(30), 637-641.

Chen, L. E., Minkes, R. K., & Langer, J. C. (2000). Pediatric surgery on the Internet: Is the truth out there. *Journal of Pediatric Surgery, 35*(8), 1179-1182.

Davies, P., Chapman, S., & Leask, J. (2002). Antivaccination activists on the World Wide Web. *Archives of Disease in Childhood, 87*(1), 22-25.

Friedlander, E. R. Opposition to immunization: A pattern of deception. *Scien. Rev. Alt. Med., 5*(1), 18-23.

Kitch, E. W., Evans, G., & Gopin, R. (1999). U.S. law. In S. A. Plotkin & W. A. Orenstein (Eds.), Vaccines (3rd ed., pp. 1165-1186). Philadelphia: W. B. Saunders Co.

Nasir, L. (2000). Reconnoitering the antivaccination Web sites: News from the front. *Journal of Family Practice, 40(8)*, 731-733.

Pew Internet and American Life Project. (2000). *The online health care revolution: How the Web helps Americans take better care of themselves.* Washington, DC: Pew Internet and American Life Project. Available at: http://www.pewinternet.org/reports/toc.asp?Report=26 [Accessibility verified August 23, 2002].

Taylor, H. (2002, April 17). *Internet penetration at 66% of adults (137 million) nationwide. Harris Poll No. 18.* Rochester, NY: Harris Interactive. Available at: http://www.harrisinteractive.com/harris_poll/index.asp?PID=295 [Accessibility verified August 23, 2002].

Taylor, H. (2002, May 1). *Cyberchrondriacs update. Harris Poll No. 21.* Rochester, NY: Harris Interactive. Available at: http://www.harrisinteractive.com/harris_poll/index.asp?PID=299 [Accessibility verified August 23, 2002].

Wolfe, R. M., Sharp, L. K., & Lipsky, M. S. (2002). Content and design attributes of antivaccination Web sites. *Journal of the American Medical Association, 287*(24), 3245-3248.

THE ROLE OF HEALTHCARE PROVIDERS

Despite the advent of the Internet, individual providers still determine, to a great extent, whether a child is immunized. A large majority of parents continue to trust and rely on their physicians for vaccine communication and decisions. Parents desire verbal input by their primary providers as a matter of trust and respect. However, a recent national study found that physicians rarely initiate discussion of vaccine risks and benefits, leaving it to office nurses or support staff; 40 percent of physicians do not discuss vaccine risks at all. This raises the question of who is informing parental consent since physicians have the responsibility of ensuring that patients are adequately informed about risks and benefits prior to any medical intervention.

Healthcare providers report the greatest barriers to effective risk communication are the lack of time, given the significant number of anticipatory guidance issues to be covered on most well-baby visits, and the increasing financial pressures of office practice. This situation is aggravated by inadequate reimbursement for immunization services, and the fact that patient education is not viewed as billable time. Generally, providers think they know what parents need to know, and communicate this information, except that half the time they do not review contraindications to vaccination. About a quarter of physicians who do not routinely discuss vaccine risks and benefits feel that were they to do so, parents might be alarmed or even refuse immunization. For others, the reluctance may be due to insufficient knowledge of current vaccine issues and practice or inadequate insight into how to deal with the concerns of a parent who questions or even refuses immunization.

Further, physicians' beliefs—including misconceptions—about vaccine risks and efficacy and their interactions with parents influence their behavior. Some physicians believe that multiple injections should be avoided due to potential psychological and physical trauma, choose not to administer live-virus vaccines to children with minor acute illness and low-grade fever, or are unaware of or ill informed about liability protections under the National Vaccine Injury Compensation Program (VICP).

Sources

Askew, G. L., Finelli, L., Lutz, F. A., et al. (1995). Beliefs and practices regarding childhood vaccination among urban pediatrics providers in New Jersey. *Pediatrics, 96*(5), 889-892.

Davis, T. C., Fredrickson, D. D., Arnold, C. L., et al. (2001). Childhood vaccine risk/benefit communication in private practice office settings: A national survey. *Pediatrics, 107*(2).

Fitzgerald, T. M., & Glotzer, D. E. (1995). Vaccine information pamphlets: More information than parents want? *Pediatrics, 95*(3), 331-334.

Freed, G. L., Bordley, W. C., Clark, S. J., & Konrad, T. R. (1993). Family physician acceptance of universal hepatitis B immunization of infants. *Journal of Family Practice, 36*(2), 153-157.

Gellen, B. G., Maibach, E. W., & Marcuse, E. K. (2000). Do parents understand immunizations? A national telephone survey. *Pediatrics, 106*(5), 1097-1102.

Taylor, J. A, Darden, P. M., Slora, E., Hasemeier, C. M., Asmussen, L., & Wasserman, R. (1997). The influence of

provider behavior, parental characteristics, and a public policy initiative on the immunization status of children followed by private pediatricians: A study from Pediatric Research in Office Settings. Pediatrics, 99(2), 209-215. [Erratum in: Pediatrics 1997 Sep; 100(3 Pt. 1), 333].

Zimmerman, R. K., Schlesselman, J. J., Mieczkowski, M. A., et al. (1998). Physician concerns about vaccine adverse effects and potential litigation. *Archives of Pediatrics & Adolescent Medicine, 152*(1), 12-19.

THE ROLE OF THE MEDIA

The media has greatly influenced vaccine risk communication over the past two decades. Following "DTP: Vaccine Roulette," continued stories about DTP vaccine safety in the electronic and print media likely contributed to a vaccine liability crisis by 1984, with shortages and pricing instability remedied only by passage of NCVIA.

The latter half of the 1990s brought more and more complex media focus on vaccine safety issues, judging by calls to CDC's National Immunization Hotline through 2000. Some were generated by research published in the United States (rotavirus vaccine and intussusception) and the United Kingdom (measles vaccine, inflammatory bowel disease, and autism); others by government-related vaccine safety activities (*Thimerosal in Vaccines: A Joint Statement of the American Academy of Pediatrics and the U.S. Public Health Service*), or in the case of hepatitis B vaccine, a change in immunization policy by the French Government. Despite being featured on national or cable news magazine programs or in prominent stories in major magazines (*Time, Consumer Reports*) and newspapers (*USA Today*), followup media interest appeared limited. In contrast, a search on "vaccine" and "risk" in the New York Times archives from 1996 through mid-July 2002 produced more than 300 articles.

Questions of media responsibility usually follow major stories on health risk. All parties are rarely satisfied. While the vast majority of vaccine stories mention benefits, when something happens, the downsides are emphasized. Reporting vaccine risk is especially challenging given that images overwhelm words and that the relevant scientific concepts are hard to simplify. Providing viewpoints on both sides of an emerging vaccine issue is imperative; investigating the credibility of sources should be as well. At the same time, evenly balanced stories may leave readers confused as to what to believe. Media experts say that one problem is the use of the word "safe" by those wishing to reassure the public. This may actually be doing the opposite since no medicine or biologic is completely safe. They suggest the alternatives "relatively safe" or "as safe as possible," which warrant empirical testing. Risk communicators emphasize the need to be frank about all risks and uncertainties, including data gaps and areas of significant disagreement among experts. To not do so imperils the trust and credibility of future communication efforts. To do so leaves the challenge of how to convey the relative magnitudes of competing risks understandably and not magnify small uncertainties where there is significant consensus.

The advent of the Internet has also transformed the ability of organized media to communicate, providing new forms of access to print and audiovisual material. It remains to be seen how Internet use will ultimately affect or incorporate other media.

Sources

Centers for Disease Control and Prevention. (1999). Withdrawal of rotavirus vaccine recommendation: Recommendations of the Advisory Committee on Immunization Practices (ACIP). *Morbidity and Mortality Weekly Report, 48*(43), 1007.

Cohn, V. (1993). Medical journals and the popular media. *New England Journal of Medicine, 392*(12), 890.

Cohn, V. (1996). Vaccines and risks: The responsibility of the media, scientists and clinicians [Editorial]. *Journal of the American Medical Association, 276*(23), 1917-1918.

Danovaro-Holliday, M. C., Wood, A. L., & LeBaron, C. W. (2002). Rotavirus vaccine and the news media, 1987-2001. *Journal of the American Medical Association, 287*(11), 1455-1462.

Dixon, B. (2002). Triple vaccine fears mask media efforts at balance. *Current Biology, 12(5),* R151-R152.

Evans, G., Bostrom, A., Johnston, R. B., Fisher, B. L., & Stoto, M. A. (Eds.). (1997). *Risk communication and vaccination: Workshop summary.* Washington, DC: National Academy Press.

Expanded Programme on Immunization: Lack of evidence that hepatitis B vaccine causes multiple sclerosis. (1997). *Weekly Epidemiological Record, 72,* 149-152.

Freed, G. L., Katz, S. L., & Clark, S. J. (1996). Safety of vaccinations: Miss America, the media and public health. *Journal of the American Medical Association, 276,* 1869-1872.

Inside the world of autism. (2002, May 6). *Time.*

Manning, A. (1999, August 3). Parents fear growing number of vaccines. *USA Today.*

Manning, A. (2000, July 18). To vaccinate or not to vaccinate: Parents worry about safety which worries health officials. *USA Today.*

Thimerosal in vaccines: An interim report to clinicians. (1999). *Pediatrics, 104*(3), 570-574.

Thompson, N. P., Montgomery, S. M., Pounder, R. E., & Wakefield, A. J. (1995). Is measles vaccination a risk for inflammatory bowel disease? Lancet, 345.

Vaccines: An issue of trust. (2001, August). *Consumer Reports.*

The Role of Government

NCVIA not only brought the Federal Government into a more prominent vaccine safety and risk communication role, it greatly enhanced information on vaccine risks and benefits. Key provisions included creation of the Vaccine Adverse Event Reporting System (VAERS), which began operation in 1990 as a national passive surveillance system for the reporting of adverse events following immunization; a call for IOM studies of adverse events from childhood vaccines, published in 1991 and 1994; and the development of vaccine information materials, currently known as Vaccine Information Statements (VISs).

Two major programs, VICP and the National Vaccine Program, were created by NCVIA. VICP is a no-fault system to compensate families of children, or individuals, thought to be injured from childhood vaccines. Its very existence implies risk, especially when the numbers of families (or individuals) compensated (more than 1,500) and overall awards (more than $1 billion) are reported in the media or on the Internet. At the same time, VICP staff and outside medical consultant analysis of medical records submitted with claims has led to a better understanding of the very limited role vaccines play in chronic illnesses thought to be vaccine related. The Advisory Commission on Childhood Vaccines (ACCV), which is composed of parents, physicians, and attorneys in equal numbers, oversees operation of VICP.

The National Vaccine Program Office (NVPO) coordinates and integrates all Federal agency activities related to immunization (Table 2). Working with its advisory body, the National Vaccine Advisory Committee (NVAC), and through special needs funding, NVPO has sponsored a number of projects and workshops relating to communication. One noteworthy example was a public workshop in October 2000 to identify more effective approaches to vaccine risk communication.

Each Federal agency contributes to communication efforts. On its Web site, the Food and Drug Administration (FDA) through the Centers for Biologics Evaluation and Research (CBER) provides information for health professionals and consumers on regulatory activities that ensure the safety and efficacy of vaccines. FDA also shares management of VAERS with CDC and provides reporting forms and research results online and accepts VAERS reports online.

The National Institute of Allergy and Infectious Diseases (NIAID) is the major source of support for vaccine research. In addition to the *Jordan Report*, a brochure on vaccine development process and testing, called *Understanding Vaccines*, and the *Task Force Report on Safer Childhood Vaccines* can be accessed at the NIAID Web site. Among the latter's major recommendations is a blueprint for educating the public and health professionals on vaccine benefit and risk.

CDC's immunization efforts are through the National Immunization Program (NIP) and the National Center for Infectious Disease (NCID). The latter is responsible for laboratory and clinical research on vaccines. NIP coordinates and promotes immunization activities nationwide and monitors vaccine safety and efficacy. Through written materials, videotapes, the National Immunization Hotline, and a Web site, NIP provides information on vaccine benefit and risk to healthcare providers, the general public, and the media. CDC through NIP is also responsible for developing and updating VISs using a process of public comment (including review by ACCV).

VISs are 1-page, 2-sided sheets written at the fifth- to seventh-grade level designed to facilitate, not replace, provider-patient communication. Providers are required to distribute them each time a vaccine covered by VICP is administered. Studies show VIS reading level is too high for some and overly simplistic and incomplete for others. Compliance with the distribution requirements has been questionable, with one self-reporting survey showing that about a third of physicians do not have VISs in their offices, and a somewhat greater percentage do not give out a VIS at every visit.

Sources

Chen, R. T., Rastogi, S. C., Mullen, J. R., Hayes, S. W., et al. (1994). The Vaccine Adverse Event Reporting System (VAERS). *Vaccine, 12*(6), 542-550.

Goodman, M., Lamm, S. H., & Bellman, M. H. (1997). Temporal relationship modeling: DTP or DT immunizations and infantile spasms. *Vaccine, 16*(2-3), 25-31.

Howson, C. P., Howe, C. J., & Fineberg, H. V. (Eds.). (1991). *Adverse effects of pertussis and rubella vaccines. Report from the Institute of Medicine.* Washington, DC: National Academy Press.

Humiston, S. G., Levine, L., Dolan, J., et al. (1996). Parental preference among polio vaccination options: A decision analytic approach [Abstract]. *Archives of Pediatric & Adolescent Medicine, 150*(Suppl.), 52.

Jozwiak, S., Goodman, M., & Lamm, S. H. (1998). Poor mental development in TSC patients: Clinical risk factors. *Archives of Neurology, 55*(3), 379-384.

Lamm, S. H., Goodman, M., Engel, A., Shepard, C. W., Houser, O. W., & Gomez, M. R. (1997). Cortical tuber count: A bio-marker indicating cerebral severity of tuberous sclerosis complex. *Journal of Child Neurology, 12,* 85-90.

Melman, S. T., Kaplan, J. M., Lee, N. C., et al. Readability of the revised childhood vaccine information statements [Abstract]. *Archives of Pediatrics & Adolescent Medicine, 149*(Suppl.), 69.

"New Vaccine Information Materials Notice" [59 FR 31889, July 20, 1994].

Stratton, K. R., Howe, D. J., & Johnston, R. B. (Eds.). (1994). *Adverse events associated with childhood vaccines: Evidence bearing on causality. Report from the Institute of Medicine.* Washington, DC: National Academy Press.

THE ROLE OF NONGOVERNMENTAL ORGANIZATIONS

Professional associations, academic institutions, and consumer groups comprise a growing list of nongovernmental organizations (NGOs) contributing to vaccine risk communication, mostly via the Internet. Target audiences for the most part are health professionals and the public; others list the media and policymakers. In addition, some organizations have developed communication resource materials, like the National Network for Immunization Information or the Immunization Action Coalition, which provides downloadable versions of the VISs in more than two dozen languages.

In their capacity as a credible independent scientific institution, IOM's reports on adverse events have helped channel discussion and debate on a number of complex and controversial vaccine policy issues. Information from IOM reports, for example, is used in development of VISs, modifications to the Vaccine Injury Table, and formulation of vaccine recommendations by CDC and AAP. Through the National Academy of Sciences Web site, more than a dozen IOM reports and workshop summaries on vaccine topics can be read or downloaded.

In 1999, near-simultaneous publicity over rotavirus vaccine and intussusception and the issue of thimerosal in vaccines raised concern that the public might be starting to doubt the safety of vaccines. To help regain any loss of confidence, CDC and NIAID contracted with IOM to perform independent, expedited scientific reviews of current and emerging vaccine safety hypotheses. In an extraordinary attempt to eliminate potential conflict of interest, membership on the new Immunization Safety Review Committee was limited to scientists without financial ties to industry, previous service on major vaccine advisory committees, or prior expert testimony or publications on issues of vaccine safety. The committee's charge went beyond past efforts of providing a plausibility assessment (biologic plausibility and causality) to include a significance assessment looking at the burden of disease, the potential vaccine adverse event, and the level of public concern; a public health response assessment of the need for a review of current policy and suggestions for future research; and an analysis of communications and, if relevant, general and crosscutting issues.

IOM held public workshops on each topic, working on a 60- to 90-day completion schedule. Four reports had been issued by the summer of 2002, covering purported associations between measles-mumps-rubella (MMR) vaccine and autism, thimerosal-containing vaccines and neurodevelopmental disorders, multiple immunizations and immune system dysfunction, and hepatitis B vaccine and neurological disorders. None of them found proven evidence for any of the vaccine safety hypotheses, although the committee, for example, was unable to conclude from the available evidence whether or not thimerosal causes certain neurodevelopmental disorders, and supported use of thimerosal-free vaccines. The reports seem to have helped reduce some of the public uncertainty about vaccine safety.

Regarding communication, IOM found barriers while looking for parent materials on government Web sites in terms of the organization and availability of information on specific topics, as well as the wording in some of the safety narratives. The committee also pointed to the lack of research on individual vaccine risk perception and decisionmaking, recommending to the government a comprehensive research agenda for knowledge leading to better design and evaluation of risk communication approaches. One report pointed out the lack of discussion of ethical issues, such as providing enough information on the more rarely occurring risks for parents living in States with compulsory immunization.

Sources

Howe, C. J., & Johnston, R. B. (Eds.). (1996). Options for poliomyelitis vaccination in the United States. Washington, DC: National Academy Press.

Howe, C. J., Johnston, R. B., & Alexander, E. R. (Eds.). (1997). *Workshop safety forum: Summaries of two workshops (Research to identify risks for adverse events following vaccination: Biological mechanisms and possible means of prevention). Report from the Institute of Medicine.* Washington, DC: National Academy Press.

Howe, C. J., Johnston, R. B., & Genichel, G. M. (Eds.). (1997). *Workshop safety forum: Summaries of two workshops (Detecting and responding to adverse events following vaccination: Workshop summary). Report from the Institute of Medicine.* Washington, DC: National Academy Press.

Howson, C. P., Howe, C. J., & Fineberg, H. V. (Eds.). (1991). *Adverse effects of pertussis and rubella vaccines. Report from the Institute of Medicine.* Washington, DC: National Academy Press.

Stratton, K., Almario, D., & McCormick, M. (Eds.). (2002). *Hepatitis B vaccine and demyelinating neurological disorders. Report from the Institute of Medicine.* Washington, DC: National Academy Press.

Stratton, K., Gable, A., & McCormick, M. (Eds.). (2001). *Thimerosal-containing vaccines and neurodevelopmental disorders. Report from the Institute of Medicine.* Washington, DC: National Academy Press.

Stratton, K., Gable, A., Shetty, P., & McCormick, M. (Eds.). (2001). *Measles-mumps-rubella vaccine and autism. Report from the Institute of Medicine.* Washington, DC: National Academy Press.

Stratton, K., Wilson, C. B., & McCormick, M. (Eds.). (2002). *Multiple immunizations and immune dysfunction. Report from the Institute of Medicine.* Washington, DC: National Academy Press.

Stratton, K. R., Howe, C. J., & Johnston, R. B. (Eds.). (1994). *Adverse events associated with childhood vaccines: Evidence bearing on causality. Report from the Institute of Medicine.* Washington, DC: National Academy Press.

Stratton, K. R., Howe, C. J., & Johnston, R. B. (Eds.). (1994). *DTP vaccine and chronic nervous system dysfunction: A new analysis.* Washington, DC: National Academy Press.

Thimerosal in vaccines: An interim report to clinicians. (1999). *Pediatrics, 104*(3), 570-574.

THE ROLE OF VACCINE COMPANIES

Vaccine companies communicate product information via written materials and their Web sites. Many companies and biotech firms promote immunization through the National Partnership for Immunization. However, the primary risk communication tool for industry remains the manufacturer's vaccine package insert. While inserts are included in the shipments to offices or pharmacies, they are probably easiest to access by reading the *Physicians Desk Reference* or going online to the company Web site. The inserts include statements on efficacy, contraindications, warnings, precautions, and adverse events associated with the use of the vaccine. Package inserts are regulated by the FDA, which determines the type of information that must be included and reviews and approves each package insert prior to marketing and whenever changes are made. Frequently, the list of adverse events associated with the vaccine includes a number of events generally thought not to be related but which are included for legal (liability) reasons. The contraindications or precautions that are listed may also differ from those of the major recommending bodies: CDC's Advisory Committee on Immunization Practices (ACIP) and AAP. These differences, plus the poor readability due to small font size, make current package inserts an understandably limited resource. Recent revisions to the requirements for package inserts may help address some of these limitations.

Sources

Evans, G., Bostrom, A., Johnston, R. B., Fisher, B. L., & Stoto, M. A. (Eds.). (1997). *Risk communication and vaccination: workshop summary.* Washington, DC: National Academy Press.

Federal Register (2001, March 30). Vol. 66, No. 62; 21 C.F.R. Part 201.

Mehta Mukesh, R. (Ed.). (2002). *Physician's desk reference (56th ed.).* New Jersey: Medical Economics.

RISK COMMUNICATION SCIENCE AND VACCINES

Over the last several decades, government and industry efforts to reassure the public about a number of technological and environmental hazards (e.g., nuclear power plants, toxic waste sites, indoor radon) have sometimes provoked unanticipated responses. Risk communication research has developed to predict and support risk management behaviors. It has interdisciplinary roots in cognitive and social psychology, behavioral decision theory, risk assessment and management, and communications.

Vaccine risk communication research is relatively new, but is rapidly acquiring its own profile. A PubMed search in mid-July 2002, showed 73 publications on "vaccine risk communication" in the last two decades, of which almost half were published in the last 5 years. While it shares features with technological and environmental risk communications aimed at supporting informed decisionmaking as a public health concern, vaccine risk communication is also often treated as an issue of how to achieve effective advocacy. A mental models approach (i.e., ascertaining people's understanding of a risk) to risk communication starts with the fact that people interpret information based on what they already know, that this must be assessed empirically, and that empirical evaluation of communications is also essential. Other approaches are concerned with catching readers' attention, increasing their belief in their ability to control (disease) risk effectively (with vaccination), or, as in fear appeals, changing their affective responses to a risk.

Vaccine messages based on mental models and other empirical methods are in the early stages of development. Building on insights from other domains, vaccine risk communicators are developing validated empirical approaches to the design and evaluation of risk communication, and a cadre of researchers and new institutional structures to assist in these efforts.

Recent risk communication research has focused on: 1) examining the role of trust in institutions and sources of risk communications, and in particular how value similarity affects risk communication; 2) gaining a better understanding of mental models of risks and their roles in risk communication; 3) examining how emotions and affect influence risk perception and communication; and 4) integrating social psychological theories of persuasion and message processing in risk communication. Vaccine risk communication research is underway in at least the first two of these four areas.

Sources

Bandura, A. (1999). Social cognitive theory: An agentic perspective. [Special Issue]. *Asian J. Soc. Psyc., 2*(1), 21-41.

Baron, J. (1994). Thinking and deciding (2nd ed.). New York: Cambridge University Press.

Bostrom, A. (1997). Vaccine risk communication: Lessons learned from risk perception, decisionmaking, and environmental risk communication research. Risk: *Health, Safety & Environment, 8,* 173-200.

Bostrom, A., Atman, C. J., Fischhoff, B., & Morgan, M. G. (1994). Evaluation of risk communications: Completing and correcting mental models of hazardous processes, *Part II. Risk Analysis, 14*(5), 789-798.

Cvetkovich, G., & Lofstedt, R. E. (Eds.). (1999). Social trust and the management of risk. *London: Earthscan.*

Finucane, M. L., Alhakami, A., Slovic, P., & Johnson, S. M. (2000). The affect heuristic in judgments of risks and benefits. *Journal of Behavioral Decision Making, 13, 1-17.*

Fischhoff, B., Bostrom, A., & Quadrel, M. J. (1993). Risk perception and communication. *Annual Review of Public Health, 14,* 183-203.

Fischhoff, B., Lichtenstein, S., Slovic, P., Derby, S. L., & Keeney, R. L. (1981). *Acceptable Risk.* Cambridge University Press.

Hadden, S. G. (1989). Institutional barriers to risk communication. *Risk Analysis, 9*(3), 301-308.

Holmes, J. G., Miller, D. T., & Lerner, M. J. (2002). Committing altruism under the cloak of self-interest: The exchange fiction. *J. Exp. Soc. Psy., 38*(2), 144-151.

Keeney, R. L., & von Winterfeldt, D. (1986). Improving risk communication. *Risk Analysis, 6*(4), 417-424. [http://www ncbi nlm nih.gov/entrez/query.fcgi?cmd=Retrieve&db=PubMed&list_uids=87262214&dopt=Abstract].

Lerner, J. S., Gonzalez, R. M., Small, D. A., & Fischhoff, B. (in press). Effects of fear and anger on perceived risks of terrorism: A national field experiment. *Psychological Science.*

Maibach, E., & Parrott, L. R. (1995). *Designing health messages: Approaches from communication theory and public health practice.* Thousand Oaks, CA: Sage Publications.

McComas, K. A., & Trumbo, C. W. (2001). Source credibility in environmental health-risk controversies application of Meyer's credibility index. *Risk Analysis, 21*(3), 467-480.

Morgan, M. G., Fischhoff, B., Bostrom, A., & Atman, C. J. (2002). *Risk communication: A mental models approach.* Cambridge University Press.

Plous, S. (1993). *The psychology of judgment and decision making.* New York: McGraw-Hill.

Siegriest, M., Cvetkovich, G., & Gutscher, H. (2002). Risk preference predictions and gender stereotypes. *Organizational Behavior and Human Decision Processes, 87*(1), 91-102.

Slovic, P. (Ed.). (2000). *The perception of risk.* London: Earthscan. [www.earthscan.co.uk].

Witte, K., Meyer, G., & Martell, D. P. (2001). *Effective health risk messages: A step-by-step guide.* Thousand Oaks, CA: Sage Publications.

FUTURE CHALLENGES

As the 20-year timeline (Table 1) shows, the trend is toward more vaccine policy events and more related communication activities and challenges. Recent and imminent changes in the political and institutional realities of public health, technological advances in communication, and molecular biology and immunology are likely to play a significant role in determining future investments in vaccine risk perception and communication research and practice.

For government agencies, new and better methods of communication through a comprehensive research strategy were outlined in the 2000 NVPO Workshop on Vaccine Risk Communication and more recent IOM Immunization Safety Review Committee reports. Gaining knowledge in the design and evaluation of vaccine risk-benefit communication approaches will enable more effective ways of communicating emerging vaccine safety hypotheses, changes in vaccine policy, and the uncertainty over gaps in information. Other needs include more user-friendly Web sites, and low-literacy and higher level communication materials that are understandable and appropriate (i.e., not judgmental or prescriptive). The "one size fits all" approach for VISs clearly has limited usefulness.

Perhaps the greatest challenge for government is to establish and maintain trust with the "organized" public (i.e., interested parents or parents of children thought harmed by vaccines), as well as parents in general. Only through dialogue can there be a better understanding and appreciation of viewpoints and misconceptions on both sides. Efforts to gather immunization stakeholders for face-to-face discussions, which began in 1995 with the IOM Vaccine Safety Forum, were being pursued once again in 2002 through a CDC/NVPO-sponsored project called the Vaccine Collaborative. In 2002, CDC added a consumer representative to ACIP to be consistent with FDA's Vaccines and Related Biological Products Advisory Committee (VRBPAC) and NVAC. While vaccine activists are the visible, vocal public, no less important are the views and values of the general public. Accessing these views on immunization risk has not been routinely attempted up to this point. Only through shared decisionmaking can the interest of the public be best served.

Unfortunately, funding for communication research and related outreach efforts is anything but certain. In a climate of competing health priorities and limited budgets, arguments for proactive measures on risk communication, although sound in principle, do not appear as compelling when vaccine safety issues regularly draw media attention and concern. Philanthropic foundations have funded vaccine registries and communication efforts in the past, and perhaps will be a viable option for future communications research and collaborative efforts with the public.

Another challenge is the elimination of barriers and promotion of effective risk communication by healthcare professionals. Generally, providers should be informed about vaccine-preventable disease, safety issues, and the practice and ethics of informing parents about vaccine risks and benefits. Today, providers should expect that some parents will question the need for or safety of vaccination, refuse certain vaccines, or even reject all immunizations for their child. The best approach is empathetic vaccine risk communication, which is essential in responding to misinformation and concerns that parents may have encountered on the Internet or have heard elsewhere. Some vaccines may be acceptable to the resistant parent. Concerns may be addressed by a variety of materials now available. If not, parents should be advised of State laws pertaining to school or childcare entry, which may require that unimmunized children stay home from school during outbreaks. Documenting such discussions in the patient's record is important, and even having a parent sign an "informed refusal" document may help to reduce any potential liability should a vaccine-preventable disease occur in the unimmunized patient. Above all, patients should not be excluded from a practice; parental questioning or refusal of a vaccine does not necessarily mean a parent does not trust the provider and will dismiss other health advice and guidance.

Events in the last year illustrate the potential for the unanticipated to drive vaccine risk perceptions and communications: Anthrax attacks, heightened concerns about smallpox and bioterrorism, new vaccine policy recommendations, increased research and publication on vaccine perception and communication, and shortages of many routine childhood and adult vaccines. Vaccine risk communicators have found themselves with more than ever to do. With sufficient resources, they should be able to marshal the advances of the past two decades to address these challenges and to improve immunization programs and policies.

ACKNOWLEDGMENTS

The author wishes to thank Kristine Sheedy; Skip Wolfe; Robert Chen, M.D., M.A.; Glen Nowak, Ph.D.; and Norman Baylor, Ph.D., for assistance in obtaining background information, and Leslie Ball, M.D., for comments on the manuscript.

Table 1: Timeline of Vaccine Risk and Risk Communication Events, 1982-2002

1982:
- "DTP: Vaccine Roulette" excerpts aired on *The Today Show*
- Parent consumer group Dissatisfied Parents Together (DPT) formed

1984: *Morbidity and Mortality Weekly Report (MMWR)* notice calling for rationing of DTP vaccine supplies due to liability crisis

1985:
- *DTP: A Shot in the Dark* (Coulter and Fisher) published
- *Phil Donahue Show* on DTP vaccine safety

1986:
- National Childhood Vaccine Injury Act signed into law
- National Vaccine Program Office created
- DPT demonstration at Advisory Committee on Immunization Practices (ACIP) meeting in Atlanta

1988: National Vaccine Injury Compensation Program (VICP) begins operation

1989:
- National Research Council report: "Improving Risk Communication"
- Resurgence of measles in preschool age children
- Second dose of measles-mumps-rubella (MMR) recommended by ACIP and the American Academy of Pediatrics (AAP)
- DPT changes name to National Vaccine Information Center

1990:
- Vaccine Adverse Event Reporting System (VAERS) begins operation
- Centers for Disease Control and Prevention (CDC)/ National Immunization Program (NIP) initiates Vaccine Safety Datalink (VSD)

1991:
- Institute of Medicine (IOM) report "Adverse Effects of Pertussis and Rubella Vaccines"
- ACIP/AAP recommend acellular pertussis vaccine for the 4th and 5th dose
- ACIP/AAP recommend routine use of hepatitis B vaccine in infants
- "Measles White Paper" on the measles epidemic published in the *Journal of the American Medical Association* (*JAMA*)

1992:
- Childhood immunization initiative target of 90-percent immunization coverage of 2-year- olds announced
- NIP moved to Office of the Director, CDC
- Vaccine safety becomes distinct activity within NIP

1993: "Standards for Pediatric Immunization Practices" published in *MMWR* and *JAMA*

1994:
- IOM report entitled "Adverse Events Associated with Childhood Vaccines"
- IOM report on the 10-year followup to the National Childhood Encephalopathy Study of whole-cell pertussis vaccine and long-term neurological effects
- Vaccines for Children (VFC) program enacted
- National Vaccine Plan is approved by the Secretary of the Department of Health and Human Services (DHHS)
- Vaccine risk communication becomes distinct activity within NIP
- Vaccine Risk Communication (VARICO) conference calls started at CDC

1995:
- *IOM Vaccine Safety Forum* Workshop on Vaccine Risk Communication
- "6 Common Misconceptions About Vaccines: And How to Respond to Them" CDC, NIP
- Varicella and hepatitis A vaccines licensed
- VICP final rule adding chronic arthritis for rubella-containing vaccines and removing shock-collapse and residual seizure disorder for DTP vaccine on Vaccine Injury Table

1996:
- ACIP recommends acellular pertussis vaccine for routine use in infants
- "Vaccination: The Issue of Our Times" in *Mothering*, summer edition
- Goal of 90-percent immunization rates for 2-year-olds is achieved
- Reverse transcriptase detected in live-attenuated virus vaccines
- Task Force on Safer Childhood Vaccines report is approved by the Secretary, DHHS
- Studies published showing evidence of simian virus 40 (SV40) in rare human tumors
- CDC issues apology for errors in obtaining informed consent for E-Z measles vaccine studies in Los Angeles

Table 1: Timeline of Vaccine Risk and Risk Communication Events, 1982-2002 (continued)

1997:
- ACIP recommends sequential inactivated poliovirus (IPV)/oral poliovirus (OPV) vaccine schedule
- Emerging Viruses: AIDS and Ebola: Nature, Accident or Intention? *(Horowitz)* published
- First International Conference on Vaccination held by National Vaccine Information Center
- Institute for Vaccine Safety established at Johns Hopkins University
- Workshop on possible association between polio vaccine-contaminated SV40 and cancer
- Food and Drug Administration (FDA) Modernization Act (includes review/assessment of all mercury-containing foods and drugs)

1998:
- *Lancet* paper suggesting association between measles vaccine and autism
- Gannett News Service series on vaccine safety and VICP
- *New England Journal of Medicine (NEJM)* paper on Guillain-Barre syndrome and influenza vaccines
- Rotavirus vaccine licensed
- Secretary of Defense orders anthrax vaccine use for all active duty military personnel
- National Network for Immunization Information established
- Bill & Melinda Gates Foundation grant of $100 million for global vaccination
- "A Shadow Falls on Hepatitis B Vaccination Efforts" *Science,* July 31
- French Government suspends middle school-based hepatitis B immunization
- Illinois Board of Health hearing on hepatitis B vaccine and mandatory immunization
- Massachusetts Public Health Council hearing on varicella vaccine and mandatory immunization
- Lyme disease vaccine licensed

1999:
- ABC News program on hepatitis B vaccine on *20/20*
- Congressional hearings on vaccine safety in general, hepatitis B and anthrax vaccines, vaccines and autism, and improving VICP
- Rotavirus vaccine use suspended, then withdrawn from marketplace
- Joint statement of AAP/Public Health Service on thimerosal preservative in childhood vaccines
- *The River* is published, links OPV clinical trials in Africa to acquired immunodeficiency syndrome (AIDS) epidemic (Hooper)

- ACIP broadens use recommendation for hepatitis A vaccine making it routine use in those States where disease is endemic
- "Parents Fear Growing Number of Vaccines" *USA Today,* August 3
- National Vaccine Advisory Committee workshop on thimerosal
- ABC News program on vaccine safety and mandatory immunization on *Nightline*
- CDC hires communication specialist to direct vaccine risk communication efforts

2000:
- ACIP recommends exclusive use of IPV
- Congressional hearings on vaccine safety and autism
- "Don't Worry about Vaccinations" *Parade* magazine, January 9
- "When Vaccines Do Harm to Kids" *Insight* magazine, February
- ABC Evening News *program: "Vaccine Victims?" (Lyme disease vaccine and adverse effects)*
- National Vaccine Program Office workshop on vaccine risk communication
- Pneumococcal conjugate vaccine licensed for routine use
- "To Vaccinate or Not to Vaccinate: Parents Worry About Safety Which Worries Health Officials" *USA Today,* July 18
- "Murder or Bad Vaccine?" *Redbook,* September
- Allied Vaccine Group launches "Web ring" of four Web sites for access to science-based information
- Vaccine Education Center at the Children's Hospital of Philadelphia established
- Tetanus vaccine supply shortage begins—shortages occur for other childhood and adult vaccines over next 2 years

2001:
- National Vaccine Program Office workshop on rotavirus vaccines
- ABC News program on MMR vaccine and autism on *20/20*
- NBC News program on MMR vaccine and autism on *Dateline*
- Congressional hearings on vaccine safety and autism/ and the VICP
- "Vaccines: An Issue of Trust" *Consumer Reports,* August
- *NEJM* papers on hepatitis B vaccine and multiple sclerosis
- *Brighton Collaboration* established to define/ analyze adverse events following immunization

Table 1: Timeline of Vaccine Risk and Risk Communication Events, 1982-2002 (concluded)

- Clinical Immunization Safety Assessment (CISA) centers funded http://www.partnersforimmunization.org/cisa.pdf)
- Class action lawsuits filed in several States alleging thimerosal-related injury
- VAERS goes online for reporting of adverse events
- 9/11 attacks in New York, Washington, and Pennsylvania
- Anthrax bioterrorist attack—supplies of anthrax and smallpox vaccine increased
- IOM reports on MMR vaccine and autism/thimerosal-containing vaccines and neurodevelopmental disorders are released

2002:
- Congressional hearings on autism and vaccine safety
- National Vaccine Program Office workshop on vaccine supply shortages
- Lyme disease vaccine distribution is discontinued by manufacturer
- ACIP recommends limiting use of smallpox vaccine to frontline response teams
- IOM reports on multiple immunizations and immune dysfunction/hepatitis B vaccine and demyelinating neurological disorders are released
- IOM report on anthrax vaccine released

Table 2: Vaccine Risk Communication Resources

Organizations/Web sites

Government

- National Vaccine Program Office, HHS (http://www.cdc.gov/od/nvpo)
- National Immunization Program, CDC (http://www.cdc nip)
- National Center for Infectious Disease (http://www.cdc.gov/ncidod)
- Centers for Biologics Evaluation and Research, FDA (http://www fda.gov/cber)
- National Institute for Allergy and Infectious Diseases (http://www niaid nih.gov/dmid.vaccines).
- National Vaccine Injury Compensation Program, HRSA (http://www.hrsa.gov/osp/vicp)
- Vaccine Adverse Event Reporting System (http://vaers.org)

Nongovernment

- American Academy of Pediatrics (http://www.aap.org)
- National Network for Immunization Information (http://www.immunizationinfo.org)
- Allied Vaccine Group (http://www.vaccine.org)
- Vaccine Education Center at the Children's Hospital of Philadelphia (http://www.vaccine.chop.edu)
- Institute for Vaccine Safety at Johns Hopkins University (www.vaccinesafety.edu)
- Every Child by Two (www.ecbt.org)
- National Coalition for Adult Immunization (http://www nfid.org/ncai)
- Immunization Action Coalition (http://www.immunize.org)

- National Partnership for Immunization (http://www.partnersforimmunization.org)
- National Healthy Mothers, Healthy Babies Coalition (http://www.hmhb.org)
- National Foundation for Infectious Diseases (http://www.nfid.org)
- Infectious Diseases Society of America (http://www.idsociety.org)
- Pediatric Infectious Diseases Society of America (http://www.pids.org)
- Sabin Vaccine Institute (http://sabin.org)
- All Kids Count (http://www.allkidscount.org)
- Children's Vaccine Program at PATH (http://childrensvaccine.org)
- Global Alliance for Vaccines and Immunization (http://www.vaccinealliance.org)
- World Health Organization (http://www.who.int/vaccines-disease/safety/)
- Brighton Collaboration (http://brightoncollaboration.org).
- Institute of Medicine (http://www.nas.edu)
- Institute of Medicine Vaccine Safety Review Committee (http://www.iom.edu/imsafety)

Consumer

- Parents of Kids with Infectious Diseases (PKids)(http://www.pkids.org/)
- National Vaccine Information Center (NVIC) (http://www.909shot.com),
- Parents Requesting Open Vaccine Education (PROVE) (http://vaccineinfo.net)
- Vaccine Information and Awareness (VIA) (http://home.san.rr.com/via)

Table 2: Vaccine Risk Communication Resources (concluded)

Books/Brochures

Parents Guide to Childhood Immunizations: CDC/NIP Web site

Six Common Misconceptions about Vaccination and How to Respond to Them: CDC/NIP Web site

Epidemiology and Prevention of Vaccine-Preventable Diseases (Pink Book)*: CDC/NIP Web site*

Guide to Contraindications to Childhood Vaccines: CDC/NIP Web site

Vaccine Information Statements: CDC/NIP & Immunization Action Coalition Web sites

Understanding Vaccines: NIAID Web site

The Baby Shot Book: HRSA/National Vaccine Injury Compensation Program (available in 2003)

What Every Parent Should Know About Childhood Immunization (1998) Paul A. Offit/ Louis M. Bell

The Consumers Guide to Childhood Vaccines (1997) National Vaccine Information Center

The Immunization Resource Guide—4th edition (2000) Diane Rozario

Telephone

Immunization Hotline: 1-800-232-2522 for English; 1-800-232-0233 for Spanish

Vaccine Adverse Event Reporting System (VAERS): 1-800-822-7967

National Vaccine Injury Compensation Program: 1-800-338-2382

Author's Biography

Dr. Evans is Medical Director of the National Vaccine Injury Compensation Program. Following private and managed care pediatric practice, he joined the Health Resources and Services Administration's Division of Vaccine Injury Compensation where he has served as a liaison member to the National Vaccine Advisory Committee, Advisory Committee on Immunization Practices, and Advisory Commission on Childhood Vaccines. It was while working on these advisory committees that Dr. Evans first became interested in health risk communication. Since then, he has authored or collaborated on journal articles covering the growing scientific discipline of vaccine risk communication. Dr. Evans also has presented at scientific meetings, co-chaired the 1995 Institute of Medicine Vaccine Safety Forum Workshop on Risk Communication and Vaccination, participated on Centers for Disease Control and Prevention (CDC) advisory panels to evaluate draft Vaccine Information Statements (VISs), and served as a consultant on vaccine safety and communication to the World Health Organization. More recently, he updated the legal requirements for use of VISs and contributed to a new section on vaccine risk communication for the *American Academy of Pediatrics' 2000* Red Book *publication.*

Author's Biography

Dr. Bostrom is Associate Professor in the School of Public Policy at Georgia Institute of Technology where she teaches quantitative methods, environmental risk, and risk communication at the graduate and undergraduate levels. She has research interests in risk perception, communication, and management, and in cognitive aspects of survey methodology. Dr. Bostrom's research focuses on mental models of hazardous processes and is funded by the National Science Foundation, National Institutes of Health, and Environmental Protection Agency. Among her current research projects are a study on how to improve informed consent for BRCA1/2 genetic screening decisions (in collaboration with researchers at Research Triangle Institute, Johns Hopkins University, Carnegie Mellon University, and other universities) and survey studies of economic and environmental risk perceptions (in collaboration with researchers at Georgia Institute of Technology). Dr. Bostrom has published in journals such as Risk Analysis, RISK: Health, Science and Environment, *and* Journal of Social Issues. *She has consulted for the Institute of Medicine on vaccine risk communication.*

Dr. Bostrom is a member of the Vaccine Risk Communication (VARICO) group of the Centers for Disease Control and Prevention (CDC). She also has been a member of the Advisory Committee for the Harvard Center for Risk Analysis.

Economics of Vaccine Development and Implementation: Changes Over the Past 20 Years

Economics of Vaccine Development and Implementation: Changes Over the Past 20 Years

Julie Milstien, Ph.D., and Brenda Candries, Ph.D.

INTRODUCTION

Twenty years ago, vaccine developers were for the most part the public-sector cousins of the pharmaceutical industry. Vaccines in use in 1980 included Bacillus de Calmette-Guerin (BCG), diphtheria and tetanus toxoids and whole-cell pertussis (DTP), measles, and oral poliovirus (OPV), all of which had been on the market for more than a decade, and some for the better part of half a century. The Food and Drug Administration (FDA) had overseen regulation of vaccines in the United States for only 8 years. The vaccine industry in the United States was feeling the impact of adverse reactions and potential liability issues with pertussis and swine flu vaccines, and prices for established vaccines were less than $1 to $3 per dose (see Table 1). Plasma-derived hepatitis B vaccine was not yet licensed, and recombinant products were still under development. The era of increased major expansion of vaccine research and development support (1) was just beginning. Good manufacturing practice (GMP) was far from an industry-wide concept.

**Table 1: U.S. Vaccine Prices —
1980 Versus 2000, U.S. $ per Dose***

Year/Product	Public Sector	Private Sector
1980		
Diphtheria and tetanus toxoids and whole-cell pertussis (DTP)	0.15	0.30
Oral poliovirus (OPV)	0.35	1.60
Measles-mumps-rubella (MMR)	2.71	7.24
2000		
Diphtheria and tetanus toxoids and acellular pertussis (DTaP)	9.25	16.64
Inactivated poliovirus (IPV)	6.99	15.42
MMR	14.69	28.19
Varicella	35.41	45.56

* B. Snyder, Centers for Disease Control and Prevention, personal communication, 2001

Today, with blockbuster products like *Haemophilus influenzae* type b (Hib) and pneumococcal conjugate vaccines, vaccines are big business. Vaccine selection has changed and prices are now much higher (see Table 1); the new seven-valent pneumococcal vaccine Prevnar® costs $232 for a four-dose series (2). The major vaccine producers are divisions of global pharmaceutical houses. Annual vaccine sales have gone from about $2 billion in 1982 (3) to an estimated $5.4 billion today (4). While still only a fraction of the $337.3 billion pharmaceutical market (4), the vaccine market is projected to increase 12 percent per year (2). This paper explores some of the major change areas in the economics of vaccine development.

COST COMPONENTS

The cost components of vaccine development include research and development, production, and regulation, including clinical trials. We have focused on patents relating to the development of or access to a particular technology, on process standardization and scale-up as an example of production costs, and on clinical trials, licensing, and testing to highlight some of the cost components of regulation.

Impact of TRIPS

When Jonas Salk developed the first polio vaccine, he was asked if he intended to patent it. He replied, "It would be like patenting the sun" (5). In the 1970s, many European countries were not giving patents on pharmaceutical products. Today, accessing intellectual property is a major factor in the product development cycle. However, for vaccines, it may not be an important barrier. With the new vaccines against acellular pertussis, hepatitis B recombinant, Hib conjugate, pneumococcal conjugates, and rotavirus, only the first two had exclusive licenses that limited access. The conjugation technology used for Hib and pneumococcal vaccines is in the public domain (6) (although alternative conjugated products exist) while the rotavirus vaccine technology, developed by the National Institutes of Health and licensed solely to Wyeth, is unlikely to be further developed.

DNA recombinant hepatitis B vaccine is produced in yeast or mammalian cells using bioengineering technology. The British firm Biogen obtained a broad patent covering all methods of making the vaccine antigens using recombinant technology. Biogen granted licenses to Merck and SmithKline Beecham (now

GlaxoSmithKline) who put the recombinant vaccine on the market by the mid-1980s for $30 to $40 per dose. By 1993, due to the competition from the plasma-derived vaccine, the price decreased to only marginally above that of the plasma-derived product—$1.25 to $2 per dose (7). Biogen started infringement procedures against Medeva (now part of Powderject) who, beginning in 1992, had wanted to market a recombinant DNA vaccine, even though it was based on a different production process. Following a counterclaim by Medeva, the House of Lords, in 1996, revoked the patent on the basis of the enablement provisions, which allow an attack on an overly broad claim: "The court stated that to grant a monopoly to the first person who has found a way of achieving an obviously desirable goal for every way of doing so would stifle further research and healthy competition in the post grant phase" (8, 9). While the price had come down significantly, access to the technology was still limited. By the mid-1990s the Biogen patent expired in many parts of the world, and this factor, coupled with the House of Lords' decision in 1996 to revoke the patent, resulted in new manufacturers entering the market. By 1999, two Korean manufacturers [KGCC (now Green Cross Vaccine Corporation) and LG Chem] were selling recombinant vaccines on the global market, and prices decreased to below $1 per dose. Currently, recombinant hepatitis B vaccine can be obtained by international bulk procurement for under $0.30 per dose (10). There are at least 10 manufacturers, 5 of which are prequalified to make sales to United Nations agencies (11).

Another case study is that of the pertactin antigen of *Bordetella pertussis* called P69. Evans Medical Limited (now part of Powderject) asserted that their P69 patent, licensed exclusively to SmithKline Beecham Biologicals, covered the pertactin antigen in Chiron's acellular pertussis vaccines. In a final nonappealable decision made in March 1998, the European Patent Office Technical Board of Appeal revoked the Evans patent (12). This decision, applicable to most European countries, ended patent infringement litigation against Chiron in the United Kingdom, Italy, and the Netherlands and cleared the way for sale of other acellular pertussis vaccines containing pertactin.

The impact of patents on technology access will now spread to most developing countries as they join the World Trade Organization and thus agree to uphold the Agreement on Trade-Related Aspects of Intellectual Property Rights (TRIPS), which established minimum universal intellectual property standards. A recent study (13) carefully analyzed the projected impact of TRIPS on the pharmaceutical industry in Thailand. The study did not reveal a price change due to the patent protection act in Thailand, but proposed a number of proactive strategies to avoid limitation of technology access and price rises.

It is not possible to predict the full impact of TRIPS on vaccine development costs. However, vaccine development requires not only the patentable technology, but also the know-how to produce consistently a safe and effective biological product. It is this dependence on know-how, not covered under TRIPS, that may attenuate its impact.

Process Standardization and Validation

In 1980, GMP was just being introduced into vaccine production. Today, investments in facilities, staff, and processes to maintain GMP compliance are driving production costs up (14). The ever increasing "GMP spiral" demands more and more investment. Each step of the production process must be documented and validated. Vaccine manufacturers now contract out parts of the process to contract manufacturers, particularly production scale-up. A recent study carried out at the World Health Organization (WHO) assessed 28 manufacturers capable of performing under contract some part of the vaccine development process (15).

Clinical Trials

Clinical trials have become a major expense in vaccine development. Following preclinical testing of a product, clinical trials of increasingly larger size are performed to establish clinical tolerance and acceptable safety, as well as to quantify immune response and demonstrate protective efficacy (16). In parallel, consistency of production must be demonstrated by showing comparable levels of clinical response to different vaccine batches. Factors impacting trial conduct and thus the costs include the characteristics of the study population, the power of the trial needed to detect potential safety problems, the increasing amount of documentation required to ensure that appropriate quality assurance and ethical procedures are in place, and the trend toward the use of contract research organizations (CROs) to manage these aspects.

Traditionally, vaccines available on the international market were developed, produced, and authorized for marketing in industrialized countries on the assumption that the data were applicable to most infant populations, at least for the traditional vaccines. For industrialized countries, this procedure seemed obvious and appropriate. But populations are changing, and even homogeneous populations have groups that may respond differently. Because of the potential differences in safety, immunogenicity, and efficacy among populations, safety and immunogenicity data should be obtained using the candidate vaccine in the specific population in which the efficacy trial will be performed (17, 18). This has applied, for example, to pneumococcal 9- and 11-valent conjugate vaccines developed in the United States and designed to benefit individuals in countries outside the United States as well as special high-risk groups (e.g., Eskimos and Native Americans) (19). The potential globalization of vaccines means that population characteristics must be even more carefully considered in developing clinical trial protocols.

A second factor impacting trial costs is the number of subjects needed to ensure sufficient power to demonstrate the potential safety and efficacy of the product. The story of RotaShield®, a tetravalent rhesus-based recombinant rotavirus vaccine licensed by the FDA on August 31, 1998, is illustrative. At that time, clinical trials included more than 10,000 vaccine recipients, sufficient for demonstration of efficacy, but not enough to demonstrate a statistically significant increase in intussusception (20). The Advisory Committee on Immunization Practices of the U.S. Centers for Disease Control and Prevention (CDC) recommended postlicensing surveillance for this adverse event (21), and by June 1999, following distribution of 1.8 million doses of vaccine (22), the CDC had noted increased reports of intussusception in recipients of the vaccine. This event could not have been picked up in any reasonably sized clinical trial. Especially for vaccines for universal use in children (23), the FDA is considering requiring expanded phase III trials with more attention to safety monitoring, a direction that could increase time to market and thus raise development costs significantly. Other regulatory authorities, for example in Europe, seem likely to impose instead more formal phase IV postmarketing safety studies to monitor carefully potential adverse events of vaccine candidates (20). There are benefits and drawbacks to either approach; both will impact costs.

In the effort to ensure the rights of clinical trial subjects, investigational review boards and ethics committees require more documentation and independent trial monitoring. This increase was considered at the Global Vaccine Research Forum held in Montreux, Switzerland, in June 2000 (24), where increased trial costs with little return on investment were cited.

Because of the complexity of complying with expanding guidelines on conduct of clinical trials, more sponsors are using CROs to conduct trials. According to PricewaterhouseCoopers (M. Burri, PricewaterhouseCoopers, personal communication, 2000), about 60 percent of big pharmaceutical manufacturers are outsourcing some part of their drug development, which adds up to a $5 billion market, growing at more than 20 percent per year and projected to account for 45 percent of the total research and development budget for drug development in 2003.

An important outcome of efficacy trials can be the determination of serological correlates of protection—the type and quantity of a specific immune response associated with vaccine protection. The identification of these determinants can facilitate future trials, as immune response is easier to measure than efficacy, and can help development of an appropriate lot release test. Although identification of such a correlate is not a requirement for U.S. licensure (17), failure to identify one adds complications and expense to subsequent trials, consistency demonstration, and lot release testing.

One approach used for acellular pertussis vaccine is to develop as a reference a large, well-characterized production lot shown to be effective or identical in all quantifiable respects to an

effective product, and to demonstrate consistency of each lot to the reference. This approach requires standardization and validation of tests, and full characterization of the reference. In any case, all final product tests for vaccine release must be appropriately standardized and validated.

Harmonization and Mutual Recognition

Preparation of applications for marketing authorization is hampered by differing requirements across countries. Many manufacturers now have huge regulatory divisions to prepare files and data in a multitude of languages and formats. Several initiatives are in place that may eventually reduce registration costs. The International Conference on Harmonisation (ICH) involves regulatory agencies of the United States, Japan, and Europe working with manufacturers to harmonize aspects of dossier requirements. So far, the ICH has addressed issues more applicable to pharmaceutical products, but more recently aspects applicable to vaccines, such as safety issues for biotechnological products, good clinical practice guidelines, viral safety evaluation of cell substrates, and a common technical document for all products including biologicals, have been addressed (25).

Mutual recognition agreements are in place between the European Union and Australia, New Zealand, United States, and Canada, and more are being developed (A. M. Georges, GSK, personal communication, 2000). The Pharmaceutical Inspection Convention, involving Australia, Austria, Belgium, Czech Republic, Denmark, Finland, France, Germany, Hungary, Iceland, Ireland, Italy, Liechtenstein, Norway, Portugal, Romania, Slovak Republic, Sweden, Switzerland, and United Kingdom, promotes joint GMP inspections, networking, training, and moving toward global harmonization of inspections (A. M. Georges, GSK, personal communication, 2000).

Many countries receiving vaccines through United Nations agency procurement use WHO prequalification (a system of ensuring a well-functioning regulatory process, coupled with assurance of compliance of the product with certain product specifications) (26) as a mechanism to fast-track national registration.

A major issue now confronting U.S. and European manufacturers of products designed for developing markets is the increasing difficulty of finding appropriate regulatory pathways. The regulatory agencies involved, the FDA and the European Medicines Evaluation Agency, have a primary responsibility to their home markets (4), and the use of scarce regulatory resources to evaluate products for different epidemiological situations is of low priority. Nevertheless, this problem must be addressed if manufacturers are to invest in the development of future vaccines against diseases such as malaria and AIDS.

PRICING CONSIDERATIONS

The pricing of vaccines has been characterized by heavy tiering across markets, which is possible because of highly scale sensitive manufacturing economics and product life cycles. The product life cycle has three distinct phases, as seen in Table 2: New product launch, market penetration, and product maturity. Most price tiering has been seen with mature products. The challenge for bringing new products to market is to ensure effective management of the life cycle (27) so that manufacturers and the market will benefit.

Table 2: Managing the Product Life Cycle (28)

Factor	New Product Launch	Market Penetration	Product Maturity
Number of producers	One	Multiple, industrialized countries	High, industrialized and developing countries
Available capacity	Low	High	Potential surplus
Market demand	Low	High, industrialized countries and private sector	High, all markets
Costs	High	Medium	Low
Prices	High uniform	Tiered within and across markets, high average	Tiered within and across markets, low average

On launch, there is typically only one producer, who owns product and process intellectual property. This phase will have limited capacity, low demand, high production costs, and high prices. During market penetration, new manufacturers will enter the market, either through their own development efforts or through licensing of the original manufacturer's patent, and capacity will increase. Limited price tiering will be possible. Once the product reaches maturity, and the intellectual property protection expires, there may be many manufacturers in the developing as well as the industrialized world. Production costs are low, and often there will be overcapacity so that availability is high and demand is global. Prices will be heavily tiered (28).

This paper will examine the impacts of capacity, market characteristics, and competition on pricing.

Capacity

A critical decision in vaccine development is that of scale. The price impacts depend on the risk inherent in the decision to make a specific capacity investment and the ultimate use of that capacity. A vaccine company will have to make the decision to invest in production capacity at an early stage, well in advance of knowing the real demand and before revenues are available to offset investment costs.

In the past in the United States, capacity decisions were fairly straightforward as U.S. manufacturers knew the U.S. market and their likely export market. The global market, however, depends on excess capacity. Manufacturers can choose between two extremes: Focus only on the core market, which implies low availability, high cost, high price, and risk of competition from manufacturers offering lower prices; or focus on the global market, with low cost and high revenues through market segmentation, but running the risk of threatening the domestic price structure through price tiering. Data analysis suggests that the most profitable route for manufacturers is to maximize production volumes, serving all segments of the market at appropriate price points (29). However, unused capacity will have a cost. Capacity decisions are relatively immutable as the GMP requirements for biologicals make capacity expansion very expensive and time consuming. Thus, capacity investments imply higher prices because of high risks incurred by manufacturers.

Markets

The vaccine market is really a series of markets, including private markets in all countries, and the public sector markets in industrialized countries and those countries that are mostly donor dependent. Managing pricing (tiered pricing) over the product life cycle will depend on the segmenting of these markets.

Recently, there has been much discussion about mechanisms that can be used to manage markets, including push mechanisms to accelerate product development for specific markets or pull mechanisms to create more attractive markets. Push mechanisms include direct financing of or tax credits for product development, and facilitation of clinical trials. They tend to reduce risk for product developers and have a proven record (4). They influence the earlier segments of product development activities and provide a credible indication of public-sector will to encourage specific research and development (1, 30). Pull mechanisms, including innovative intellectual property rights protection and market assurances, are stronger later in the value chain (4). They are a safer form of intervention for the funder because they are not given until the product is available, and can be of larger direct value to the product developers. On the other hand, they tend to lock the funder into an outcome, and they are currently untried. Both types are needed.

Competition

We touched earlier on the role of competition in reducing prices. There are two competing tensions in play that impact competition: The consolidation of large multinational vaccine producers, and the growing importance of vaccine manufacturers in developing countries and emerging economies. Table 3 shows the impact this has on the number of manufacturers serving United Nations procurement agencies.

Table 3: United Nations Agency Purchase —
Changing Mix of Suppliers (14)

Year	Number of Vaccines	Number of Suppliers	Percent Located in Developing Countries or Emerging Economies
1986	4	7	0
1996	5	14	50
2001	6	12	58

Note: BCG not included

The extent to which this mix of manufacturers can positively impact new product development depends on their ability to develop research and development capacity or to access technologies. Recent developments indicate that developing-country and emerging-economy (DC/EE) manufacturers will play an increasingly important role:

The Developing Country Vaccine Manufacturers Network, a new alliance of manufacturers, represented on the Board of the Global Alliance for Vaccines and Immunization, is comprised of manufacturers, private and public sector, meeting or on track to meet international standards of quality and viability.

A limited number of joint ventures have been initiated between multinational manufacturers and developing-country manufacturers, and more are under consideration. While some of these are for the express purpose of leveraging market access or regulatory pathways, their existence will enhance the impact of DC/EE manufacturers.

FUTURE CHANGES IMPACTING THE ECONOMICS OF VACCINE DEVELOPMENT

A number of potential changes will impact vaccine development activities in the future:

Product Lines — In the past, vaccines have been produced in industrialized countries and used on a global basis. In the future, many vaccines are likely to be developing market or at least region specific, which will in turn impact capacity decisions and market sizes.

Regulatory Spiral — There is a trend toward substantially increasing regulation. This will increase product development costs with uncertain gains. Moreover, it could impact possible regulatory pathways.

Increasing Role of Outsourcing — The current product development model, where a large pharmaceutical company carries out the entire process, may be outmoded. Product development in the future may be coordinated by virtual organizations, with more emphasis on outsourcing at all stages—basic research, early preclinical and clinical work, manufacture, and even sales.

Competition — Any vision of the future must take into account the changing vaccine production industry, from increasingly consolidated global manufacturers to a new breed of developing country manufacturers reaching high standards of excellence. This group is already a major source for production of existing products; time will tell if it will also serve as a source for innovative, developing market products as well.

New Funding Sources — With the formation of the Global Alliance for Vaccines and Immunization, and increasing investment into the Vaccine Fund, there is likely to be a large funding increase for vaccine development, especially those for developing markets. Many of these are being implemented by public-private partnerships, a new mechanism for accelerating research and development. Current vaccine developers are watching these initiatives closely.

References

1 Hilleman, M. R. (1999). The business of science and the science of business in the quest for an AIDS vaccine. *Vaccine, 17,* 1211-1222.

2 Siwolop, S. (2001, July 25). Big steps for vaccine industry. *The New York Times.*

3 Milstien, J. B., Evans, P., & Batson, A. (1994). Discussion on paper vaccine development in developing countries. In F. T. Cutts & P. G. Smith (Eds.), *Vaccination and world health* (p. 62). Chichester, United Kingdom: John Wiley & Sons.

4 Glass, S. N., Batson, A., & Levine, R. (2001). *Issues paper: Accelerating new vaccines.* Paper written for the Global Alliance for Vaccines and Immunization Financing Task Force.

5 Smith, J. S. (1990). *Patenting the sun: Polio and the Salk vaccine.* New York: W. Morrow.

6 Robbins, J. B., & Schneerson, R. (1990). Polysaccharide-protein conjugates: A new generation of vaccines. *Journal of Infectious Diseases, 161,* 821-832.

7 DeRoeck, D. (2001). *Immunization financing in developing countries and the international vaccine market.* Manila, Philippines: Asian Development Bank. http://www.adb.org/documents/books/immunization_financing/default.asp.

8 European & UK case law review in the area of biotechnology. (1999, October 4). *World Biotech Supplement.*

9 Takenaka, T. (1997). *Highly anticipated UK decision of Biogen v. Medeva about validity of biotechnology patents.* Seattle, WA: University of Washington, School of Law.

10 UNICEF Supply Division. (2000). *Vaccines & immunization products guideline for countries eligible for support from the Global Fund for Children's Vaccines.*

11 UN prequalified vaccines. World Health Organization. (2001). http://www.who.int/vaccines-access/vaccines/vaccine_quality/UN_prequalified/unhepBproducers html.

12 Chiron Corporation. (1998, March 18). *Chiron successful in revocation of Evans' pertactin patent throughout Europe* [Press Release]. Emeryville, CA: Author. http://www.shareholder.com/chiron/news/19980318-4050 htm.

13 Supakankunti, S., Janjaroen, W. S., Tangphao, O., Ratanawijitrasin, S., Kraipornsak, P., & Pradithavanij, P. (2001). Impact of the World Trade Organization TRIPS Agreement on the pharmaceutical industry in Thailand. *Bulletin of the World Health Organization, 79,* 461-470.

14 Milstien, J. B., Glass, S. N., Batson, A., Greco, M., & Berger, J. (2001). *Divergence of vaccine product lines in industrialized and developing countries.* Paper presented to the Strategic Advisory Group of Experts of the World Health Organization's Department of Vaccines and Biologicals. http://www.vaccinealliance.org/reference/resourcecentre html.

15 Database on contract manufacturers. World Health Organization. (2001). http://www.who.int/vaccines-access/CMProject/Index.html.

16 André, F. E., & Foulkes, M. A. (1998). A phased approach to clinical testing: Criteria for progressing from phase I to phase II to phase III studies. In S. Plotkin, K. Brown, & F. Horaud (Eds.), *Preclinical and clinical development of new vaccines.* [Special Issue]. *Developments in Biological Standardization (Basel), 95,* 57-60.

17 Goldenthal, K. L., Vaillancourt, J. M., Lucey, D. R. (1998). Preventive HIV type 1 vaccine clinical trials: A regulatory perspective. *AIDS Research and Human Retroviruses, 14* (Suppl. 3), S333-S340.

18 Future access to HIV vaccines. Report from a WHO-UNAIDS consultation, Geneva, 2-3 October 2000. (2001, May). *AIDS, 15,* W27-W44.

19 Klein, D. (2000). Development and testing of *Streptococcus pneumoniae* conjugate vaccines. In M. A. Gerber (Ed.), *Jordan report* (pp. 111-130). Bethesda, MD: National Institutes of Health.

20 Jacobson, R. M., Adegbenro, A., Pankratz, V. S., Poland, G. A. (2001). Adverse events and vaccination: The lack of power and predictability of infrequent events in pre-licensure study. *Vaccine, 19,* 2428-2433.

21 Centers for Disease Control and Prevention. (1999). Rotavirus vaccine for the prevention of rotavirus gastroenteritis among children: Recommendations of the Advisory Committee on Immunization Practices (ACIP). *Morbidity and Mortality Weekly Report, 48,* 1-20.

22 Centers for Disease Control and Prevention. (1999). Intussusception among recipients of rotavirus vaccine – United States, 1998-1999. *Morbidity and Mortality Weekly Report, 48,* 577-581.

23 Ellenberg, S. S. (2000, November 14-15). Safety considerations for new vaccine development. *Evaluation of New Vaccines: How Much Safety Data?* Workshop. http://www fda.gov/cber/summaries/111400se htm.

24 World Health Organization. (2001). *Proceedings of the First Global Vaccine Research Forum, WHO/V&B/01.21, 6.*

25 Web site of the International Federation of Pharmaceutical Manufacturers Associations. ich@ifpma.org.

26 World Health Organization. (1997). *Procedure for assessing the acceptability in principle of vaccines for purchase by United Nations organizations, WHO/VSQ/97.06.*

27 Batson, A. (1998). Win-win interactions between the public and private sectors. *Nature Medicine, 4* (Vaccine Supplement), 487-491.

28 Whitehead, P. (1999, October 28). *Public sector procurement approaches.* Presentation to the Board of the Global Alliance for Vaccines and Immunization, New York (pp. 47-49). (GAVI 99.02). http://www.vaccinealliance.org/resource/ny2810.pdf.

29 Milstien, J. B., & Batson, A. (1998). Accelerating availability of new vaccines: The role of the international community. *Drug Information Journal, 32,* 175-182.

30 Esparza, J., & Bhamarapravati, N. (2000). Accelerating the development and future availability of HIV-1 vaccines. Why, when, where and how? *The Lancet, 355,* 2061-2066.

Author's Biography

Dr. Milstien is Team Coordinator in the Access to Technologies Team, Department of Vaccines and Biologicals, World Health Organization (WHO). The team mission is to remove technical and financial barriers to vaccines and immunization-related technologies. Dr. Milstien's responsibilities include planning and coordinating activities related to supply, financing, and quality of vaccines and immunization-related technologies in global immunization programs, including establishing mechanisms to facilitate availability of new vaccines and technologies. Prior to 1994, she was with the Biologicals Unit in the same organization, where her responsibilities included advising UNICEF and national authorities on the quality of vaccines used in national immunization programs.

Before joining WHO in 1988, Dr. Milstien worked for the Food and Drug Administration for 14 years, first directing laboratory research on the molecular biology of measles and polio vaccines, and later developing and implementing a surveillance system to monitor adverse reactions to vaccines and other biological products.

Author's Biography

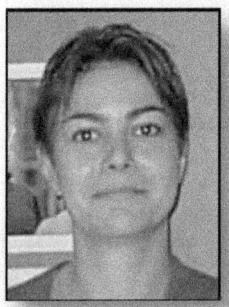

Brenda Candries, Ph.D.

Dr. Candries' background is in economics and she is currently an independent consultant. She worked for the World Health Organization on the financial sustainability of immunization in Geneva.

Previously, Dr. Candries worked as an economic advisor for the European Commission in Kenya and Suriname and covered programs in health, private sector development, and institutional strengthening.

Vaccine Research and Development: The Key Roles of the National Institutes of Health and Other United States Government Agencies

Vaccine Research and Development: The Key Roles of the National Institutes of Health and Other United States Government Agencies

Gregory K. Folkers, M.S. and Anthony S. Fauci, M.D.
National Institute of Allergy and Infectious Diseases, National Institutes of Health

INTRODUCTION

The impact and importance of vaccines cannot be overstated—they provide safe, cost effective and efficient means of preventing illness, disability and death from infectious diseases. Vaccines, along with the availability of improved medical care, living conditions, and sanitation, helped reduce mortality from infectious diseases in the Unites States more than 14-fold in the 20th century.

The United States government agencies charged with protecting and improving health traditionally have long made vaccine research and development a top priority. Together with partners in the public and private sectors, government-supported scientists have helped develop many of our most useful vaccines, including new or improved vaccines that protect against invasive *Haemophilus influenzae* type b (Hib) disease, pneumococcal pneumonia and meningitis, pertussis, influenza, measles, mumps, rubella, chickenpox, and hepatitis A and B. In addition to developing vaccines against classic infectious diseases, the National Institutes of Health (NIH) and other government agencies are working to develop new and improved vaccines against potential agents of bioterrorism, chronic diseases with infectious origins, as well as autoimmune diseases and other immune-mediated conditions. In this volume of *The Jordan Report,* several articles describe the many promising vaccine candidates currently being developed against a wide range of human diseases.

PROGRESS AND CHALLENGES

Safe and effective vaccines, along with the operational expertise and political commitment to administer them, have led to some of the greatest triumphs in public health, including the eradication of naturally occurring smallpox and the near-eradication of poliomyelitis. Each year, immunization programs save 3 million lives worldwide, and more widespread administration of currently available vaccines could prevent at least another 3 million deaths every year.

A notable "success story" is the development and widespread use of polysaccharide-protein conjugate vaccines against Hib, developed by NIH and partners in the public and private sectors. Before these vaccines were licensed, approximately 20,000 cases of invasive Hib disease occurred among children each year, and Hib was the leading cause of childhood bacterial meningitis and postnatal mental retardation. The use of Hib conjugate vaccines has virtually eliminated invasive Hib

diseases among children in the United States and other developed countries. Studies have confirmed the effectiveness of these vaccines in low-income countries, and widespread distribution of Hib vaccines could significantly reduce the global burden of this infection, which leads each year to 2-3 million cases of invasive diseases and at least 450,000 deaths worldwide. Ultimately, global vaccination programs could lead to the eradication of this terrible disease. Furthermore, the utilization of the polysaccharide-protein conjugate technology for improved pneumococcal vaccines has proven extremely promising.

Other examples of triumph in the field of vaccinology abound. For instance, vaccines that protect against Hepatitis B virus (HBV) have dramatically reduced the incidence of serious hepatic disease in countries where HBV vaccines are routinely used. As with conjugate Hib vaccines, NIH and multi-sector partners worked together to develop HBV vaccines. Efforts to increase global coverage with HBV vaccines hold great promise in significantly reducing the mortality associated with the virus, estimated to be about 900,000 deaths per year worldwide.

Despite significant progress in the development and distribution of vaccines, much remains to be accomplished. Infectious diseases remain the second leading cause of death and the leading cause of disability-adjusted life years worldwide (one disability-adjusted life year is one lost year of healthy life). Among children aged 0 to 4 years, infectious diseases cause approximately two thirds of all deaths worldwide. In 2001, approximately six million deaths were attributed to three diseases, for which no effective vaccines are available: AIDS, tuberculosis and malaria. Effective vaccines also are lacking for many other serious infectious diseases that exact an enormous toll worldwide, such as sexually transmitted diseases (other than hepatitis B), many parasitic diseases, respiratory pathogens such as respiratory syncytial virus, as well as a host of enteric diseases that contributed to more than two million diarrhea-related deaths in 2001.

In addition to endemic diseases, the world must cope with the ongoing threat of new and re-emerging diseases and the widespread development of antimicrobial resistance. More than 50 newly recognized infectious diseases and syndromes have been identified since 1980, including AIDS and its etiologic agent, the human immunodeficiency virus (HIV). HIV has now infected well over 60 million people worldwide, of whom more than a third of have died. Certain other emerging infections, such as Ebola virus and Nipah virus, are highly virulent but have so far involved relatively small numbers of people in restricted geographic areas, and have yet to become global public health threats. Other re-emergent diseases, including vector-borne pathogens such as dengue virus and West Nile virus, continue to spread. The epidemic of West Nile Virus infections in the United States in 2002, which has markedly outstripped the initial encounter with this disease in 1999, is a stark reminder of the public health implications of re-emerging infections. In addition, the recent anthrax attacks in the United States underscore our vulnerability to infections that "emerge" because of an intentional human act.

Resistance to antimicrobial agents has been observed in virtually all classes of organisms, resulting in a diminished capacity to treat many serious infections. The world is faced with the continuing threat of antimicrobial resistance on a wider scale than ever before, with the emergence of resistant strains of a number of important microbes, including pneumococci, enterococci, staphylococci, as well as the malaria parasite *Plasmodium falciparum*, and the tuberculosis bacillus *Mycobacterium tuberculosis*. The development of viral resistance is also a major problem in the treatment of HIV-infected individuals, many of whom have been treated with all available class of antiretroviral drugs and harbor virus that that is multi-drug resistant.

Unfortunately, safe and effective vaccines are lacking for most emerging and re-emerging diseases, as well as many endemic infections that are increasingly more difficult to treat because of antimicrobial resistance. The development of vaccines to prevent these conditions—with a particular focus on HIV/AIDS, tuberculosis, malaria, and potential agents of bioterrorism—is a critical priority of the NIH and other U.S. government agencies involved in biomedical research. Clearly, preventing an infection is preferable to attempting to treat it, especially in resource-poor settings where even rudimentary medical care is unavailable.

COLLABORATIONS AND COMMITMENT

The process whereby a vaccine is developed and tested is complex and requires many steps. The various partners in vaccine development bring perspectives, resources and skills that are sometimes unique, but more often productively overlapping and complementary. Industry provides expertise in product development and manufacturing, while many government efforts have traditionally focused on creating and expanding the scientific base in disciplines that underlie product development, a role sometimes described as "priming the pump."

Most currently available vaccines, as well as those in the development "pipeline," have resulted from collaborations between partners in the public and private sector, including federal and state governments, global organizations, small and large companies, academic research institutions and non-governmental organizations (Figure 1).

Figure 1.

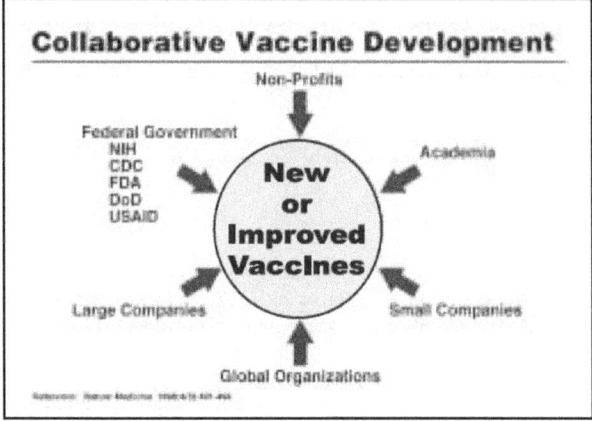

A prototypic example of successful partnerships across sectors is the development of "acellular" pertussis vaccines, based on individual components of *Bordetella pertussis*, rather than the whole bacterium. Basic research in government and university laboratories provided the insights that enabled industry to develop candidate acellular pertussis vaccines. Phase I and Phase II clinical trials of these products, supported by industry and government, were conducted at academic medical centers, notably within the National Institute of Allergy and Infectious Diseases' nationwide network of Vaccine and Treatment Evaluation Units (see Figure 2). International efficacy trials, funded and overseen by government and industry, and facilitated by public health officials through intergovernmental channels, helped provide the data that led to the licensure of acellular pertussis vaccines in the United States and abroad. These new vaccines are considerably less reactogenic than older whole-cell products and their availability has helped remove a major disincentive to vaccination against pertussis.

Figure 2.

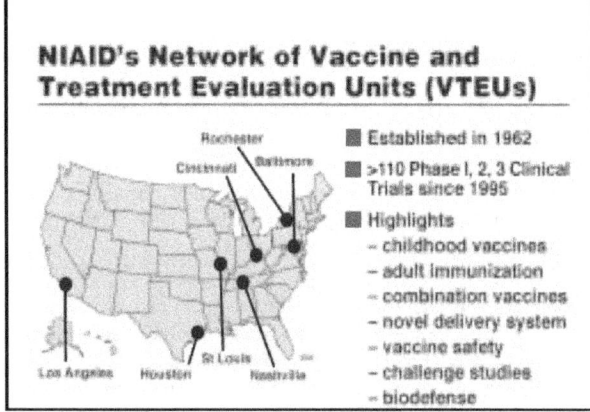

The importance of vaccine development and the necessity for strong cross-sector partnerships have been recognized at the highest levels of government, both in the U.S. and internationally. For example, in 2001 the United Nations General Assembly convened a special session on HIV/AIDS and adopted a resolution calling for increased investment to accelerate HIV/AIDS vaccine research. In the United States, both the executive and legislative branches have made immunization, including vaccine research and development, a top priority. In 2000, the Administration unveiled a Millennium Vaccine Initiative to promote delivery of existing vaccines in developing countries and accelerate development of new vaccines. The President's Fiscal Year 2003 Budget for vaccine research and development at the NIH calls for $1.3 billion, up more than x percent from 1990 (see Figure 3). In the US Congress, numerous legislative proposals are being pursued to support the discovery and to facilitate the delivery of vaccines (see http://thomas.loc.gov).

Figure 3.

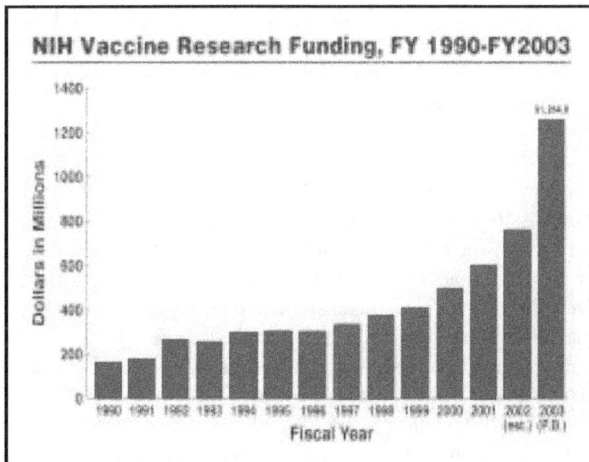

In addition, the NIH, the Centers for Diseases Control and Prevention and other national research agencies participate in the development and/or support of public-private partnerships such as the Global Alliance for Vaccines and Immunization (GAVI), the International AIDS Vaccine Initiative, and the Malaria Vaccine Initiative, which combine the resources and skills of a wide range of collaborators. Such partnerships, which build on previous cross-sector collaborations for the donation and distribution of existing health-enhancing products, also play an important role in the research and development of new and improved vaccines. GAVI is a prototypic example; its partners include not only US government agencies, but also numerous other national governments in both rich and poor countries, pharmaceutical manufacturers, philanthropies and foundations such as the Bill and Melinda Gates Foundation, the World Health Organization, the United Nations Children's Fund (UNICEF), and non-governmental organizations.

The private sector also has demonstrated a renewed commitment to vaccine development. Recent advances in gene cloning and expression, peptide synthesis and other technologies have created new opportunities for developing patentable

"bioengineered" vaccines with the potential for a substantial return on research and development cost. In addition, new initiatives such as the NIH Challenge Grant Program, which provides matching funds to companies who will commit their own dollars and resources toward developing new vaccines and other medical interventions, have helped engage the private sector and spur vaccine research and development. NIH Challenge Grants are milestone-driven awards, meaning that recipients must achieve predetermined product goals during the development process. Progress is assessed at each milestone, at which time decisions are made regarding continuing project funding.

THE GOVERNMENT PLAYERS IN VACCINE RESEARCH

Within the federal government, more than 20 different agencies have a role in vaccine research. Among these, NIH, CDC, the Department of Defense (DoD), the Food and Drug Administration (FDA), and the United States Agency for International Development (USAID) have the largest investment in vaccine development. The roles of these different agencies in vaccine development are related and complementary, and range from the support and conduct of basic research to licensure activities and program implementation. Table 1 lists examples of key roles for selected U.S agencies involved in vaccine research and development. In addition, the National Vaccine Program Office has important coordinating functions with regard to research, licensing, production, distribution and use of vaccines.

Table 1: Government Players in Vaccine Research

- **CDC** has a myriad of roles related to vaccines. Among them, the agency conducts the epidemiological studies and surveillance needed to define health priorities. In addition, CDC develops recommendations for vaccine use through the Advisory Committee for Immunization Practices (ACIP).

- **DoD** supports research into vaccines that likely will protect against pathogens that military personnel are likely to encounter.

- **USAID** supports research on vaccines of particular relevance to young children in developing countries.

- **FDA** establishes standards for the processes, facilities, and pre- and post-licensure activities needed to insure the safety and efficacy of vaccines.

- **NIH** supports, through its extramural and intramural programs, much of the basic research in microbiology and immunology that underpins vaccine development. NIH also provides research resources such as reagent repositories, genomic databases, and clinical trials support to identify vaccine targets and move candidates along the pathway to licensure.

Sources: Folkers/Fauci, 1998; National Vaccine Advisory Committee, 1997

THE KEY ROLE OF BASIC RESEARCH

Basic biomedical research funded by NIH and other agencies underpins vaccine development. Historically, scientific advances in microbiology and related disciplines have led to the development of new vaccines. For example, the identification of microbial toxins, as well as methods to inactivate them, allowed the development of some of our earliest vaccines, including those for diphtheria and tetanus. In the 1950s, new tissue culture techniques ushered in a new generation of vaccines, including those for polio, measles, mumps and rubella. In recent years we have seen rapid advances in our understanding of the immune system and the complex interactions between pathogens and the human host, as well as extraordinary technical advances such as recombinant DNA technology, gene sequencing and peptide synthesis. These developments have created opportunities for identifying new vaccine candidates to prevent diseases for which no vaccines currently exist; improving the safety and efficacy of existing vaccines; and designing novel vaccine approaches, such as new vectors and adjuvants.

NIH and other agencies actively pursue research portfolios that involve interaction with industry and academia and the transfer of technology to the private sector for commercialization. Historically, an important focus of these efforts has been to further explore concepts that may not be of immediate financial interest, including those for which the principal market might be less developed nations, but nonetheless are of great potential public health importance. The government also plays a critical role in vaccine development by providing scientists with reagents that might not otherwise be shared because of proprietary interests. Of growing importance are research resources such as reagent repositories, genomic databases, animal models, and clinical trials support, as well as milestone-driven partnerships and contracts. Increasingly, government agencies such as NIH have sought to overcome challenges to vaccine development by conducting translational research that takes basic research findings through the process of target identification, and preclinical and clinical development.

The use of the new technologies in the 21st century promises to provide a renaissance in the already vital field of vaccinology. In particular, the availability of the annotated sequences of the entire genomes of microbial pathogens will allow for the identification of a wide array of new antigens for vaccine targets. A number of government agencies, including NIH and DoD, support projects to sequence the genomes of medically important pathogens. Sequence information can be used in many ways, including identifying antigens to incorporate into vaccines. The success of the first microbe sequencing project—the delineation of the complete *Haemophilus influenzae* genome in 1995—encouraged the current government-sponsored efforts to sequence the full genomes of many other pathogens. NIH has made a significant investment in the growing field of microbial genomics, and has funded the genomic sequencing of more than

60 medically important microbes. Approximately 20 of these projects have been completed, including the sequencing of bacteria that cause tuberculosis, gonorrhea, chlamydia, cholera, the parasite that causes malaria, as well as the mosquito that transmits malaria. These sequencing efforts have been facilitated by technologies such as DNA chip technology and microarrays that enable the rapid, simultaneous analysis of tens of thousands of genes.

ADDRESSING THE THREAT OF BIOTERRORISM

The anthrax attacks of 2001 in the eastern United States revealed significant gaps in our overall preparedness against bioterrorism, giving a new sense of urgency to biodefense efforts, especially with regard to vaccine development. NIH has significantly bolstered research efforts on vaccines against many of the pathogens considered to be bioterrorist threats, with an eye toward producing products that are safe and effective in civilian populations of varying ages and health status. Recently, a clinical trial conducted by several of NIAID's Vaccine and Treatment Evaluation Units demonstrated that existing stocks of the smallpox vaccine known as Dryvax could successfully be diluted at least five-fold and retain its potency, effectively expanding the number of individuals who could be immediately vaccinated against smallpox using existing stocks if a smallpox attack were to occur. In addition, a second-generation smallpox vaccine is now being produced in cell culture, and large supplies of this product are scheduled to be available by the end of 2002. This new product, as well as more than 75 million additional doses of smallpox vaccine that have been stored by a pharmaceutical company since 1972, will be tested for safety and immunogenicity by NIH-supported investigators. In the long-term, basic research promises to provide a third generation of smallpox vaccines that could be used in all segments of the population, including pregnant women and people with weakened immune systems. One such vaccine nearing phase I clinical trials is based on Modified vaccinia Ankara (MVA), which is related to the current smallpox vaccine strain, but may cause fewer adverse reactions. Additional bioterrorism vaccines also are in various stages of development. To name just two, a new anthrax vaccine, based on a bioengineered component of the anthrax bacterium called recombinant protective antigen (rPA), will soon enter human trials. On the NIH campus, researchers at the NIAID Dale and Betty Bumpers Vaccine Research Center have developed a DNA vaccine that protected monkeys from infection with Ebola virus, and that will undergo testing in human volunteers beginning in early 2003. In each of these endeavors, NIH is working closely with partners in the public and private sectors.

As we prepare for the public health challenges of endemic, emerging and re-emerging infectious diseases, it is imperative that a robust commitment to basic research and cross-sector collaboration be maintained. Only with such collaborations can we successfully translate basic research findings and technological advances into improved health through immunization.

Sources

Armstrong GL, Conn LA, Pinner RW. Trends in infectious disease mortality in the United States during the 20th century. *JAMA* 1999; 281(1): 61-6.

Chang MH et al. Universal hepatitis B vaccination in Taiwan and the incidence of hepatocellular carcinoma in children. Group. *N Engl J Med* 1997; 336:18559.

Fauci AS. Biomedical research in an era of unlimited aspirations and limited resources. *Lancet* 1996; 348(9033):1002-3.

Fauci AS. Infectious diseases: considerations for the 21st century. *Clin Infect Dis* 2001; 32(5): 675-85.

Folkers GK, Fauci AS. The AIDS research model: implications for other infectious diseases of global health importance. *JAMA* 2001;286(4):458-61.

Folkers GK, Fauci AS. The role of US government agencies in vaccine research and development. *Nat Med* 2001;4(5 Suppl):491-4.

Frey SE et al. Clinical responses to undiluted and diluted smallpox vaccine. *N Engl J Med* 2002; 346(17):1265-74.

Global Alliance for Vaccines and Immuniation (GAVI). A promise to every child. Geneva, 2002. Available at http://www.VaccineAlliance.org.

Hilleman MR. Vaccines in historic evolution and perspective: a narrative of vaccine discoveries. *Vaccine* 2000; 18:143647.

Joint United Nations Programme on AIDS (UNAIDS). The Report on the Global HIV/AIDS Epidemic. Geneva, 2002. Available at http://www.unaids.org/barcelona/presskit/report.html

National Institute of Allergy and Infectious Diseases. NIAID biodefense research agenda for CDC category A agents. Bethesda, Maryland, 2002. Available at: http://www.niaid.nih.gov/dmid/pdf/biotresearchagenda.pdf

National Institute of Allergy and Infectious Diseases. NIAID global plan for HIV/AIDS, malaria and tuberculosis. Bethesda, Maryland, 2001. Available at http://www.niaid.nih.gov/publications/globalhealth/global.pdf

National Vaccine Advisory Committee. United States vaccine research: a delicate fabric of public and private collaboration. *Pediatrics* 1997; 100(6), 1015–1020.

Sullivan NJ. Development of a preventive vaccine for Ebola virus infection in primates. Nature 2000;408(6812):605-9

Wheeler C, Berkley S. Initial lessons from public-private partnerships in drug and vaccine development. *Bull World Health Organ.* 2001; 79(8):728-34.

World Health Organization (WHO). World Health Report 2001. Geneva, 2001.

WHO. World Health Organization report on infectious diseases: removing obstacles to healthy development. Geneva, 1999. Available at http://www.who.int/infectious-disease-report/index-rpt99.html.

Author's Biography

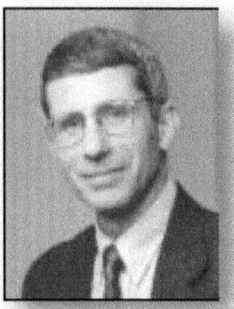

Anthony S. Fauci, M.D.

Since 1984, Dr. Fauci has been Director of the National Institute of Allergy and Infectious Diseases (NIAID) of the National Institutes of Health (NIH). He also is Chief of the Laboratory of Immunoregulation at NIAID.

Dr. Fauci has made many contributions to basic and clinical research on the pathogenesis and treatment of immune-mediated diseases. He has pioneered the field of human immunoregulation, making a number of scientific observations that serve as the basis for current understanding of the regulation of the human immune response. Dr. Fauci has made seminal contributions to the understanding of how the acquired immunodeficiency syndrome (AIDS) virus destroys the body's defenses.

At major medical centers throughout the country, Dr. Fauci has served as Visiting Professor. He has lectured throughout the world and is the recipient of numerous awards.

Dr. Fauci is a member of the National Academy of Sciences; Royal Danish Academy of Science and Letters; American College of Physicians; American Society for Clinical Investigation; Infectious Diseases Society of America; American Academy of Allergy, Asthma and Immunology; and other professional societies. He serves on many editorial boards and is author, coauthor, or editor of more than 1,000 scientific publications

Author's Biography

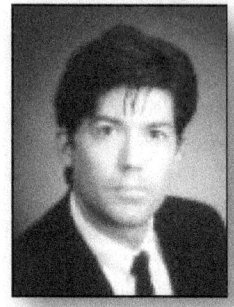

Gregory K. Folkers, M.S.

Gregory K. Folkers is Special Assistant to the Director, NIAID. A 1981 graduate of Dartmouth College, Folkers holds an MPH from Johns Hopkins University and an MS in science journalism from Boston University. He has written extensively about HIV/AIDS and other global health issues.

Vaccine Updates

Enteric Infections

Image © Jean-Yves Sgro

Enteric Infections

OVERVIEW

Diarrheal diseases are a major cause of morbidity in developed countries and of morbidity and mortality in developing countries. The large number of bacterial and viral pathogens that cause diarrheal disease complicates surveillance and accurate diagnosis and presents formidable challenges to the application of vaccination strategies for public health. Even when the most sophisticated methods and diagnostic reagents are used, greater than half of the cases of diarrheal illness cannot be ascribed to a particular agent. Certainly, there are enteric pathogens that have not been discovered yet.

Pharmaceutical companies do not see a large market for enteric vaccines in the United States. For the most part, these enteric pathogens do not induce life-threatening illness in this country. The U.S. vaccine market is often targeted toward travelers and deployed military personnel. Unfortunately, most people who could benefit from these vaccines are in countries that cannot afford to pay for them.

The focus of the National Institute of Allergy and Infectious Diseases' (NIAID's) enteric diseases program will continue to be basic research needed to better characterize pathogenesis of the organisms responsible for diarrheal diseases, definition of the protective immune responses, and testing of prevention and therapeutic strategies in clinical trials. Tremendous gains in understanding pathogenesis have come from these research efforts, and that information has been essential for the creation of vaccine candidates. The recent sequencing of the genome of some of these pathogens, and significant progress on others, promises to give new insights on pathogenesis and additional targets for deletion from vaccine candidates. Many of the enteric vaccines are early in clinical development and have yet to enter scaleup production and testing in large clinical trials. The availability and future use of these vaccines for improving public health around the world remains a long-term goal.

CHOLERA

Cholera remains an important disease in areas where poor sanitation is common (developing countries, refugee camps, etc.). Two significant events have altered the epidemiologic picture of cholera in the last 20 years. One was the emergence of a new epidemic serotype O139 that appeared in India in 1992 and that continues to cause disease in Asia, where it coexists with the more common O1 serotype. The other was the appearance in 1991 of cholera in the Western Hemisphere for the first time in 100 years. Hundreds of thousands of individuals in South and Central America were affected by that epidemic. The organism associated with that event was the O1 El Tor strain, which also has been responsible for most of the disease associated with

refugee camps in Africa and the Middle East. While the organism continues to cause disease in South and Central America, many fewer cases have been reported in recent years.

There are at present two cholera vaccines that have been licensed in many countries (but not yet in the United States). One is the killed whole cell plus recombinant cholera toxin B (rCTB) formulation produced by SBL Vaccin AB in Sweden. This vaccine (Dukoral®) is administered orally in two doses spaced 1 to 2 weeks apart and protects against O1 and O139 strains. It has been approved for use in Sweden, Norway, Estonia, El Salvador, Guatemala, Honduras, Mexico, Nicaragua, Peru, Mauritius, Madagascar, and Kenya. Protective efficacy has been in the range of 50 to 85 percent in field trials, and protection seems to diminish after the first 2 years. The rCTB component in this vaccine also affords partial protection against enterotoxigenic strains of *Escherichia coli* expressing heat labile toxin (LT). A vaccine modeled after this killed SBL vaccine has been produced and tested in Vietnam with good results. Dukoral® would appear to be available for use as a cholera vaccine for travelers (although not in the United States), in refugee settings, or following natural disasters where large numbers of people may be in areas where clean water and good sanitation are not available.

The other vaccine is CVD-103HgR produced by Berna Biotech, Ltd., (formerly Swiss Serum and Vaccine Institute Berne) in Switzerland. This is a live-attenuated product that is given as a single oral dose in buffer. It has been approved in some European countries and Canada, but has yet to be licensed in the United States. The vaccine recently has shown outstanding protection from experimental challenge in a double-blind multicenter study in U.S. volunteers. Therefore, it may be quite useful as a travelers' vaccine. However, it did not show efficacy in a large field trial conducted in Indonesia, bringing into question its usefulness for public health in endemic regions. Current manufacturing problems have limited the supply of this vaccine and are holding up application for U.S. license.

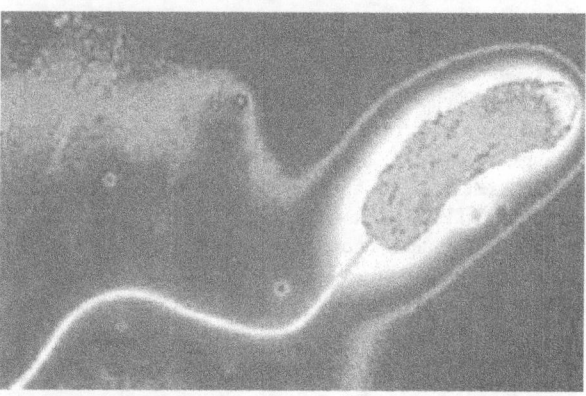

Cholera

Other vaccines are in the early phases of clinical testing. Peru 15 is another live-attenuated strain directed against O1 cholera, which is being developed by Avant Immunotherapeutics, Inc., of Massachusetts. Peru 15 has shown outstanding protection of volunteers against experimental challenge in a trial conducted recently in the United States and supported by NIAID. The vaccine will be tested in field trials in Bangladesh. Live-attenuated vaccines directed against O139 cholera are being developed independently by Berna Biotech, Ltd., and Avant Immunotherapeutics, Inc. Intramural scientists of the National Institute of Child Health and Human Development (NICHD) of the National Institutes of Health have tested, in animals, a parenteral cholera vaccine consisting of O antigen conjugated to recombinant mutant diphtheria toxin.

SHIGA TOXIN-PRODUCING *E. COLI* (STEC) AND ENTEROPATHOGENIC *E. COLI* (EPEC)

STEC, also referred to as enterohemorrhagic *E. coli*, primarily of the O157:H7 serotype, is usually transmitted by contaminated food or water or direct contact with infected animals in developed countries. Interestingly, STEC does not contribute significantly to the diarrheal disease burden in developing countries. STEC expresses one or both of the Shiga toxins (Stx-I and Stx-II). The Centers for Disease Control and Prevention estimates that as many as 100,000 cases per year occur in the United States. Clinical symptoms can include mild diarrhea, severe abdominal cramping, and bloody diarrhea. Children, the elderly, and immunocompromised individuals are at particular risk of developing severe complications, including kidney failure due to hemolytic uremic syndrome (HUS). Contaminated food products, such as undercooked ground beef, unpasteurized apple juice, raw milk, sausages, lettuce, and sprouts, as well as swimming pools and well water have all been identified as sources of infection. Outbreaks caused by sorbitol fermenting O157:H- (Germany) and Shiga toxin-producing O111 (United States) emphasize the need to consider strains other than O157:H7 as potentially dangerous and capable of producing HUS. Recently, STEC infection of the urinary tract has been linked to the development of HUS in children.

The sporadic and relatively rare occurrence of infections due to STEC limits the usefulness of a vaccine for humans. Potential uses of an effective vaccine could be in a large community outbreak to prevent secondary spread or in institutional or childcare settings. If a vaccine could protect against STEC and EPEC, a stronger case for a preventive vaccine strategy could be made, particularly if EPEC is shown to contribute a significant disease burden in the United States.

Current vaccine development efforts for STEC are focused on livestock cattle and other ruminants known to asymptomatically carry these organisms and shed them in their feces. Vaccine

approaches target the colonization factor intimin, the protein required for attachment of STEC and EPEC. If intimin proves to be a good immunogen, it would be useful against both groups of pathogenic *E. coli*. The expression of the B subunit of Stx-I in vaccine strains of *Vibrio cholerae* protects rabbits challenged with Stx-I toxin. The expression of intimin in canola, alfalfa, or other animal feed crops is also being evaluated as an edible animal vaccine. Of course, if this strategy were to be successful in animals, it also could define a new approach for an edible human vaccine. Conjugate vaccines targeting the bacterial lipopolysaccharide have been developed by Dr. John Robbins' group at NICHD, and these are in early clinical development.

Therapeutics for treatment of individuals infected with STEC are also under development. Toxoids, if safe and immunogenic in human volunteers, could provide protection against STEC strains and *Shigella dysenteriae* 1. Antitoxin antibodies also could be purified from donor serum and assessed for their ability to prevent the development of HUS and other serious sequelae in patients presenting with STEC infection. NIAID-supported investigators, in collaboration with corporate partners, have produced "humanized" monoclonal reagents of mouse monoclonals that have been shown to neutralize Stx-I and II. These hybrid antibodies, which contain the specific binding variable regions of the original mouse monoclonals with the constant regions of human antibodies, also would be tested for efficacy in preventing the development of the systemic effects of STEC infection. Phase I trials of this treatment strategy are planned. Another group of NIAID investigators is producing completely "human" monoclonals against the Shiga toxins in transgenic mice. These products also should be ready for clinical trials in the near future.

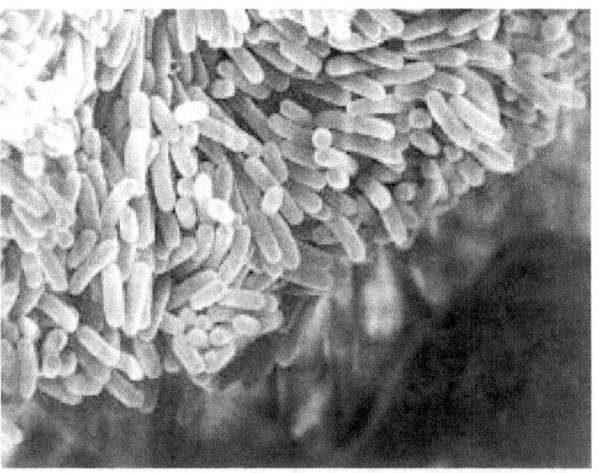

E. Coli

ENTEROTOXIGENIC *E. COLI* (ETEC)

As with cholera, a safe and effective vaccine against ETEC would be of potential public health benefit to young children living in areas of the world where ETEC is endemic, and to travelers visiting these areas. ETEC is second only to rotavirus as the cause of severe dehydrating diarrhea in young children throughout the world. Volunteer studies have shown that infection with ETEC generates protective immunity against rechallenge with the same strain.

Swedish investigators at SBL Vaccin AB have produced a vaccine composed of a mixture of five formalin-inactivated ETEC strains, which together express the major colonization factor antigens (CFAs) important in human disease, combined with rCTB, which will elicit antibodies that neutralize the ETEC LT. Clinical studies in more than 500 volunteers have demonstrated that this vaccine is safe, immunogenic, and capable of generating antibody-secreting cell (ASC) responses equivalent to natural infection in Bangladeshi adults. In studies conducted in Egypt, this vaccine was found to be safe and immunogenic and to induce ASC and immunoglobulin (Ig) G responses in adults. A large randomized blinded study is underway in U.S. travelers.

NIAID-funded investigators have used attenuated strains of Shigella and Salmonella to express ETEC CFAs. Animal experiments with the Shigella construct have indicated that an immune response to the expressed CFAs is generated following oral or intranasal administration.

Dr. Charles Arntzen and Dr. John Clements have teamed up on a novel edible vaccine approach. Phase I safety and immunogenicity studies in volunteers have been completed at the University of Maryland Vaccine Treatment and Evaluation Unit (VTEU). The trial demonstrated that this vaccine was safe and immunogenic. Dr. Arntzen's long-term goal is to express antigens in a plant that people find appetizing, such as tomatoes or bananas.

NIAID plans to sponsor a phase I trial of another edible vaccine designed and produced by ProdiGene, Inc., of Texas. This vaccine consists of transgenic corn expressing LTB. It would seem to have the advantages of a stable shelf life at room temperature, a homogeneous distribution of antigen in a palatable product produced by standard corn processing methodology, and a level of antigen produced that is sufficiently high to allow convenient consumption.

Investigators at Walter Reed Army Institute of Research (WRAIR) have developed and tested in small numbers of volunteers a vaccine containing ETEC CFAs CS1 and CS3 (CFA/II) encapsulated in biodegradable microspheres. Trials are being planned that will use this antigen preparation in combination with a nontoxic mutant LT as a mucosal adjuvant to try and improve immunogenicity and protective efficacy. Recent studies on a similar CS6 product showed that the antigen administered in microspheres alone induced a rather poor immune response.

Scientists at Acambis, United Kingdom and Massachusetts, in collaboration with investigators at the Navy Medical Research Center; Johns Hopkins University; and the International Centre for Diarrheal Diseases Research, Bangladesh (ICDDR,B) have

developed a series of live-attenuated ETEC, tox(-) strains that show promise in phase I studies. Lack of reactogenicity, as well as good immunogenicity have encouraged investigators to pursue this approach. Phase I testing of these attenuated strains expressing engineered (nontoxic) LT and heat stable toxin antigens is planned.

HELICOBACTER PYLORI

It is now well recognized that *H. pylori* is the main cause of gastric and duodenal ulcers as well as gastritis and is a contributing factor for the development of cancers of the stomach worldwide. In some developing countries, the infection rate approaches 100 percent of the population, while in the United States, as much as 40 percent of the adult population is infected with this organism. Not all infected individuals are symptomatic. *H. pylori* disproportionately affects individuals of Hispanic and African-American decent. There remains an intensive effort to educate the public and healthcare providers about the association between *H. pylori* and ulcer disease and to stress that this is an infectious disease that can be cured by antibiotic therapy.

A vaccine to prevent infection with *H. pylori* is worthy of consideration. The organism has been shown to be extremely heterogeneous at a genetic level and may make the development of a preventive vaccine difficult. On the other hand, animal experiments have demonstrated that a vaccine composed of purified urease or other antigens can be protective and therapeutic if coadministered with cholera toxin, the potent mucosal adjuvant. Of course, cholera toxin cannot be used in humans, but the use of nontoxic mutants of either cholera toxin or *E. coli* heat LT could be useful as adjuvants. In addition to urease, combinations of antigens, and killed whole cells or cell extracts are being evaluated by a number of investigators and companies including: Acambis and Astra in Massachusetts, Antex Biologics in Maryland, IRIS Chiron Biocene in Italy, and Commonwealth Serum Labs in Australia.

Other approaches include the expression of *H. pylori* antigens in live-attenuated orally delivered vectors. NIAID is working with Acambis and Iomai Corporation on a transcutaneous vaccination strategy that will use the *H. pylori* urease as antigen with LT as an adjuvant. It is hoped that phase I studies will begin within the next year.

POLIO

As worldwide polio eradication efforts accelerate, the number of countries that are free of polio continues to increase. Globally, health officials now are optimistic that polio can be eradicated by the end of 2005. Since 1988, the number of reported polio cases has decreased by greater than 99 percent from an estimated 350,000 to less than 1,000. In 2001, 537 confirmed polio cases (as of April 2002) were reported. This is down from 2000 when a total of 2,971 cases were reported. Only 10 countries documented indigenous transmission of wild poliovirus during

2001, and wild type 2 poliovirus has not been detected worldwide since October 1999. In 2000, reported global vaccination coverage with three doses of oral poliovirus (OPV) vaccine (children less than 12 months of age) was 82 percent.

In the Western Hemisphere, the Pan American Health Organization (PAHO) documented that the last case of paralytic poliomyelitis associated with a wild-virus isolate was in Peru on August 23, 1991. The successful methods developed during this pioneering regional eradication effort led to a now-standard worldwide eradication strategy of 1) achieving and maintaining high routine vaccine coverage, 2) giving supplemental vaccine doses during National Immunization Days (NIDs) to interrupt wild poliovirus transmission, 3) developing sensitive systems for surveillance, and 4) conducting mopping-up immunization campaigns.

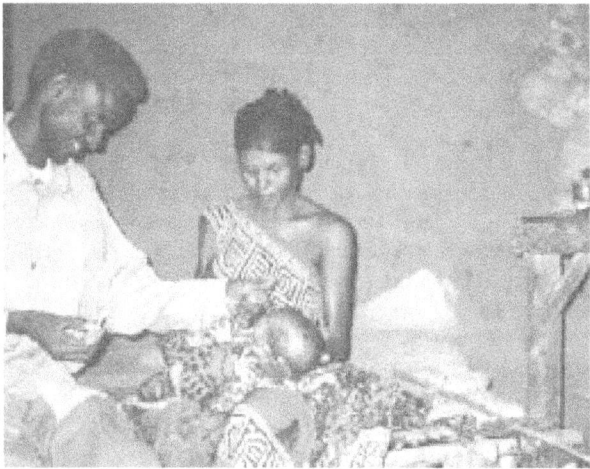

Oral Polio Vaccination courtesy of CDC

Worldwide immunization is being coordinated by an international coalition of partners, including the World Health Organization (WHO), the Rotary International, the Centers for Disease Control and Prevention (CDC), the United Nations International Children's Fund, a number of national governments, and many nongovernmental organizations. During 1996 alone, two-thirds of the world's children younger than 5 years of age received oral polio vaccine. A new WHO/partner plan for acceleration of polio eradication emphasizes rounds of NIDs pulse immunizations in India, and sub-NIDs in other key countries.

With two regions of the world now polio free, and three other regions close to polio elimination, global eradication appears to be feasible. Laboratory confirmation of cases is available through a global laboratory network for poliomyelitis eradication, which includes national, regional, and specialized laboratories. However, the need for repeated contacts with infants to administer the three doses required to immunize fully, and the heat sensitivity of the vaccine remain challenges to the global eradication effort.

The problems of controlling polio in developed countries are different from those in developing countries. Although polio is controlled in developed areas, a small number of cases occur each year, and these appear to be associated with use of the live-attenuated vaccine.

During 2000-2001, a cluster of polio cases attributed to circulating vaccine-derived poliovirus (cVDPV) type 1 was found in Haiti and the Dominican Republic and in the Philippines. The virus in these outbreaks had greater than 2 percent genetic sequence difference from the parent Sabin virus. The revertant virus probably circulated for 2 years before the outbreak. It is hypothesized that low vaccination coverage is allowing cVDPVs to circulate and revert to a more virulent, wild-type virus. Vaccination campaigns with OPV are underway to control these outbreaks.

Wild poliovirus transmission has been interrupted in the United States since 1979, and in 1997, to reduce the risk for vaccine-associated paralytic poliomyelitis (VAPP), increased use of inactivated poliovirus (IPV) vaccine was recommended. In 1999, to eliminate the risk for VAPP, exclusive use of IPV was recommended for routine vaccination in the United States. However, because of superior ability to induce intestinal immunity and to prevent spread among close contacts, OPV remains the vaccine of choice for areas where wild poliovirus is still present. Until worldwide eradication of poliovirus is accomplished, continued vaccination of the U.S. population against poliovirus will be necessary.

Current challenges to global polio eradication efforts include ongoing intense transmission in heavily populated countries (e.g., India, Pakistan, Nigeria), continued importations of wild poliovirus into polio-free areas, and the detection of cVDPV.

As the world approaches eradication of polio, there have been preliminary meetings to discuss whether there will be a time when all polio immunization could be stopped. This issue is controversial, with some experts recommending continuing OPV, others recommending continuing indefinitely only with IPV, and still others seeing a possibility of stopping all immunization after a period of only IPV. This issue is unresolved and will remain the focus of intense debate.

Another issue for the posteradication era is the safety of performing research on wild poliovirus strains in less than biosafety level 4 containment facilities. After eradication, there is concern that the laboratory or the vaccine manufacturing facility would become a potential source of reintroduction of wild poliovirus into the community. The seed virus for production of IPV is a high-yielding, wild-type poliovirus, and recently there was a case of accidental transport of the strain from a production facility into the community via an infected but immunized worker. Eventually, if poliovirus immunization is stopped, all poliovirus strains, including vaccine-derived strains, might have to be contained or destroyed. Other unresolved issues about the posteradication era include: 1) Whether reintroduction is possible from immune-suppressed individuals persistently shedding vaccine strain virus, 2) whether the persistent shedding could be controlled with immune globulins or antivirals, 3) which vaccine would be used if a reemergence occurred, 4) which vaccine(s) will be needed in the posteradication age, 5) how these vaccines will be produced if all stocks are destroyed or high-containment production facilities are required, and 6) whether polio bioterrorism will become an important concern.

NIAID currently funds several extramural basic research projects on the virological and immunological aspects of polio. One goal of this work is to apply the knowledge obtained to make better vaccines that will be genetically stable and not revert to a more neurovirulent form, and more efficient and efficacious, especially when used in tropical and developing regions of the world.

Several major NIAID-supported discoveries have added greatly to the knowledge about polioviruses, as well as other RNA viruses. Molecular studies have been advanced substantially by the development of quick, reliable nucleic acid sequencing methods and the construction of a cDNA infectious clone of poliovirus. The changes in viral nucleic acid that occur during vaccine reversion to virulence have been defined, and a number of studies are examining the basis of viral virulence and attenuation.

The detailed study of viruses always has been hindered by the fact that viruses must invade a host and replicate within living cells; however, research supported by NIAID shows that it is possible to induce the *de novo* synthesis of infectious poliovirus in a cell-free, test-tube system. This system has provided a number of new research approaches to the study of virus replication.

Another major breakthrough was the ability to insert into mice the human gene responsible for producing the receptor for human poliovirus. Because such transgenic mice are able to make the receptor for poliovirus, they become susceptible to infection and develop a paralytic-like disease. These new mice have helped advance research focusing on the pathogenesis of viruses.

These discoveries are of great significance not only for the study of poliovirus, but for research on other viruses. As a model, polio research has led to major breakthroughs, particularly in other RNA viral systems. Nonpolio enteroviruses will remain a problem even after eradication. In a recent study of more than 3,200 cases between 1993 and 1996 in the United States, echoviruses 9, 30, 6, and 11 were commonly isolated, as were coxsackieviruses B5, A9, and B2. Enterovirus 71 has been increasingly linked to neurologic disease, and evidence continues to mount implicating certain enteroviruses in the etiology of diabetes. This group of viruses requires intensified research. The knowledge derived from poliovirus studies will be of great value in the development of new vaccines or antiviral drugs against many other RNA viruses that are now difficult to study.

Sources

American Academy of Pediatrics Committee on Infectious Diseases. (1997). Poliomyelitis prevention: Recommendations for use of inactivated poliovirus vaccine and live poliovirus vaccine. *Pediatrics, 99*(2), 300-305.

Centers for Disease Control and Prevention. (1997). Nonpolio enterovirus surveillance—United States, 1993-1996. *Morbidity and Mortality Weekly Report, 46*(32), 748-750.

Centers for Disease Control and Prevention. (1997). Poliomyelitis prevention in the United States: Introduction of a sequential vaccination schedule of inactivated poliovirus vaccine followed by oral poliovirus vaccine. Recommendations of the Advisory Committee on Immunization Practices. *Morbidity and Mortality Weekly Report, 46*(RR-3), 1-25.

Centers for Disease Control and Prevention. (1997). Prolonged poliovirus excretion in an immunodeficient person with vaccine-associated aparalytic poliomyelitis. *Morbidity and Mortality Weekly Report, 46*(28), 641-643.

Centers for Disease Control and Prevention. (1997). Status of global laboratory network for poliomyelitis eradication, 1994-1996. *Morbidity and Mortality Weekly Report, 46*(30), 692-694.

Centers for Disease Control and Prevention. (2002). General Recommendations on Immunization: Recommendations of the ACIP and AAFP. *Morbidity and Mortality Weekly Report, 51*(RR02), 1-36.

Centers for Disease Control and Prevention. (2002). Progress toward global eradication of poliomyelitis, 2001. *Morbidity and Mortality Weekly Report, 51*(12), 253-256.

Dove, A., & Raccaniello, V. (1997). The polio eradication effort: Should vaccine eradication be next. *Science, 277*(5327), 779-780.

Dowdle, W., & Birmingham, M. (1997). The biologic principles of poliovirus eradication. *Journal of Infectious Diseases, 175*(Suppl. 1), S286-S292.

Hill, W. M. (1996). Are echoviruses still orphans? *British Journal of Biomedical Science, 53*(3), 221-226.

Hull, H., & Aylward, R. (1997). Ending polio immunization. *Science, 277*(5327), 780.

Hull, H., Birmingham, M., Melgaard, B., & Lee, J. (1997). Progress toward global polio eradication. *Journal of Infectious Diseases, 175*(Suppl. 1), S4-S9.

Melnick, J. L. (1996). Current status of poliovirus infections. *Clinical Microbiology Reviews, 9*(3), 293-300.

Robbins, F., & deQuadros, C. (1997). Certification of the eradication of indigenous transmission of wild poliovirus in the Americas. *Journal of Infectious Diseases, 175*(Suppl. 1), S281-S285.

Sutter, R., & Cochi, D. (1997). Ethical dilemmas in worldwide polio eradication programs. *American Journal of Public Health, 87*(6), 913-916.

Taylor, C., Cutts, F., & Taylor, M. (1997). Ethical dilemmas in current planning for polio eradication. *American Journal of Public Health, 87*(6), 922-925.

ENTERIC VIRUSES

Rotavirus is the leading cause of severe diarrheal disease of infants in developed and developing countries. Although Wyeth-Ayerst has licensed the RotaShield® vaccine, which was developed by NIAID intramural scientists, the increased incidence of intussusception among infants who had received this vaccine resulted in its withdrawal from the market. Two other vaccines are in active phase III trials. The first is a WC3 bovine reassortant vaccine being tested by Merck. The second is a human nursery strain being tested by SmithKline Beecham (SKB). Both of these trials are underway in the United States. The SKB trial is also recruiting subjects in Europe and in some developing countries. Clearly, a vaccine against rotavirus is needed and would find application worldwide.

Two additional nursery strains that were isolated in India and have been manufactured in the United States under NIAID contract have been in early phase I trials in adults and seropositive children at the Cincinnati VTEU. There is hope about the prospects of further testing of these two strains in seronegative children and in phase I trials to be conducted in the United States and by collaborators in India. One advantage that these weakened human viruses may have is the lack of vaccine-induced fever, a side effect seen in a small percentage of recipients of the rhesus or bovine-based reassortant vaccines.

At a more experimental stage, a NIAID grantee has succeeded in assembling virus-like particles (VLPs) from the products of baculovirus-expressed rotavirus genes. The resultant particles are noninfectious and can be designed to contain structural proteins from multiple serotypes. This recombinant particle vaccine would be given parenterally, and the results obtained thus far in animals have been promising. Oral vaccination with VLPs could also be considered with or without mucosal adjuvants.

Animal studies performed by a NIAID grantee have indicated that VP6 may be a good vaccine target. IgA monoclonal antibody directed against this protein provides protective immunity against rotavirus in mice. Efforts are also underway to produce subunit vaccines expressed in bacteria to a number of rotavirus proteins. Another NIAID grantee is testing the possibility of using gene gun-administered DNA vaccines to induce protection against rotavirus in animals. The DNA vaccines, which were also administered orally after the DNA was encapsulated in microspheres, were shown to be immunogenic and protective in mice. Studies of this nucleic acid vaccine approach are proceeding in pigs.

Caliciviruses have been shown recently to be significant contributors to diarrheal disease burden in children and adults [(2000). *Journal of Infectious Diseases, 181*(Suppl. 2), S249-S391.]. The capsid proteins from a number of caliciviruses have been expressed in baculovirus-infected insect cells and in human cells. When the protein accumulates in high concentration, VLPs self-assemble and can be purified. These VLPs are immunogenic and protective as vaccines in animals. In a phase I human trial, Norwalk VLPs showed rather modest immunogenicity when orally delivered. Addition of a mucosal adjuvant is planned for future studies. Measurement of vaccine efficacy is also planned and will require administration of wild Norwalk virus in a challenge protocol. NIAID is characterizing a new challenge pool to serve as a reference for future Norwalk virus vaccine efficacy studies.

Development of an edible vaccine strategy for Norwalk virus has also begun. Transgenic potatoes expressing Norwalk capsid protein (some of which forms VLPs) have been found to be immunogenic in human volunteers. Further studies to measure the protective efficacy of such edible vaccines await availability of the challenge model.

SHIGELLA

Shigellosis (bacillary dysentery) is endemic throughout the world. More than 90 percent of all cases reported in the United States were caused by *Shigella sonnei*. Although there are 30 serotypes of shigellae, usually only 2 or 3 serotypes predominate in a given area. *S. sonnei* predominates in industrialized countries, whereas *Shigella flexneri* is most commonly found in developing countries; both are associated with endemic disease. *Shigella dysenteriae* causes epidemic outbreaks of dysentery, as well as significant endemic disease. Therefore, a comprehensive vaccine approach to controlling shigellosis must include components of all three species. There are currently no licensed vaccines available against Shigella.

Early studies showed that the O somatic antigens of Shigella are major immunogens and that the most effective attenuated vaccines were those that transport these immunogens to mucosal tissues where they can generate a local or mucosal immune response. Limited tissue invasion of the vaccine strain would also likely generate a better cell-mediated immune response, thought to be important for protection against invasive pathogens such as Shigella. The main problem in developing Shigella vaccines is the very small safety margin that exists between a strain that is too reactogenic and one that is overattenuated and sufficiently immunogenic.

Investigators at WRAIR have developed an attenuated *S. sonnei* vaccine WRSS1, which was tested recently in NIAID-supported phase I trials at the Center for Vaccine Development at the University of Maryland in Baltimore. The strain is attenuated by deletion of a portion of the *vir*G gene. It was only mildly reactogenic, while exhibiting good antigenicity. The Department of Defense plans further field testing of this very promising vaccine candidate.

Investigators at the Pasteur Institute have made a *vir*G, *iuc*A deletion mutant of *S. flexneri* 2a (strain SC602) that demonstrated 100-percent protection against severe shigellosis in seven North American volunteers when they were challenged with virulent *S. flexneri* 2a. However, this strain still induced shigellosis at higher doses. Auxotrophic mutants are also being evaluated as attenuating deletions in *S. flexneri* 2a. Researchers at the Center for Vaccine Development have created deletions in *aro*A and *vir*G (strain CVD 1203), *gua*BA and *vir*G (CVD 1205). Deletion of the *gua*BA genes alone (CVD 1204) or *gua*BA and the genes encoding two enterotoxins (CVD 1208) have also been created and will be tested in NIAID-supported studies in the near future.

Efforts also are underway in the laboratory of Dr. Robbins at NICHD to develop parenteral vaccines composed of detoxified Shigella lipopolysaccharide-protein conjugate. A randomized, double-blind study has been conducted in Israeli military volunteers, and it demonstrated 74-percent protection. A recent study of O-specific polysaccharide conjugates from *S. sonnei* and *S. flexneri* 2a demonstrated safety and immunogenicity in children 4 to 7 years old.

TYPHOID

Typhoid fever remains a serious public health problem throughout the world, with an estimated 16 to 33 million cases and 500,000 deaths annually. It also is a serious threat to travelers visiting endemic areas. In the United States, approximately 12,000 cases were reported in 2001. In virtually all endemic areas, the incidence of typhoid fever is highest in children from 5 to 19 years old, which is important since school children can be immunized readily through school-based immunization programs.

Parenteral whole-cell vaccines are licensed for typhoid fever, though they are rarely used because they are only marginally effective and they produce adverse reactions in many vaccinees. Oral killed whole-cell preparations, though not reactogenic, are also not protective against *Salmonella typhi*. Therefore, efforts are now directed at the use of purified virulence (Vi) antigens (see below) or live, orally administered preparations of demonstrable efficacy.

An important advance for the control of typhoid fever has been the development of the attenuated *S. typhi* strain Ty21a from strain Ty2. This strain was extensively tested in Egypt and Chile, and although its efficacy may vary widely from site to site and

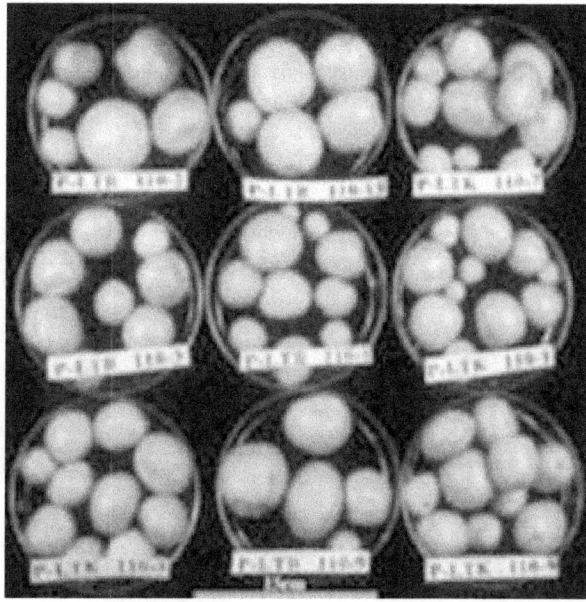

Edible Vaccine in Potatoes

with vaccine formulation, the Ty21a vaccine has been remarkably safe and reasonably immunogenic. It was licensed in the United States in 1991 and is presently being used primarily as a vaccine for travelers. Ty21a is produced by Berna Biotech, Ltd.

In collaboration with the Pasteur Institute, NICHD has developed a parenteral, nonreactogenic, immunogenic, purified Vi vaccine. Clinical trials in Nepal and South Africa demonstrated that a single injection of the Vi vaccine has an efficacy of about 72 to 80 percent. Since the Vi vaccine is effective after only one immunizing dose, it appears to offer some advantages over the Ty21a vaccine, which requires at least three doses and a strict cold chain. The Vi vaccine has been licensed in France and several countries in Africa; the manufacturer is currently assembling data to apply for a license in the United States. The Vi vaccine also is being considered for local production in developing countries. Through the efforts of the Diseases of the Most Impoverished Program being conducted by the International Vaccine Institute (Seoul, South Korea), the technology for producing this vaccine has been transferred already to China and Vietnam. Locally produced vaccine should be tested in the region in the near future.

Of a more experimental nature, several groups of investigators have been developing attenuated deletion mutants as live oral typhoid vaccines. Metabolic pathways and genes critical to virulence expression have been targeted. These include the double *aro* mutants, *aro/pur* mutants, *cya/crp*, and *phoP/phoQ* mutant. Several of these mutants have been used in early clinical trials with varying degrees of success. The focus of this discussion will be on recent efforts.

The Center for Vaccine Development has been pursuing double *aro* mutants derived from wild-type strain Ty2. CVD 908 was shown to be incompletely attenuated because it induced bacteremia in 6 of 12 volunteers at a dose of 5×10^7 colony-forming units. The additional deletion of *htr*A made it clinically more acceptable. These vaccine strains are being developed by Acambis in the United Kingdom.

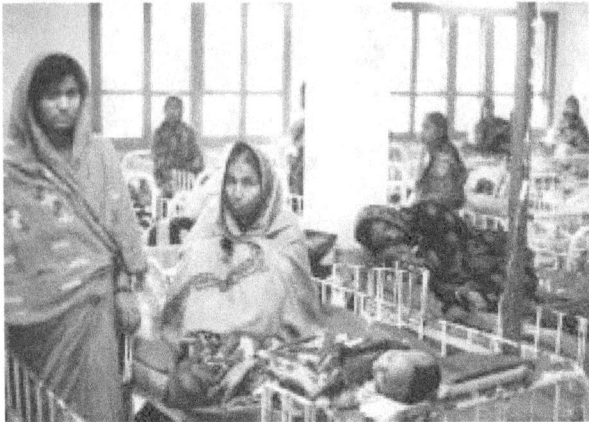

Cholera Clinic in Bangaladesh courtesy Stephen Calderwood

Another vaccine candidate developed by investigators at Washington University, St. Louis, is the *cya/crp/cdt* triple deletion mutant of Ty2. The *cya/crp* double mutant was found in clinical trials to be incompletely attenuated. Therefore, a portion of the gene adjacent to the *crp* locus was deleted. This gene was designated *cdt* since its apparent function is to control dissemination of Salmonella out of the intestinal tract and *GALT* to visceral organs in animals infected with *Salmonella typhimurium* or *Salmonella choleraesuis*. The strain of *S. typhi* containing equivalent deletions has been named $_x4073$. This strain or derivatives thereof containing the balanced lethal plasmid expression vector have been used in two different clinical trials and shown to be well tolerated and immunogenic. Most of the vaccines studied to date have employed strain Ty2 as the parent. Because this strain has been maintained in the laboratory since 1918 and probably contains a number of unknown mutations, a recent clinical isolate (ISP 1820) has been similarly attenuated in an attempt to define more clearly the genes contributing to virulence. Strain $_9$8110 ?cya-27[crp-cdt] was tested recently in volunteers at the NIAID-supported St. Louis University VTEU, but was found to be unacceptably reactogenic.

The other strain being actively pursued as a vaccine against typhoid is TY800, a *pho*P/*pho*Q deletion mutant of Ty2. The *pho*P/*pho*Q virulence regulon is a two-component system composed of a membrane-bound kinase (PhoQ) and a cytoplasmic

transcriptional regulator (PhoP). This system regulates a number of genes that contribute to Salmonella pathogenesis, and its deletion from Ty2 has created a vaccine candidate that appears to be well tolerated and highly immunogenic (high antibody-secreting cell response) in an admittedly small number of volunteers to date. NIAID is hopeful that phase I and II trials with this strain can be conducted in the near future in its VTEU facilities. Avant Immunotherapeutics, Inc., is developing this vaccine.

The recent demonstration of the attenuating effects of a DNA adenine methylase (*dam*) deletion on *S. typhimurium* pathogenesis in a mouse model has identified another virulence factor that could be targeted for deletion in human vaccine strains. This gene, which may be another global regulator, also may be an important contributor to virulence in other bacterial pathogens, including other enteric pathogens.

Because *S. typhi* is an invasive organism, it is expected that a significant cell-mediated immune response will be an important component of protection. Additionally, it is still assumed that Salmonella vectors can be developed to express foreign antigens and serve as multivalent vaccines capable of protecting against more than one disease by oral immunization. Although encouraging results have been demonstrated in animals, this concept has yet to be demonstrated convincingly in humans.

CAMPYLOBACTER

Campylobacter is the leading cause of bacterial foodborne gastroenteritis in the United States, with an estimated 2.5 million cases occurring annually [Mead, et al. (1998). *Emerging Infectious Diseases, 5*, 607-625.]. There is no vaccine currently available.

A whole-cell killed vaccine developed and tested in animals and in a small number of volunteers at the Navy Medical Research Institute is now being developed along with Antex Biologics and SKB. This Campylobacter vaccine consists of inactivated Campylobacter whole cells plus a mutant toxin adjuvant. Earlier studies with this adjuvanted vaccine indicated that it was safe and immunogenic in a small number of volunteers challenged postvaccination with a pathogenic Campylobacter strain. Data from animal models showed that the vaccine provides protective immunity against live infections and illness. This vaccine has been developed by the military because of the incidence of Campylobacter infection in their deployed personnel. If available, it also may be of use as a travelers' vaccine.

Fungal Infections

Fungal Infections

OVERVIEW

Infections caused by systemic fungal pathogens are a significant health problem in the immunocompetent and the immunocompromised host. Fungi that regularly infect and cause disease in otherwise healthy hosts are termed primary pathogens. These include *Coccidioides immitis, Histoplasma capsulatum, Blastomyces dermatitidis, Paracoccidioides brasiliensis*, and, on occasion, *Cryptococcus neoformans*. Opportunistic fungal pathogens, which more typically require immunosuppression to infect the human host, include *Candida albicans*, which is a normal inhabitant of the human gut, and *Aspergillus fumigatus*, which is ubiquitous in the environment. The primary fungal pathogens each occupy a discrete ecological niche. *C. immitis* is found in the soil of the Southwestern United States, Mexico, Central America, and South America. *H. capsulatum* can be found in soils enriched with guano from bats, chickens, and starlings, with a highly endemic focus along the Mississippi River, but with documented occurrence throughout the world. *B. dermatitidis* is believed to be present in microfoci of soil worldwide, but is primarily in geographic regions of North America that overlap those of *H. capsulatum*. Historically, it has been difficult to isolate *B. dermatitidis* from the environment, but it probably occupies a different niche than does *H. capsulatum*. Recent studies have found *B. dermatitidis* in moist, rich soil at the banks of rivers and waterways in endemic regions. *P. brasiliensis*, the etiologic agent of paracoccidioidomycosis (South American blastomycosis), is restricted to South and Central America. It has an affinity for shady areas and moist vegetation, particularly near rivers and lakes, with microniches in the armadillo's hole or in the soil rich in organic matter where this animal usually feeds. Virulent strains have been isolated frequently from naturally infected armadillos (*Dasypus novemcinctus*). The increasing incidence of paracoccidioidomycosis in the Amazon region can be associated with recent agricultural settlements, deforestation, and soil churning. Worldwide, roughly 10 million people may be infected with *P. brasiliensis*, and as many as 1 to 2 percent of these people may develop the disease. *C. neoformans* can be found in soil contaminated with pigeon guano and is prevalent worldwide. Infection is initiated by inhalation of microscopic forms of each fungus from a point source in nature.

The true incidence of infection by these agents is difficult to assess because the diseases are not reported nationally and can be difficult to diagnose. With the exception of the latex agglutination test for cryptococcal capsular polysaccharide antigen, there are few widely available serologic tests to facilitate rapid laboratory identification of the systemic mycoses. Definitive diagnosis usually depends on culture of the etiologic agent. Recent developments in molecular studies of *C. immitis*, which

include cloning and expression of the diagnostic complement fixation (CF) antigen, as well as reports of a sensitive polymerase chain reaction-based method for detecting coccidioidal DNA in patient sputum, provide the basis for new clinical methods of rapid and inexpensive diagnosis of coccidioidomycosis.

Frequency of major fungal infections in organ transplant recipients			
	Incidence of invasive fungal infections*, %	Infections due to *Aspergillus*, %	Infections due to *Candida*, %
Renal	1.4 - 14	0 - 10	2.0 - 100
Heart	5 - 21	77 - 91	8 - 23
Liver	7 - 42	9 - 34	35 - 91%
Lung and heart-lung	15 - 35	25 - 50	43 - 72
Small-bowel	40 - 59	0 - 3.6	80 - 100
Pancreas	18 - 38%	0 - 3	97 - 100

Courtesy of Mycology Research Units

It has been estimated, based on the results of skin tests, that there are between 25,000 and 100,000 new infections with *C. immitis* each year. The respiratory disease, known as Valley Fever, can occur in epidemic proportions; 1,500 seroconversions were documented in one county in California in 1991, whereas the number of officially reported cases for the entire State was less than 1,300. This finding emphasizes the problem of underreporting for these diseases. The epidemic in California resulted in more than 3,000 cases occurring in Kern County alone in 1992. It was estimated that the epidemic resulted in more than $45 million in medical costs in Kern County between 1991 and 1993. The California Department of Health sponsored a conference on coccidioidomycosis in 1993. The development of a vaccine was considered to be a promising approach for the prevention of the disease. The Valley Fever Research Foundation, a private foundation incorporated in 1993, commissioned a vaccine feasibility study. The study concluded that a vaccine effort should go forward. Current efforts focused on the development of a vaccine against coccidioidomycosis involve a consortium of seven laboratories funded by research grants from the National Institute of Allergy and Infectious Diseases (NIAID) and the California HealthCare Foundation.

The number of cases of Valley Fever in the Tucson and Phoenix areas increased by 66 percent between 1991 and 1992. A serious complication of the infection is meningitis, a life-threatening disease that is difficult to treat. Primary infections that apparently have resolved spontaneously may leave dormant but persistent fungal elements in lung tissue. Relapse with fungal diseases, such as Valley Fever, is viewed as a potential crisis among immunocompromised patients, such as those with acquired immunodeficiency syndrome (AIDS). One prospective study documented a prevalence of 25 percent in one cohort of human immunodeficiency virus (HIV)-infected patients over a 41-month period in highly endemic areas.

Histoplasmosis also is associated with epidemics in immunocompetent hosts. However, it is becoming an increasingly important infection in immunocompromised hosts, such as those with AIDS, where the incidence of this fungal disease can be as high as 27 percent. Histoplasmosis can resemble tuberculosis and has been misdiagnosed as such. In one study, 19 percent of the patients with histoplasmosis also had tuberculosis. The disease is geographically widespread, with reports from every continent except Antarctica, and 500,000 new infections are estimated to occur annually in the United States. It is estimated that 99 percent of these infections resolve spontaneously; the remaining 1 percent progress to chronic or disseminated disease. The reasons for this progression in otherwise healthy individuals remain unknown. Clinical disease can be classified as mild, moderate, and severe, with the latter category being the most difficult to treat with available chemotherapy. Given the widespread distribution of disease, the inability to prevent acquisition from a point source in nature, and the remaining problems with antifungal therapy, a vaccine for this disease would have obvious public health benefits.

Blastomycosis occurs mainly as a sporadic infection in immunocompetent hosts, but many cases of opportunistic infection among AIDS patients and other immunocompromised hosts have been described. The true incidence and prevalence of blastomycosis are unknown, but appear to be lower than those of the other systemic mycoses described here. A distinguishing feature of blastomycosis is the high proportion of clinically significant disease among infected persons, highlighting the organism's pathogenicity. Another feature of blastomycosis is that it is a common infection among dogs that reside in endemic areas. The severity of most canine infections also is evidence of the potential of *B. dermatitidis* as a primary pathogen.

Although immunosuppressive therapy and infection with HIV are recognized risk factors for the development of severe, progressive coccidioidomycosis and histoplasmosis, they are not prerequisites for human infection with these fungi. Both are primary pathogens. In addition, subclinical infection with these fungi and with *C. neoformans* poses a threat of subsequent reactivation to a progressive form of disease with the advent of immunosuppression. Cryptococcosis (cryptococcal meningitis) is a worldwide problem for immunosuppressed patients. Subclinical infection with *C. neoformans* may be more prevalent than previously estimated. Based on recent findings of Casadevall's group, exposure to *C. neoformans* occurs regularly as evidenced by seroconversion in young children in New York City. In the

United States, cryptococcosis is a well-known AIDS-defining illness and occurs in 7 to 11 percent of patients with AIDS. A hospital survey in New York City documented more than 1,200 cases of cryptococcosis in 1991 that were primarily associated with HIV-infected patients, resulting in a yearly prevalence of 6 to 8 percent in this population. Cryptococcal meningitis is also prevalent in HIV-infected individuals in Africa, where the costs of antifungal therapy can be prohibitive. Even with the advent of newer antifungal drugs, such as the triazoles, treatment remains suboptimal, and no existing treatment is curative. The situation for coccidioidomycosis and histoplasmosis in patients with AIDS is similar.

Mechanisms of virulence for the pathogenic fungi are poorly defined. The fungi considered above lack toxins that could serve as good targets for a rationally designed vaccine. In addition, they possess a complex, eukaryotic genome that makes elucidation of their molecular biology more difficult than that for either their viral or bacterial counterparts. However, fungi do present numerous effective antigens as demonstrated by the host's response to infection. In general, cell-mediated immunity is thought to be more important in recovery from infection than the antibody response. One possible exception is cryptococcosis, in which antibody specific for the capsular polysaccharide has an opsonizing effect on the encapsulated fungus. With an ever-expanding immunocompromised host population at risk for all of these fungal infections, and with the inability of even new antifungal agents to eradicate fungi from infected patients, serious consideration must be given to the preventive or therapeutic role of antifungal vaccines. The past 20 years of progress in vaccine development for the medically important fungi can be viewed as a time of transformation of the field in preparation for achieving the goal of licensed, effective, and safe vaccines for these complex microbes. The best characterized and largest efficacy trial for a vaccine for a systemic fungal infection was conducted 20 years ago with the evaluation of the killed *C. immitis* spherule vaccine (conducted between 1980 and 1985 and published in 1993). That effort, described below, fell short of the goal and was confounded by the need to dilute the protein concentration of the whole-spherule vaccine by 1:1,000 relative to the protective dose in mice to circumvent the problems of swelling and discomfort at the injection site observed with undiluted doses. The authors concluded, "A different physical form other than the whole spherules must be sought to increase the tolerability of the immunogenic component. .... If the immunogenic material is protein, the active epitopes may be determined by peptide sequencing, which may permit synthesis *in vitro* by recombinant methods. This may provide a vaccine with a minimum of other irritant components present in the whole spherule." During the ensuing two decades, the field of medical mycology gained substantially in technology and is now poised to return to the challenge with the renewed tools necessary to confront the design of vaccines for these eukaryotic pathogens. The important scientific advance in the field of medical mycology of significance to vaccines was, therefore, the noteworthy development of the field itself.

NIAID encouraged the development of research with an ultimate goal of developing vaccine approaches to the invasive mycoses, particularly over the last decade. The NIAID Workshop in Medical Mycology series focused on the following areas in each of five separate events: Molecular medical mycology, diagnosis and treatment, fungal vaccines (antigenic peptides and glycobiology), immunology (parts 1 and 2), and epidemiology (see http://www.niaid nih.gov/dmid/meetings). Additionally, recent solicitations also provided for vaccine research opportunities (PA 96-061, Modern Vaccines for Mycoses and Measles; RFA AI 98-002, Mycology Research Units). Vaccine-related applications were funded under both solicitations (e.g., one program project, P01AI037232, Kirkland, T., Principal Investigator, Molecular Strategies Toward a Coccidioidomycosis Vaccine; and one research project, R01AI025780, Levitz, S., Principal Investigator, Immune Responses to Cryptococcal Infections). Additionally, investigator-initiated research proposals focusing on vaccine approaches were funded (e.g., R01AI034361, Deepe, G., Principal Investigator, Protective Antigens From *Histoplasma capsulatum*; and grants were awarded to the work noted in the fungal section sources). Therefore, the community has succeeded in following the consensus of the third workshop in the NIAID mycology series where it was noted: "Leading researchers studying a variety of fungal pathogens say that there is a major shift in thinking regarding vaccines. Thus, the prevailing question of whether vaccines should be considered as a practical way of preventing fungal diseases is being challenged by the questions of which ones and when."

The challenges that lie ahead are much the same in medical mycology as for parasitology, or oncology, where the design issues must address the complexity of eukaryotic systems relative to the smaller genome-sized bacteria or viruses, and must address the related issue of eukaryotic target in the context of a eukaryotic host. With the beginning of the new century, there still are no fungal vaccines licensed for use in the United States, and the field has not yet moved the newer technologies from the research bench into the target populations. Yet, there is continued advancement toward this goal as evidenced by two representative examples. First, the NIAID Mycoses Study Group launched a phase I clinical trial on July 5, 2000, "A Phase I Evaluation of the Safety and Pharmacodynamic Activity of a Murine Derived Anticryptococcal Antibody 18B7 in HIV-Infected Subjects Who Have Responded to Therapy for Cryptococcal Meningitis." That monoclonal was generated by stimulation with a glycoconjugate vaccine for *C. neoformans* (see below). Also, in work described below, a live attenuated vaccine for *B. dermatitidis* was described and tested in mice. Blastomycosis is an attractive model disease for fungal vaccine development because of the prevalence of canine disease in the endemic areas, and the potential for validating a fungal vaccine in naturally occurring mammalian hosts.

Sources

Dixon, D. M., Casadevall, A., Klein, B., Mendoza, L., Travassos, L., & Deepe, G. S., Jr. (1998). Development of fungal vaccines and their use in the prevention of fungal infections. *Medical Mycology, S1,* 57-67.

Dixon, D. M., Cox, R. A., Cutler, J., & Deepe, G. (1996). Researchers use molecular immunology and technology to combat fungal pathogens. *ASM News, 62,* 81-84.

Goldman, D. L., Khine, H., Abadi, J., Lindenberg, D. J., Pirofski, L., Niang, R., & Casadevall, A. (2001). *Pediatrics, 107*(5), E66.

BLASTOMYCOSIS

Spores are inhaled into the lungs and converted into budding yeasts, which are large and relatively resistant to phagocytosis and killing by the neutrophils and mononuclear effector cells that constitute the early inflammatory response. Within several weeks after infection in humans and experimental animals, the host develops acquired immunity to *B. dermatitidis* as evidenced by the appearance of delayed-type hypersensitivity, proliferation of lymphocytes *in vitro*, and circulating antibodies in response to antigens of the fungus. In a murine model of blastomycosis, T lymphocytes but not serum passively transferred from immune to naive animals conferred protection, suggesting that immunity resides chiefly with antigen-specific T cells.

A 120-kD protein, designated *Blastomyces* adhesin 1 (BAD1) (formerly termed WI-1), is displayed on the surface of *B. dermatitidis* yeasts and is an immunodominant antigen during human, canine, and experimental murine infection. Human patients develop strong antibody and T-lymphocyte responses to determinants of BAD1. BAD1 has been cloned and sequenced and shown to contain 30 copies of a repetitive domain of 25 amino acids similar in sequence to a bacterial adhesin, invasin. This so-called tandem repeat mediates binding of the yeast to integrin receptors on human cells, and the expression of BAD1 is altered on genetically related strains of *B. dermatitidis* that differ in virulence for mice, suggesting that BAD1 plays a role in the pathogenesis of blastomycosis. Human, murine, and canine infection are associated with the development of high antibody titers directed against the tandem repeat. The functional role of monoclonal anti-BAD1 antibodies is under study, and some appear to enhance infection. T lymphocytes from human patients with blastomycosis respond strongly to BAD1 *in vitro*. At the clonal level, these cells are directed chiefly toward epitopes displayed in a short segment of amino acids at the N-terminus. BAD1 is immunogenic in mice, where protective efficacy has been shown. This supports its vaccine potential, although harmful and beneficial segments of the antigen may need to be separated.

A gene transfer system is available in *B. dermatitidis*, and BAD1 has been disrupted by homologous recombination. BAD1 knockout yeast bind poorly to host tissue and are nonpathogenic in a murine model of pulmonary blastomycosis, emphasizing the role of this adhesin in virulence. BAD1 is phase regulated, expressed in yeast but not mold, linking morphology with pathogenicity. Animals that clear BAD1 knockout yeast can resist a lethal pulmonary challenge with wild-type yeast. Therefore, BAD1 knockout yeast serve as a live attenuated vaccine. Antigens responsible for this resistance are under study. The considerable clinical importance of canine blastomycosis in veterinary medicine provides a unique target population of dogs for initial clinical investigation of novel vaccine formulations, such as naked DNA or attenuated strains.

Sources

Brandhorst, T., Wuethrich, M., Warner, T., & Klein, B. S. (1999). Targeted gene disruption reveals an adhesin indispensable for pathogenicity of *Blastomyces dermatitidis*. *Journal of Experimental Medicine, 189,* 1207-1216.

Hogan, L. H., Josvai, S., & Klein, B. S. (1995). Genomic cloning, characterization, and functional analysis of the major surface adhesin WI-1 on *Blastomyces dermatitidis* yeasts. *Journal of Biological Chemistry, 270,* 30725-30732.

Newman, S. L., Chaturvedi, S., & Klein, B. S. (1995). The WI-1 antigen on *Blastomyces dermatitidis* yeasts mediates binding to human macrophage CD18 and CD14 receptors. *Journal of Immunology, 154,* 753-761.

Rooney, P., Sullivan, T., & Klein, B. S. (2000). Selective expression of the virulence factor BAD1 upon morphogenesis to the pathogenic yeast form of *Blastomyces dermatitidis*: Evidence for transcriptional regulation by a conserved mechanism. *Molecular Microbiology, 39,* 875-889.

Wuethrich, M., Chang, W. L., & Klein, B. S. (1998). Immunogenicity and protective efficacy of the WI-1 adhesin of *Blastomyces dermatitidis*. *Infection and Immunity, 11,* 5443-5449.

Wuethrich, M., Fillutowicz H.I., & Klein, B. S. (2000). Mutation of the WI-1 gene yields an attenuated *Blastomyces dermatitidis* strain that induces host resistance. *Journal of Clinical Investigation, 106,* 1381-1389.

CANDIDIASIS

Candidiasis is a leading group of opportunistic mycoses caused by any of several species of the genus *Candida*. Most noteworthy examples include *C. albicans, C. tropicalis,* and *C. krusei.* These and other *Candida* species are normal inhabitants of humans and usually live in harmony with the mammalian host. Factors predisposing to disease include chemical immunosuppression, surgical trauma, and underlying diseases such as diabetes and AIDS. Neutropenia is a major risk factor; patients undergoing immunosuppression to prevent rejection of bone marrow or organ transplantation are particularly vulnerable to infection from either endogenous or exogenous sources.

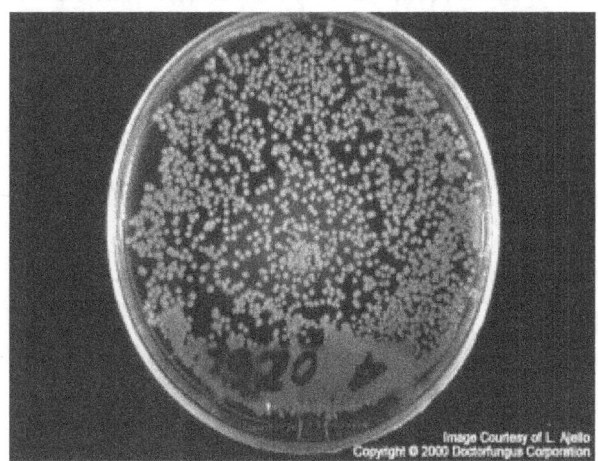

Candida Albicans

Novel advances in the identification of protective antibody in models of cryptococcosis described in this report have given hope that analogous situations may pertain to other opportunistic mycoses, including candidiasis. Indeed, a protective antibody has been identified for *C. albicans* in an animal model system. Antigen delivery was key to demonstrating that a mannan adhesin from the fungus could generate immunoprotection. Liposome encapsulation of a mannan adhesin fraction of yeast cells, and conjugation of the mannan to a carrier protein have been used to generate protective antibodies that are functional in vaccinated mice and could be passively transferred to protect normal and immunocompromised mice. Protective and nonprotective antibodies were identified. The latter can be useful in addressing the controversy generated in previous studies where circulating antibodies did not correlate with protection. Two murine monoclonal antibodies, an immunoglobulin (Ig) M antibody B6.1 and an IgG3 antibody C3.1, have been demonstrated to be protective in passive transfer experiments, and there is considerable interest in examining the role of immunotherapy as an alternative to chemotherapy in human candidiasis. Because of the newly acknowledged problem of antifungal drug resistance in *Candida*, these findings are of special relevance.

Sources

Goins, T., & Cutler, J. E. (2000). Relative abundance of oligosaccharides in *Candida* species as determined by fluorophore-assisted carbohydrate electrophoresis. *Journal of Clinical Microbiology, 38,* 2862-2869.

Han, Y., & Cutler, J. E. (1995). Antibody response that protects against disseminated candidiasis. *Infection and Immunity, 63,* 2714-2719.

Han, Y., & Cutler, J. E. *Protection against candidiasis by IgM and IgG monoclonal antibodies specific for the same mannan epitope.* Manuscript in preparation.

Han, Y., Kanbe, T., Cherniak, R., & Cutler, J. E. (1997). Biochemical characterization of *Candida albicans* epitopes that can elicit protective and nonprotective antibodies. *Infection and Immunity, 65,* 4100-4107.

Han, Y., Riesselman, M., & Cutler, J. E. (2000). Protection against candidiasis by an immunoglobulin G3 (IgG3) monoclonal antibody specific for the same mannotriose as an IgM protective antibody. *Infection and Immunity, 68,* 1649-1654.

Han, Y., Ulrich, M. A., & Cutler, J. E. (1999). *Candida albicans* mannan extract-protein conjugates induce a protective immune response against experimental candidiasis. *Journal of Infectious Diseases, 179,* 1477-1484.

Han, Y., et al. (2001). Complement is essential for protection by an IgM and an IgG3 monoclonal antibody against experimental hematogenously disseminated candidiasis. *Journal of Immunology, 167,* 1550-1557.

COCCIDIOIDOMYCOSIS

Spores of *C. immitis* are inhaled into the lungs, where they undergo a morphological conversion to a parasitic, spherule form of growth. The spherule enlarges and subdivides into propagative units that are released to repeat the cycle. Patients develop delayed-type hypersensitivity as a consequence of infection. Although complement-fixing and precipitating antibodies are produced during the course of infection, they do not seem to be protective. In fact, high titers of complement-fixing antibodies are a poor prognostic sign. In experimental infections, immunity is transferred by thymus-derived lymphocytes (T cells), but not by serum.

An experimental vaccine has been prepared from formalin-killed spherules of the fungus grown *in vitro*. After it was demon-

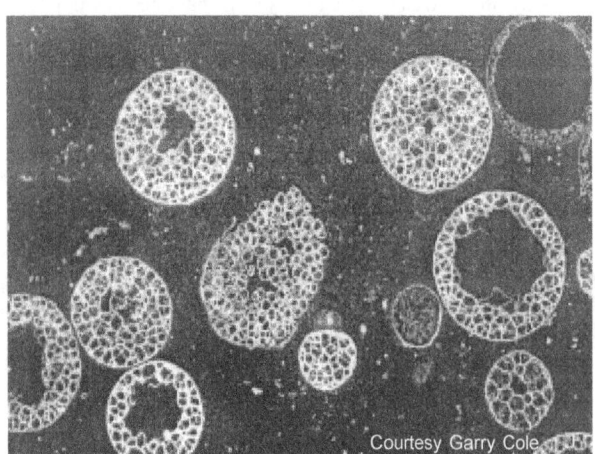

Coccidioidomycosis Immitis

strated that the vaccine increased survival in animals after a lethal experimental challenge, a phase III trial was undertaken in human volunteers. The study groups were from Arizona and California and were demonstrated to be skin test negative to spherule antigen and to coccidioidin before vaccination. A total of 1,400 subjects received the formalin-killed spherulin vaccine (1.75 mg per injection, with a total of 3 injections), and 1,400 others received placebo. The results of the trial indicate that the vaccine did not prevent clinically apparent coccidioidomycosis. In experimental trials in mice, the vaccine did not prevent infection, but did prevent progressive disease and death. Because progressive disease did not occur in either the control or vaccinated human groups, it was not possible to evaluate these potential protective effects. Failure of this trial could have been caused by dose-limiting irritation at the injection site from toxic components of the fungus. That is, the dose used in the human trial was reduced to less than 1/400 of the amount of the spherule vaccine needed to protect mice on a body-weight basis.

Disruption of the whole-spherule vaccine and centrifugation of the homogenate at 27,000 X gravity yielded a supernatant preparation (designated 27 K) that was as protective in mice as the killed-spherule vaccine. Cell walls from mechanically disrupted spherules have also shown to produce protection, and when the walls were incubated in phosphate-buffered saline containing 1-percent chloroform as a preservative, a soluble fraction was obtained that induced strong protection against challenge. Alkaline extraction of cell walls has also been reported to yield a soluble fraction (designated C-ASWS), which protects mice against challenge with *C. immitis*. The protective component of the C-ASWS extract was shown to be a glycosylated protein having antigenic identity with the polymeric antigen in coccidioidin that had been designated Antigen 2 (Ag2). In other studies, a 33-kDA peptide was isolated from a chemically deglycosylated lysate of spherules. The 33-kDA peptide expressed T and B-cell epitopes and, when examined by tandem immunoelectrophoresis, showed complete fusion with the anodal precipitin peak of the Ag2 polymer; hence, its antigenic identity with the protein moiety of Ag2. The gene that encodes Ag2 has been cloned by two groups of investigators and, when expressed in *Escherichia coli*, yielded a proline-rich antigen (PRA) having a molecular size of 19.4 kDA. Immunization of mice with the recombinant Ag2(PRA) protein induced protection against challenge, but a significantly greater level of protection was induced in mice immunized with Ag2(PRA) cDNA. The protective effects of recombinant Ag2(PRA) or the Ag2(PRA) gene vaccine were associated with, and thought to be attributable to, the induction of T helper 1 (Th1) responses, evidenced by the acquisition of a delayed footpad hypersensitivity response in mice, and increased production of interferon gamma (IFNg).

Additional vaccine-related research is underway with various fractions of *C. immitis*. A 48-kDA T-cell-reactive protein (TCRP), which is expressed in the cytoplasm of spherules, was shown to stimulate proliferation and IFNg production by T cells of spherule-immunized mice. The gene encoding this antigen was cloned and found to have 70 percent homology with mammalian 4-hydroxyphenylpyruvate dioxygenase. Mice immunized with the recombinant TCRP had approximately 1.5 log lower burden of *C. immitis* in their lungs after intraperitoneal infection. Similar experiments were performed with a recombinant protein expressed by the gene that encodes *C. immitis* heat shock protein 60 (*HSP60*). The recombinant HSP60 induced proliferation of T cells from HSP60-immunized mice, but did not induce protection against challenge. More recently, two additional T-cell-reactive antigens have been isolated and cloned [a spherule outer wall glycoprotein (SOWgp) and urease (URE)]. Both have been shown to confer immunoprotection in mice against coccidioidal infection.

Although recombinant antigens and gene vaccines have induced protection against challenge with *C. immitis*, none of these vaccines have induced a level of protection comparable to that of vaccines using either the killed spherule or native antigens obtained from *C. immitis* cells or cell walls. The reduced efficacy of the recombinant and gene vaccines could be attributable to inadequate presentation or processing by antigen presenting cells. It is also possible that a multivalent vaccine comprised of several T-cell-reactive molecules expressed during different stages of the parasitic cycle and conserved among different isolates of the pathogen will be needed for optimal vaccination against this fungal pathogen.

Sources

Cole, G. T., Thomas, P. W., & Kirkland, T. N. (1995). Molecular strategies for development of a vaccine against coccidioidomycosis. In S. Suzuki & M. Suzuki (Eds.), *Fungal cells in biodefense mechanisms* (pp. 307-317). Tokyo: Saikon Publishing Company, Ltd.

Dugger, K. O., Villareal, K. M., Ngyuen, A., Zimmermann, C. R., Law, J. H., & Galgiani, J. N. (1996). Cloning and sequence analysis of the cDNA for a protein from *Coccidioides immitis* with immunogenic potential. *Biochemical and Biophysical Research Communications, 218*, 485-489.

Jiang, C., Magee, D. M., Quitugua, T. N., & Cox, R. A. (1999). Genetic vaccination against *Coccidioides immitis*: Comparison of vaccine efficacy of recombinant Antigen 2 and Antigen 2 cDNA. *Infection and Immunity, 67*, 630-635.

Kirkland, T. N., Finley, F., Orsborne, K. I., & Galgiani, J. N. (1998). Evaluation of the proline-rich antigen of *Coccidioides immitis* as a candidate vaccine in mice. *Infection and Immunity, 66*, 3519-3522.

Kirkland, T. N., Thomas, P. W., Finley, F., & Cole, G. T. (1998). Immunogenicity of a 48-kilodalton recombinant T-cell-reactive protein of *Coccidioides immitis*. *Infection and Immunity, 66*, 424-431.

Lecara, G., Cox, R. A., & Simpson, R. B. (1983). *Coccidioides immitis* vaccine: Potential of an alkali-soluble, water-soluble cell wall antigen. *Infection and Immunity, 39*, 473-475.

Pappagianis, D., & Valley Fever Vaccine Study Group. (1993). Evaluation of the protective efficacy of the killed *Coccidioides immitis* spherule vaccine in humans. *American Review of Respiratory Disease, 148*, 656-660.

Peng, T., Osborn, K. I., Orbach, M. J., & Galgiani, J. N. (1999). Proline-rich vaccine candidate antigen of *Coccidioides immitis*: Conservation among isolates and differential expression with spherule maturation. *Journal of Infectious Diseases, 179*, 518.

Wyckoff, E. E., Pishko, E. J., Kirkland, T. N., & Cole, G. T. (1995). Cloning and expression of a gene encoding a T-cell-reactive protein from *Coccidioides immitis*: Homology to 4-hydroxyphenylpyruvate dioxygenase and the mammalian F antigen. *Gene, 161*, 107-111.

Yu, J.-J., Smithson, S. L., Thomas, P. W., Kirkland, T. N., & Cole, G. T. (1997). Isolation and characterization of the urease gene (*URE*) from the pathogenic fungus *Coccidioides immitis*. *Gene, 198*, 387-391.

Zhu, Y., Yang, C., Magee, D. M., & Cox, R. A. (1996). Molecular cloning and characterization of *Coccidioides immitis* Antigen 2 cDNA. *Infection and Immunity, 64*(7), 2695-2699.

Zimmermann, C. R., Johnson, S. M., Martens, G. W., White, A. G., Zimmer, B. L., & Pappagianis, D. (1993). Protection against lethal murine coccidioidomycosis by a soluble vaccine from spherules. *Infection and Immunity, 66*, 2342-2345.

CRYPTOCOCCOSIS

Yeast cells of *C. neoformans* are thought to be the infectious form of the fungus. Inhalation of these cells establishes a primary pulmonary infection that is often not apparent. Meningitis is the typical manifestation of disease. Early diagnosis and treatment can arrest but not cure infection in AIDS patients; lifetime suppressive therapy is required.

C. neoformans is delimited by a polysaccharide capsule and, therefore, is unique among the major fungal pathogens of humans. The antibody response to the capsular polysaccharide is minimal in clinically apparent infections. Because most patients with cryptococcal meningoencephalitis have soluble capsular polysaccharide in serum or cerebrospinal fluid, testing for antigen is useful in the diagnosis of this infection. The capsule of *C. neoformans* is a known virulence factor, and attempts have been made to induce a protective immune response against capsular polysaccharide. Injection of mice with capsular polysaccharide

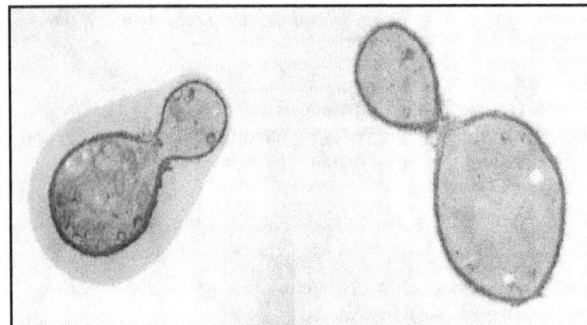

Electronmicrograph of C. Neoformans Showing the Characteristic Polysaccharide Capsule

alone or with adjuvants does not appear to result in sustained or high-titer antibody response. However, conjugation of crypto-coccal capsular polysaccharide to protein carriers may improve the antibody response. Cryptococcal glucuronoxylomannan conjugated to tetanus toxoid has been shown to be immuno-genic in mice. Preliminary clinical trials with a glycoconjugate vaccine have been conducted to determine safety and antigenic-ity. The ultimate goal is to develop a vaccine that will protect patients at high risk of developing cryptococcosis.

Antibody administration has been shown to enhance the effi-cacy of amphotericin B, fluconazole, and 5-fluorocytosine in mouse models of infection. Studies of antibody efficacy in mice have shown that antibody specificity and isotype are important characteristics for antibody effectiveness. Vaccines that elicit primarily protective antibodies may be effective in preventing infection even if the role of naturally occurring antibody in pro-tection is uncertain.

Confirmation of the protective role of antibody also comes from studies showing that the infusion of monoclonal antibody can prolong life and decrease fungal burden in mice challenged with fungi by the intraperitoneal, intravenous, or intracranial routes. Several protective murine monoclonal antibodies have been used to construct mouse-human chimeric antibodies to the cryptococcal polysaccharide; the goal of clinical studies, in this case, is to determine the efficacy of passive immunization as an adjunct to chemotherapy in cryptococcal meningitis.

Sources

Devi, S. J. N. (1996). Preclinical efficacy of a glucuronoxylomannan-tetanus toxoid conjugate vaccine of *Cryptococcus neoformans* in a murine model. *Vaccine, 14,* 841-844.

Devi, S. J. N., Schneerson, R., Egan, W., Ulrich, T. J., Bryla, D., Robbins, J. B., & Bennett, J. E. (1991). *Cryptococcus neoformans* serotype A glucuronoxylomannan-protein conjugate vaccines: Synthesis, characterization, and immunogenicity. *Infection and Immunity, 59,* 3700-3707.

Gomez, A. M., Rhodes, J. C., & Deepe, G. S., Jr. (1991). Antigenic-ity and immunogenicity of an extract from the cell wall and cell membrane of *Histoplasma capsulatum* yeast cells. *Infection and Immunity, 59,* 330-336.

Gomez, F. J., Allendoerfer, R., & Deepe, G. S., Jr. (1995). Vaccina-tion with recombinant heat shock protein 60 from *Histoplasma capsulatum* protects mice against pulmonary histoplasmosis. *Infection and Immunity, 63,* 2587-2595.

Gomez, F. J., Gomez, A. M., & Deepe, G. S., Jr. (1991). Protective efficacy of a 62-kilodalton antigen, HIS-62, from the cell wall and cell membrane of *Histoplasma capsulatum* yeast cells. *Infection and Immunity, 59,* 4459-4464.

Williamson, P. R., Bennett, J. E., Robbins, J. B., & Schneerson, R. (1993). Vaccination for prevention of cryptococcosis. *Second International Conference on Cryptococcus and Cryptococcosis, Abstract L22,* p. 60.

HISTOPLASMOSIS

Spores of *H. capsulatum* are inhaled into the lungs and con-verted into budding yeasts that proliferate within cells of the macrophage lineage. The importance of T-cell-mediated immu-nity in infection is implicit in the emergence of this fungus as a significant pathogen in AIDS. As with coccidioidomycosis, antibodies can be diagnostic, but are not thought to play a major protective role. Delayed-type hypersensitivity develops, and immunity can be demonstrated following transfer of T cells in experimental models. These models have shown the expansion of suppressor and helper cell lines in response to challenge with fungal antigens. The recent development of a transformation system for *H. capsulatum*, and an increased knowledge of its molecular biology should facilitate studies on pathogenesis and virulence and provide at least the methodological basis for vac-cine development.

HIS-62 is a 62-kD glycoprotein antigen isolated from cell wall and cell membrane extracts of yeast cells of *H. capsulatum*. This antigen induces cell-mediated immune responses in C57BL/6, BALB/c, and CBA/J mice. Vaccination with 80 micrograms of HIS-62 significantly protects all three strains of mice against lethal challenge with viable cells of this fungus. In addition, lymphocytes from humans exposed to *H. capsulatum* respond *in vitro* to this antigen. The gene encoding this antigen has been cloned and sequenced; it has a high homology with the gene that encodes for HSP60. Recombinant antigen has been gener-ated from *E. coli*, and it stimulates monoclonal populations of antigen-reactive T cells and polyclonal T cells from mice immu-nized with *H. capsulatum* yeast cells. Vaccination with the re-combinant antigen protects mice against pulmonary histoplas-mosis. A fragment spanning amino acids 172-443 contained the protective activity of HSP60, although it was not as effective as the full-length protein. Studies are currently underway to determine the mechanisms by which this protein confers protection and to determine the family of T cells engaged by the protein.

H antigen from *H. capsulatum* has been identified as a ß-glucosidase. Until recently, its utility has been restricted to serologic detection of infection. In a previous study, immunization with this antigen failed to induce protective immunity in a model of systemic histoplasmosis induced by intravenous injection of yeast cells. However, a serendipitous finding prompted a reinvestigation of the utility of H antigen as a vaccine in a pulmonary model of histoplasmosis. C57BL/6 mice were immunized with H antigen and infected intranasally with either a sublethal or lethal inoculum of yeasts 4 weeks later. Vaccination reduced colony-forming units in animals and promoted survival in a lethal challenge. The effect of H was durable since vaccination protected mice if they were challenged 3 months postimmunization. The efficacy of H antigen was associated with production of IFN? and granulocyte-macrophage colony-stimulating factor, interleukin (IL)-4, and IL-10 by spleen cells from vaccinated mice. Hence, H may be an additional target for development of a candidate vaccine.

Sources

Allendoerfer, R., Maresca, B., & Deepe, G. S., Jr. (1996). Cellular immune responses to recombinant heat shock protein 70 from *Histoplasma capsulatum*. *Infection and Immunity, 64,* 4123-4128.

Deepe, G. S., Jr., & Durose, G. G. (1995). Immunobiological activity of recombinant H antigen from *Histoplasma capsulatum*. *Infection and Immunity, 63,* 3151-3157.

Deepe, G. S., Jr., & Gibbons, R. (2001). Protective efficacy of H antigen from *Histoplasma capsulatum* in a murine model of pulmonary histoplasmosis. *Infection and Immunity, 69*(5), 3128-3134.

Deepe, G. S., Jr., Gibbons, R., Brunner, G. D., & Gomez, F. J. (1996). A protective domain of heat-shock protein 60 from *Histoplasma capsulatum*. *Journal of Infectious Diseases, 174,* 828-834.

Henderson, H. M., & Deepe, G. S., Jr. (1992). Recognition of *Histoplasma capsulatum* yeast-cell antigens by human lymphocytes and human T-cell clones. *Journal of Leukocyte Biology, 51,* 432-436.

PARACOCCIDIOIDOMYCOSIS

Natural infection with *P. brasiliensis* is assumed to occur through the respiratory route. Lungs are involved in the majority of patients with paracoccidioidomycosis. Alveolar lesions are exudative or granulomatous. The granulomatous inflammatory response with formation of epithelioid tubercles is the most effective defense against the invading fungus. In the acute lymphatic forms, the fungus reaches the lymph nodes by the afferent lymphatics. The earlier and more severe the lymph node involvement, the worse the prognosis. In the chronic progressive forms, dissemination of the fungus to mucocutaneous sites and other organs is accompanied by a vigorous cellular immune response. As the infection becomes more severe, a depression of cellular immunity may occur, leading to the anergic state. This anergy can be reversed with successful treatment. Antibody titers typically rise, but do not confer protection in natural infection.

Given the similarities between paracoccidioidomycosis and coccidioidomycosis and blastomycosis, it would be predicted that native antigens exist that can be used to generate a protective immune response. Investigations are underway that support this prediction. Most actively studied is an exocellular 43-kD antigen (gp43) from yeast cell cultures. It represents the major diagnostic antigen and is immunodominant. The gene for gp43 has been cloned and sequenced, and the immunodominant T-cell epitope mapped to a 15 aa.peptide (P10). The immune response elicited by either the gp43 or P10 involves T-CD4[+], Th1 lymphocytes producing IFNg, which is a key cytokine in the immune protection against *P. brasiliensis*. Mice knockout for IFNg receptor challenged intratracheally with virulent *P. brasiliensis* are extremely susceptible to the infection, with rapid dissemination and high mortality. Immunization with the gp43 or P10 markedly protects Balb/c mice against the intratracheal challenge, with a 200-fold reduction in colony-forming units in the lungs, and little or no dissemination to the liver or spleen. Recently, the DNA fragment corresponding to the mature gp43 cDNA and signal peptide was cloned into the VR1012 vector, and Balb/c mice were injected with this plasmid to elicit an immune protection. A type-1 cellular immune response was obtained that was protective against intratracheal *P. brasiliensis* infection. By using the TEPITOPE algorithm, eight 15-mer peptide sequences of the gp43 antigen, predicted to bind to multiple human histocompatibility leukocyte antigen (HLA)-II alleles with high avidity, were tested in proliferation assays with peripheral blood mononuclear cells from treated and cured patients. P10 was recognized by 71 percent of responders, and the combination of this peptide with three other gp43 peptide sequences covered 100 percent of peptide responders. The number of HLA alleles predicted to bind, as well as the relative avidity predicted by TEPITOPE for each peptide, correlated with the rank of T-cell proliferation frequency, magnitude, and avidity. These results suggest that a tetravalent vaccine including P10 and three other peptides of the gp43 could be tested against human paracoccidioidomycosis.

Sources

Bagagli, E. (1999). Occurrence of *Paracoccidioides brasiliensis* in armadillos. Importance to the ecology of the fungus. *Seventh International Meeting on Paracoccidioidomycosis, Abstract MR-01,* p. 37. Campos de Jordao, Sao Paulo, Brazil.

Campos de Jordao, Sao Paulo, Brazil. (1999). Abstract E-24, p.160.

Cisalpino, P.S., Puccia, R., Yamauchi, L. M., et al. (1996). Cloning, characterization, and epitope expression of the major diagnostic antigen of *Paracoccidioides brasiliensis*. *Journal of Biological Chemistry, 271*, 4553-4560.

Iwai, L. K., Yoshida, M., Marin, M. L., Juliano, M. A., Hammer, J., Shikanai-Yasuda, M. A., Juliano, L., Goldberg, A. C., Kalil, J., Travassos, L. R., & Cunha-Neto, E. (2001). Selection of potential vaccine T-cell epitopes from gp43 of *Paracoccidioides brasiliensis* based on prediction of peptide binding to multiple HLA molecules. *Scandanavian Journal of Immunology, 54*(Suppl. 1), A5.Mon.5.1/1270 (Abstract).

McEwen, J. G., Garcia, A. M., Ortiz, B. L., et al. (1995). In search of the natural habitat of *Paracoccidioides brasiliensis*. *Archives of Medical Research, 26*, 305-306.

Pinto, A. R., Puccia, R., Diniz, S. N., Franco, M. F., & Travassos, L. R. (2000). DNA-based vaccination against murine paracoccidioidomycosis using the gp43 gene from *Paracoccidioides brasiliensis*. *Vaccine, 18*, 3050-3058.

Puccia, R., Schenkman, S., Gorin, P. A. J., et al. (1986). Exocellular components of *Paracoccidioides brasiliensis*. Identification of a specific antigen. *Infection and Immunity, 53*, 199-206.

Rodrigues, E. G., & Travassos, L. R. (1994). Nature of the reactive epitopes in *Paracoccidioides brasiliensis* polysaccharide antigen. *Journal of Medical and Veterinary Mycology, 32*, 77-81.

Taborda, C. P., Juliano, M. A., Puccia, R., et al. (1998). Mapping of the T-cell epitope in the major 43-kilodalton glycoprotein of *Paracoccidioides brasiliensis*, which induces a Th-1 response protective against fungal infection in BALB/c mice. *Infection and Immunity, 66*, 786-793.

PYTHIOSIS

Pythium insidiosum is a filamentous eukaryotic organism, previously classified in the Oomycetes of kingdom fungi, but recently moved to kingdom Stramenopila (Protoctista). The organism is aquatic and has a flagellated stage. Cutaneous, subcutaneous, and systemic disease can result in humans and horses and other animals as a consequence of traumatic implantation. When left untreated, the mortality rate is 100 percent. Choices of chemotherapy are limited, and antifungal drugs are generally not effective. At least two different groups of investigators have generated promising results with therapeutic vaccines consisting of hyphal extracts. Three immunodominant proteins (28, 30, and 32 kD) have been identified. Rates of 53-percent efficacy have been reported following injections of such extracts into infected horses. Refinement of extracts by supplementation with purified protein derivatives has increased efficacy to as much as 70 percent with chronic pythiosis, which is the form least responsive to treatment. This vaccine was effective in curing more than 300 horses with the disease. Three cases of vaccination have been described in individuals from Thailand with pythiosis in their arteries refractory to multiple courses of antifungal and surgical therapy. The infection resolved following vaccination in all cases. Recent studies in experimental rabbits, 35 horses with the infection from Texas, and 2 cases in humans from Thailand have shown that immune modulation from Th2 to Th1 response is behind the curative properties of this vaccine. Investigators have found that IL-4, IL-5, IgE, IgG isotypes (in study), and eosinophils (all features of Th2 response) are present during pythiosis infections. Although IL-2, INFg, IgG isotypes (different from the one detected before vaccination), T cytotoxic lymphocytes, and macrophages (all features of Th1 response) are in place 7 to 20 days after successful vaccination, in successfully vaccinated humans and horses, IL-4, IL-5, IgE, and the eosinophilia of the original immune response had vanished. These data suggest that the modulation of the immune system by curative vaccines is feasible. Similar data from therapeutic vaccines used to treat cancer, allergic diseases, and infections caused by *Leishmania* spp. strongly support this idea. Characterization of relevant proteins in *P. insidiosum* in a rabbit model is under investigation.

Sources

Cohen, E. P., de Zoeten, E. F., & Schatzman, M. (1999). DNA vaccines as cancer treatment. *American Scientist, 87*, 328-335.

Mendoza, L., Nicholson, V., & Prescott, J. F. (1992). Immunoblot analysis of the humoral immune response to *Pythium insidiosum* in horses with pythiosis. *Journal of Clinical Microbiology, 30*, 2980-2983.

Mendoza, L., Villalobos, J., Calleja, C. E., & Solis, A. (1992). Evaluation of two vaccines for the treatment of pythiosis insidiosi in horses. *Mycopathologia, 119*, 89-95.

Miller, R. I. (1981). Treatment of equine phycomycosis by immunotherapy and surgery. *Australian Veterinary Journal, 57*, 377-382.

Thitithanyanont, A., Mendoza, L., Chuansumrit, A., Pracharktam, R., Laothamatas, J., Sathapatayavongs, B., Lolekha, S., & Ajello, L. (1998). Use of an immunotherapeutic vaccine to treat a life-threatening human arteritis infection caused by *Pythium insidiosum*. *Clinical Infectious Diseases, 27*, 1394-1400.

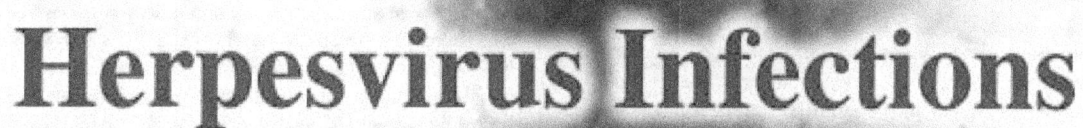

Herpesvirus Infections

Herpesvirus Infections

OVERVIEW

The eight human herpesviruses—herpes simplex virus types 1 and 2 (HSV-1 and HSV-2); Epstein-Barr virus (EBV); human cytomegalovirus (HCMV); varicella-zoster virus (VZV); and human herpesviruses 6, 7, and 8 (HHV-6, HHV-7, and HHV-8)— are a significant public health problem in the United States. Most of the population has been infected with several of these herpesviruses, and therefore has lifelong latent infections.

Clinical Manifestations

Primary infections are not usually severe or life threatening in healthy persons, but many of the human herpesviruses can produce severe or chronic active infections in certain individuals. While primary infection of young children with most herpesviruses is often unrecognized or mild, primary infection of adults with VZV or EBV can be severe. HSV and HCMV pose a particular threat to newborns whose mothers have had a primary infection during pregnancy.

Reactivation-associated disease is often more severe than primary infection. HSV-1, HSV-2, and VZV are associated in some individuals with frequent and/or painful recurrences that manifest themselves as cold sores, genital herpes, and shingles, respectively. Reactivation of herpesviruses in individuals with compromised or waning immunity may result in severe and life-threatening illnesses such as HCMV pneumonia and EBV-associated lymphomas. Therefore, herpesviruses can pose a particular threat to acquired immunodeficiency syndrome (AIDS) patients, cancer patients, organ transplant recipients, and the elderly. Induction of immunity that could withstand immunosuppressive regimens would bring significant benefit to these patients. An additional concern with reactivation is that asymptomatic individuals shedding reactivated virus may serve as reservoirs for herpesvirus transmission.

Herpesvirus infection also can have long-term consequences. In certain geographical areas and in certain populations, EBV is associated with nasopharyngeal carcinoma and with Burkitt's lymphoma. More recently, the association of EBV with Hodgkin's lymphoma, T-cell lymphomas, and some gastric carcinomas has been suggested. HHV-8 is now recognized as the herpesvirus associated with Kaposi's sarcoma. There also has been suggestion of an association between herpesviruses and certain chronic diseases, including HHV-6 and multiple sclerosis, and HCMV and heart disease.

Challenges in Developing Herpesvirus Vaccines

Clinically, the goals of immunization against herpesviruses include reducing the severity of disease associated with primary infection, reducing the frequency of reactivation of latent virus, limiting the severity of reactivated disease, and restricting the transmission of virus associated with either primary or reactivated infection. For most human herpesviruses, there is reason to believe that at least some of these goals should be achievable. One effective herpesvirus vaccine, VZV vaccine, is already licensed and in use. For other herpesviruses, there is evidence that natural infection can provide at least partial protection against subsequent infection by different viral strains. Further, there are several effective herpesvirus vaccines in use in domestic animals (e.g., pseudorabies virus, Marek's disease virus, feline herpesvirus, equine herpesvirus, and bovine herpesvirus). Experimental vaccination also can provide protection in herpesvirus animal models. Nevertheless, there are several aspects of vaccine research and development that are complicated by unique properties of herpesviruses and their interactions with their hosts.

Immune Correlates of Protection

Defining the nature of protective immunity for herpesvirus infections is complex because different specificities and types of responses may be needed to prevent primary disease, prevent or limit the establishment of latency, prevent or limit reactivation, control the severity of reactivation disease, and minimize the shedding of infectious virus. In primary infections, the role of antibody is generally limited, with CD8$^+$ T cells and/or CD4$^+$ (T helper 1) acting foremost in clearing virus. Cellular responses also appear to be essential for limiting the replication and/or spread of reactivated virus. Considerably more work is needed to delineate more precisely the protective responses unique to each of the human herpesviruses. New approaches for measuring specific immune responses, such as flow cytometric assessment of intracellular cytokine production and tetramer analysis, are expected to be valuable in this regard.

Mucosal Immunity

Most human herpesviruses infect via mucosal surfaces; reactivated infection may occur at such sites, and free virus is typically shed from such sites. Thus, systemic immunity may not provide adequate protection against initial or recurrent infection, or virus shedding and transmission; antibody at mucosal surfaces and/or cell-mediated response within mucosal tissues may be required. While the nature of mucosal immune responses is not well understood, it is clear that immunization protocols that successfully induce systemic immunity may not induce adequate humoral and cellular responses at mucosae. Therefore, a major area of interest in herpesvirus vaccine research is the development of strategies for inducing such responses.

Latency

A hallmark of herpesvirus infections, latency presents a dilemma for vaccine development: While it is desirable to prevent latency and thus reactivation disease, latent infection may in some cases be beneficial if periodic subclinical reactivation and immunologic stimulation lead to more durable immunity. In any case, preventing the establishment of latency is likely to be difficult. Few or no viral proteins are produced during latent infection, eliminating targets for recognition by the immune system. Rapid establishment of latency thus makes it difficult for a herpesvirus vaccine to provide "sterilizing" immunity, although restriction of initial replication may not only mitigate primary disease, but also reduce the extent of latent infection and thereby the frequency or severity of reactivated replication and disease. If latency is established following vaccination, then a second concern is that the vaccine must induce an immune response of appropriate type and sufficient duration to provide long-term protection against reactivated replication. Durable immunity may depend upon periodic boosting by endogenous (subclinically reactivated) virus, as noted above, or by exogenous (wild-type) infection. If wild-type boosting is important for durability, it is possible that a vaccination program leading to a significant reduction in circulating virus could actually shorten the duration of immunity and increase the frequency of reactivated infection.

Immune Evasion

In addition to avoiding immune recognition through latency, herpesviruses have developed a diverse array of strategies for manipulating and outmaneuvering host immune responses (1). Specific means include interference with antigen processing, transport, and presentation; negative regulation of cytokine activity; inhibition of cytotoxic T lymphocyte (CTL)-induced apoptosis; interference with natural killer cell-mediated clearance; and inhibition of complement-mediated antibody attack. The role of these processes in modulating the level of vaccine-induced immunity (for live vaccines), or in blocking the vaccine-induced immune response to a challenge infection, is not well understood.

Animal Models

Animal models play a critical role in assessing the potential safety, immunogenicity, and efficacy of new human vaccines, but the testing of herpesvirus vaccines in animals is frequently problematic. One major consideration is the host range of the virus. While the alphaherpesviruses (HSV, VZV) have a variable host range and can infect rodents and primates as model hosts, the gammaherpesviruses (EBV, HHV-8) infect only species in the same family or order as the natural host, and the betaherpesviruses (HCMV, HHV-6, and HHV-7) replicate little if at all in species other than their natural hosts. For this last group, alternative models have included humanized severe combined immunodeficient (SCID-hu) mice, and the use of related viruses of rodents or primates (e.g., murine and guinea pig CMVs). While these systems are useful for some studies of pathogenesis and immune response, they cannot be used for preclinical evaluation of vaccine safety and efficacy. A further concern is the relevance to humans of immunogenicity and protection studies done in animals. For example, the immune

responses and efficacy obtained with an experimental vaccine can vary between mouse strains (2), and an HSV subunit vaccine that was very effective in protecting mice was not found to be effective in subsequent human trials.

Vaccination Approaches for Herpesviruses

Most of the approaches for vaccination available today have been applied to one or more of the human herpesviruses. For each of these approaches, there are advantages and potential obstacles that derive from the unique nature of herpesviruses and their infections.

Live-Attenuated Virus

This vaccination approach has enjoyed the greatest success against herpesviruses to date. The live-attenuated Oka strain of VZV used for the prevention of chickenpox is the only human herpesvirus vaccine presently licensed by the Food and Drug Administration (FDA). In addition, the U.S. Department of Agriculture (USDA) licenses effective modified-live vaccines for five different herpesviruses infecting domestic animals. Live vaccines offer a theoretical advantage over other approaches in that the full spectrum of viral proteins is presented in its natural context and abundance. However, by using live vaccines for herpesviruses, latency may be established, and thus there is the potential for reactivation-associated or other chronic disease. These concerns are tempered somewhat by the lack of problems seen in long-term followup of healthy and leukemic children who received the VZV vaccine, as well as renal transplant recipients immunized with the attenuated Towne strain of HCMV. In fact, establishment of latency by an attenuated vaccine virus may in some cases be desirable for ensuring durable immunity. A technical problem with traditional attenuation approaches for herpesviruses has been the difficulty of achieving an acceptable reduction in virulence while maintaining adequate immunogenicity. Thus, efforts are underway to engineer new attenuated vaccines for HSV and HCMV by identifying and manipulating regions of the genome or specific viral genes that control latency, reactivation, and virulence.

Disabled Virus

One approach that may address some of the problems of live herpesvirus vaccines involves engineering replication-defective strains of virus. Mutations have been introduced into essential genes to prevent the formation of progeny virions (3, 4), or into structural protein genes so that only noninfectious progeny virions are produced (5). This strategy requires a good understanding of the genes controlling a virus's replication and virulence and has thus far been applied only to HSV, although it is being considered for VZV. Disabled virus vaccines have been able to protect mice against challenge with virulent HSV and appeared to be safe and immunogenic in a phase I trial (6), suggesting that it may be possible to induce protective immune responses in humans without complete virus replication. An unexpected potential advantage of at least one disabled HSV strain is an apparent inability to establish latency (4).

Vectored Subunits

Delivery of one or more herpesvirus proteins via a viral vector (replicating or not) could address concerns with pathogenicity and latency while delivering adequate quantities of viral antigens and presenting them in a suitable context. The potential of recombinant vaccinia virus has been demonstrated by the successful oral rabies vaccine used for wildlife, and highly attenuated versions of mammalian and avian poxviruses are available for use in humans (7). Several poxvirus constructs expressing proteins from HCMV, EBV, and HSV have demonstrated immunogenicity or efficacy in experimental animals, but the immune responses observed in human trials of HCMV and EBV recombinants have been relatively modest. Poxvirus recombinants also may be useful for augmenting immune responses through a prime-boost regimen (8), as has been described for HCMV.

Inactivated Virus

The classical strategy of using inactivated virus has a history of yielding safe and effective viral vaccines, but it has several potential limitations for herpesviruses. Viral proteins are not presented in a natural context, and only structural proteins are presented, thereby limiting the type and breadth of the immune response obtained. Several vaccines derived from inactivated virions—either complete preparations or partially purified proteins—of HSV and VZV have been evaluated clinically. None of the HSV vaccines have proven effective, and heat-inactivated VZV provides significantly poorer protection against varicella as compared to the live Oka vaccine.

Recombinant Subunits

Subunit vaccines containing purified viral proteins are a relatively safe alternative to live vaccines. Most studies have focused on the external viral glycoproteins; however, early viral antigens also have been shown to induce T cell-mediated immunity. To date, clinical experience with subunit vaccines for herpesviruses has not been encouraging. While those subunits evaluated in phase I and II trials have been safe and immunogenic, a recent phase III trial of an HSV-2 gB+gD subunit vaccine failed to prevent or delay outbreaks in infected individuals (9). Approaches for improving subunit immunogenicity, such as novel adjuvants or incorporation of subunits into structures such as virus-like particles (VLPs) or immunostimulating complexes (ISCOMs), have received some attention, but no clinical evaluation to date.

Peptides

Delivery of specific T-cell epitopes as peptides has the potential to be safe and exquisitely specific in the immune response induced. Its utility is limited, however, by the need to identify the immunogenic epitopes and by the major histocompatibility complex (MHC) specificity of the response. The approach has been tested only to a limited extent *in vitro* and in animals for HSV, HCMV, and EBV; recent results suggest that protection can be achieved with an HSV peptide conjugate (10), and an EBV peptide vaccine has been tested in clinical trials.

Purified DNA

The advantages of DNA vaccines for herpesviruses include no risk of disease or latency, presentation of the viral proteins in their native form and context, ability to induce cytotoxic-T-cell responses, and potential for induction of long-lived immunity (11). Promising results in animal models have been reported for HSV, HCMV, and VZV; and at least one HSV DNA vaccine has moved into phase I trials.

References

1 Ploegh, H. L. (1998). Viral strategies of immune evasion. *Science, 280*, 248-253.

2 Manickan, E., Francotte, M., Kuklin, N., et al. (1995). Vaccination with recombinant vaccinia viruses expressing ICP27 induces protective immunity against herpes simplex virus through CD4+ Th1 + T cells. *Journal of Virology, 69*, 4711-4716.

3 Nguyen, L. H., Knipe, D. M., & Finberg, R. W. (1992). Replication-defective mutants of herpes simplex virus (HSV) induce cellular immunity and protect against lethal HSV infection. *Journal of Virology, 66*, 7067-7072.

4 De Costa, X. J., Jones, C. A., & Knipe, D. M. (1999). Immunization against genital herpes with a vaccine virus that has defects in productive and latent infection. *Proceedings of the National Academy of Sciences of the United States of America, 96*, 6994-6998.

5 Farrell, H. E., McLean, C. S., Harley, C., et al. (1994). Vaccine potential of a herpes simplex virus type I mutant with an essential glycoprotein deleted. *Journal of Virology, 68*, 927-932.

6 Cantab Pharmaceuticals. (1999, September 23). *Cantab reports positive phase I clinical trial results for DISC HSV genital herpes vaccine* [Press Release]. Cambridge, United Kingdom.

7 Paoletti, E. (1996). Applications of pox virus vectors to vaccination: An update. *Proceedings of the National Academy of Sciences of the United States of America, 93*, 11349-11353.

8 Tartaglia, J., Excler, J. L., El Habib, R., et al. (1998). Canarypox virus-based vaccines: Prime-boost strategies to induce cell-mediated and humoral immunity against HIV. *AIDS Research and Human Retroviruses, 14*(Suppl. 3), S291-S298.

9 Corey, L., Langenberg, A. G. M., Ashley, R., et al. (1999). The Chiron HSV Vaccine Study Group. Recombinant glycoprotein vaccine for the prevention of genital HSV-2 infection: Two randomized controlled trials. *Journal of the American Medical Association, 282*, 331-340.

10 Rosenthal, K. S., Mao, H., Home, W. I., et al. (1999). Immunization with a LEAPS heteroconjugate containing a CTL epitope and a peptide from beta-2-microglobulin elicits a protective and

DTH response to herpes simplex virus type I. *Vaccine, 17,* 535-542.

11 Robinson, H. L., Ginsberg, H. S., Davis, H. L., et al. (1997). *The scientific future of DNA for immunization.* Washington, DC: American Academy of Microbiology.

CYTOMEGALOVIRUS

Background

Approximately 50 percent of the U.S. population is seropositive for CMV. Seropositivity varies with socioeconomic status and geographic location: 40 to 60 percent in middle-income groups, and up to 80 percent in lower socioeconomic groups. The outcome of CMV infection is highly dependent on the immune status of the host. Primary infection in healthy individuals is likely to be asymptomatic, or may cause a mild mononucleosis-like syndrome. However, in patients with deficient or immature immune systems, CMV infection can be a serious, even life-threatening problem.

Congenital Cytomegalovirus

Congenital CMV is the most common intrauterine infection in the United States, occurring in 0.4 to 2.3 percent of all infants born alive. It is estimated that 37,000 to 40,000 infants in the United States are born with congenital CMV each year. About 3,000 to 4,000 infected newborns per year have symptomatic CMV disease; of those who survive, most suffer from profound progressive deafness and/or mental retardation. An additional 4,500 to 6,000 children who are asymptomatic at birth also develop serious handicaps. The highest risk for congenital CMV infection is among infants born to mothers who have had primary infection during pregnancy. In the United States, congenital CMV may be the cause of 20 to 40 percent of congenital deafness, and is as frequent a cause of mental retardation as the fragile X chromosome. The cost of custodial care for severely affected children in the United States is estimated at $1.86 billion annually.

Organ Transplants

CMV is the single most important infectious agent affecting recipients of organ transplants, with at least two-thirds of these patients developing CMV infection or reactivation 1 to 4 months after transplantation. Also, about 15 percent of bone marrow transplant recipients develop CMV pneumonia; without treatment, such infections are fatal about 80 percent of the time. Although less severe, active CMV infection occurs in 20 to 60 percent of all liver transplant recipients. CMV also causes five distinct neurological syndromes in patients with AIDS.

Current Status and Key Issues in Research and Development

Although the correlates of CMV immunity are not precisely known, clinical observations suggest that preexisting humoral

and/or cellular immunity may reduce the severity of disease. Maternal antibody in seropositive women appears to reduce significantly the incidence and severity of congenital infection, and passive immunoglobulin therapy may benefit some transplant recipients. In addition, infusion of *ex vivo* expanded CMV-specific CTLs appears to reconstitute immunity and provide protection against disease in bone marrow transplant recipients. The major CMV immunogenic protein appears to be the surface glycoprotein gB. This protein induces the development of virus-neutralizing antibodies and T cell-mediated immunity, and the T helper cell response to gB is human leukocyte antigen (HLA) class II restricted. The viral tegument protein (pp65, from the UL83 gene) has been shown to be a major target for CD8[+] CTLs during natural infections. Other viral antigens, including the surface glycoprotein gH and additional early antigens, also are being considered for use in vaccines. Despite the presence of gB-neutralizing antibodies, virus can be reactivated and infections caused by other strains of CMV can occur; indeed, multiple strains of CMV have been identified. An additional concern in vaccine design is that CMV employs several strategies that prevent the host immune system from recognizing infected cells, and that could potentially interfere with the ability of a live-attenuated vaccine to stimulate a protective cellular immune response.

Several CMV vaccination strategies have been evaluated in humans. A live-attenuated strain (Towne) stimulates humoral and cellular immunity, although less than natural infection. The efficacy of Towne has been evaluated in several clinical studies: Protection has been documented in seronegative women and transplant recipients, but is less than that afforded by a natural infection, and complete protection has been achieved against only low doses of challenge virus. Further efforts are needed to improve the immunogenicity of live-attenuated vaccines (see below for the approach taken by MedImmune, Inc.). Subunit vaccines have been shown to induce humoral and cellular immune responses, but to date have not been able to prevent infection or disease. Evaluations of alternative vaccine formulations and antigens are underway. A subunit vaccine developed by Chiron Corporation (Emeryville, CA) and now produced by Aventis-Pasteur, consisting of recombinant gB [produced in Chinese hamster ovary (CHO) cells] and the adjuvant MF59, has been evaluated in phase I and II trials. The vaccine is well tolerated and highly immunogenic in seronegative adults and toddlers, and stimulates high levels of neutralizing antibody that cross-neutralize clinical isolates. Additional approaches are being evaluated in animal models. Delivery of gB via a canarypox vector has been tested in guinea pigs and is capable of inducing humoral and cell-mediated responses. DNA immunization holds the promise of improving the presentation of individual viral proteins to the host immune system. Immunization with DNA plasmids encoding gB and the matrix protein pp65 has been evaluated in mice and induces neutralizing antibody and CTL responses.

Recent Accomplishments and Developments

Engineering an Improved Live-Attenuated Cytomegalovirus Vaccine

As noted above, the attenuated vaccine strain of CMV (Towne), while immunogenic, did not stimulate as high a level of immunity as that produced in a natural infection. Investigators at MedImmune, Inc., are attempting to make Towne more immunogenic by replacing selected parts of its genome with sequences from nonattenuated strains of CMV. They have identified numerous differences between the genome of the Towne strain and that of wild-type CMV, including a large DNA segment present in the genomes of a virulent laboratory strain (Toledo) and of five clinical isolates, but not in the Towne genome. The extensive variation in genome sequence observed between these strains may explain the differences that they exhibit in virulence and tissue tropism. The investigators used this information in conjunction with a unique method they developed to engineer changes in the CMV genome to construct hybrid viruses that replace defined portions of the Towne genome with corresponding segments of a nonattenuated strain of CMV. Initial vaccine candidates have been created, and MedImmune, Inc., will soon complete a phase I clinical trial using four chimeric vaccine candidates.

Cytomegalovirus Employs Multiple Mechanisms to Evade Cell-Mediated Immune Responses

For a viral vaccine to stimulate a cell-mediated immune response, viral proteins must be broken down into peptides, which are then transported into the endoplasmic reticulum and displayed on the surface of the infected cell in conjunction with MHC molecules. Multiple strategies employed by CMV to subvert this process could interfere with the ability of a live-attenuated vaccine to induce a protective, cell-mediated immune response. Recent work has dissected out the mechanisms by which at least three CMV proteins act to interfere with the processing and MHC class I-associated presentation of viral peptides. One approach used by CMV is to downregulate expression of class I MHC molecules by facilitating the degradation of newly synthesized class I heavy chains. Hidde Ploegh and coworkers have shown that CMV expresses at least two genes—US11 and US2—that encode a product that causes the dislocation of newly synthesized class I heavy chains from the lumen of the endoplasmic reticulum to the cytosol. The US11 and US2 gene products have different specificities for class I molecules, suggesting that CMV has responded to the polymorphism of the MHC by evolving a diversity of functions that interfere with class I-restricted antigen presentation. A second point in the MHC/peptide presentation process is targeted by the product of the US6 gene. This glycoprotein has been shown to bind the transporter associated with antigen processing (TAP)-dependent translocation of peptide from the cytosol to the endoplasmic reticulum. The importance of these proteins in modulating the cell-mediated immune response to a live CMV vaccine remains to be determined.

Maintenance and Reactivation of Latent Cytomegalovirus

Following initial infection, CMV remains latent in the host and, under conditions of immune suppression such as organ or bone marrow transplantation, can reactivate and produce significant disease. Knowledge of the mechanisms of maintenance and reactivation of latent infection is important to developing vaccines that protect against reactivation disease and that do not contribute to such disease themselves. Studies have shed new light on several important aspects of CMV latency. Edward Mocarski and colleagues have characterized latent CMV transcripts in human granulocyte-macrophage progenitors. Sense and antisense transcripts with the potential to encode small proteins are expressed in culture and in bone marrow aspirates from seropositive individuals. Antibodies reactive with two of these potential gene products are also detected in seropositive individuals. Overall, these results suggest that bone marrow-derived myeloid progenitors are an important natural site of viral latency. These cells are also the source of circulating monocyte-derived macrophages (MDMs). Jay Nelson and colleagues have shown that allogeneic stimulation (similar to what would occur during a transplant) is required for productive CMV infection in these cells. They also have used allogeneic stimulation to show for the first time that latent virus can be reactivated from MDMs isolated from seropositive individuals. Monocytes are therefore also a natural site of CMV latency from which the virus can be reactivated under conditions of allogeneic stimulation.

Next Steps and Challenges Ahead

Further work is needed to define more precisely the key antigens and epitopes important for protection against infection, primary disease, and reactivation. The role of immune evasion in the induction of and response to host immunity needs to be clarified. Clinical testing of DNA vaccines is also on the horizon.

Sources

Adler, S. P., Starr, S. E., Plotkin, S. A., Hempfling, S. H., Buis, J., Manning, M. L., & Best, A. M. (1995). Immunity induced by primary human cytomegalovirus infection protects against secondary infection among women of childbearing age. *Journal of Infectious Diseases, 171,* 26-32.

Bale, J. F., Jr., Petheram, S. J., Souza, I. E., & Murph, J. R. (1996). Cytomegalovirus reinfection in young children. *Journal of Pediatrics, 128*(3), 347-352.

Boppana, S. B., & Britt, W. J. (1995). Antiviral antibody responses and intrauterine transmission after primary maternal cytomegalovirus infection. *Journal of Infectious Diseases, 171,* 1115-1121.

Boppana, S. B., Miller, J., & Britt, W. J. (1996). Transplacentally acquired antiviral antibodies and outcome in congenital human cytomegalovirus infection. *Viral Immunology, 9*(4), 211-218.

Borysiewicz, L. K., Hickling, J. K., Graham, S., Sinclair, J., Cranage, M. P., Smith, G. L., & Sissons, J. G. (1988). Human cytomegalovirus-specific cytotoxic T cells. Relative frequency of stage-specific CTL recognizing the 72-kD immediate early protein and glycoprotein B expressed by recombinant vaccinia viruses. *Journal of Experimental Medicine, 168*(3), 919-931.

Britt, W. J., Vugler, L., Butfiloski, E. J., & Stephens, E. B. (1990). Cell surface expression of human cytomegalovirus (HCMV) gp55-116 (gB): Use of HCMV-recombinant vaccinia virus-infected cells in analysis of the human neutralizing antibody response. *Journal of Virology, 64*(3), 1079-1085.

Cha, T. A., Tom, E., Kemble, G. W., Duke, G. M., Mocarski, E. S., & Spaete, R. R. (1996). Human cytomegalovirus clinical isolates carry at least 19 genes not found in laboratory strains. *Journal of Virology, 70*, 78-83.

Chou, S. W., & Dennison, K. M. (1991). Analysis of interstrain variation in cytomegalovirus glycoprotein B sequences encoding neutralization-related epitopes. *Journal of Infectious Diseases, 163*(6), 1229-1234.

Conti, D., Freed, B., Gruber, S., & Lempert, N. (1994). Prophylaxis of primary cytomegalovirus disease in renal transplant recipients. A trial of ganciclovir vs. immunoglobulin. *Archives of Surgery, 129*, 443-447.

Demmler, G. J. (1991). Infectious Diseases Society of America and Centers for Disease Control and Prevention. Summary of a workshop on surveillance for congenital cytomegalovirus disease. *Reviews of Infectious Diseases, 13*(2), 315-329.

Dobbins, J. G., Stewart, J. A., & Demmler, G. J. (1992). Surveillance of congenital cytomegalovirus disease, 1990-1991. Collaborating Registry Group. *Morbidity and Mortality Weekly Report. CDC Surveillance Summaries, 41*, 35-39.

Dummer, J. S. (1990). Cytomegalovirus infection after liver transplantation: Clinical manifestations and strategies for prevention. *Reviews of Infectious Diseases, 12*(Suppl. 7), S767-S775.

Fowler, K. B., & Pass, R. F. (1991). Sexually transmitted diseases in mothers of neonates with congenital cytomegalovirus infection. *Journal of Infectious Diseases, 164*(2), 259-264.

Fowler, K. B., Stagno, S., Pass, R. F., Britt, W. J., Boll, T. J., & Alford, C. A. (1992). The outcome of congenital cytomegalovirus infection in relation to maternal antibody status. *New England Journal of Medicine, 326*(10), 663-667.

Frey, S., Harrison, C., Pass, R., Boken, D., Sekulovich, R., Percell, S., Hirabayashi, S., & Duliege, A. M. (1997, March 5-9). *Biocine CMV gB/MF59 vaccine induces antibody responses when given at two dosages and three immunization schedules* [Abstract 156]. Sixth International Cytomegalovirus Workshop, Perdido Beach, AL.

Gershon, A. A., Gold, E., & Nankervis, G. A. (1997). Cytomegalovirus. In A. S. Evans & R. A. Kaslow (Eds.), *Viral infections of humans: Epidemiology and control* (pp. 229-251). New York: Plenum Press.

Gilbert, M. J., Riddell, S. R., Plachter, B., & Greenberg, P. D. (1996). Cytomegalovirus selectively blocks antigen processing and presentation of its immediate-early gene product. *Nature, 383*, 720-722.

Gonczol, E., Berensci, K., Pincus, S., Endresz, V., Meric, C., Paoletti, E., & Plotkin, S. A. (1995). Preclinical evaluation of an ALVAC (canarypox)-human cytomegalovirus glycoprotein B vaccine candidate. *Vaccine, 13*(12), 1080-1085.

Gonczol, E., Endresz, V., Kari, L., Berencsi, K., Kari, C., Jeney, C., Pincus, S., Rodeck, U., Meric, C., & Plotkin, S. A. (1997, March 5-9). *DNA immunization induces human cytomegalovirus (HCMV)-glycoprotein B (gB)-specific neutralizing antibody as well as phosphoprotein 65 (pp-65)-specific cytotoxic T lymphocyte responses and primes immune responses to HCMV proteins* [Abstract 47]. Sixth International Cytomegalovirus Workshop, Perdido Beach, AL.

Griffiths, P. K., & Baboonian, C. (1984). A prospective study of primary cytomegalovirus infection during pregnancy: Final report. *British Journal of Obstetrics and Gynaecology, 91*(4), 307-315.

Kemble, G., Duke, G., Winter, R., Evans, P., & Spaete, R. (1997, March 5-9). *Derivation of novel, recombinant, live, attenuated CMV vaccine strains* [Abstract 49]. Sixth International Cytomegalovirus Workshop, Perdido Beach, AL.

Kemble, G., Duke, G., Winter, R., & Spaete, R. (1996). Defined large-scale alterations of the human cytomegalovirus genome constructed by cotransfection of overlapping cosmids. *Journal of Virology, 70*(3), 2044-2048.

Kondo, K., Xu, J., & Mocarski, E. S. (1996). Human cytomegalovirus latent gene expression in granulocyte-macrophage progenitors in culture and in seropositive individuals. *Proceedings of the National Academy of Sciences of the United States of America, 93*(20), 11137-11142.

Laughon, B. E., Allaudeen, H. S., Becker, J. M., Current, W. L., Feinberg, J., Frenkel, J. K., Hafner, R., Hughes, W. T., Laughlin, C. A., Meyers, J. D., et al. (1991). From the National Institutes of Health. Summary of the workshop on future directions in discovery and development of therapeutic agents for opportunistic infections associated with AIDS. *Journal of Infectious Diseases, 164*(2), 244-251.

Lehner, P. J., Karttunen, J. T., Wilkinson, G. W., & Cresswell, P. (1997). The human cytomegalovirus US6 glycoprotein inhibits transporter associated with antigen processing-dependent peptide translocation. *Proceedings of the National Academy of Sciences of the United States of America, 94*, 6904-6909.

Li, L., Coelingh, K. L., & Britt, W. J. (1995). Human cytomegalovirus neutralizing antibody-resistant phenotype is associated with reduced expression of glycoprotein H. *Journal of Virology, 69*(10), 6047-6053.

Liu, H., Chou, S., Sekulovich, R., Duliege, A. M., & Burke, R. L. (1997, March 5-9). *A CMV glycoprotein gB subunit vaccine elicits cross neutralizing antibodies that cross neutralize clinical isolates* [Abstract 43]. Sixth International Cytomegalovirus Workshop, Perdido Beach, AL.

Liu, Y. N., Curtsinger, J., Donahue, P. R., Klaus, A., Optiz, G., Cooper, J., Karr, R. W., Bach, F. H., & Gehrz, R. C. (1993). Molecular analysis of the immune response to human cytomegalovirus glycoprotein B. I. Mapping of HLA-restricted helper T cell epitopes on gp93. *Journal of General Virology, 74*(Pt.10), 2207-2214.

Machold, R. P., Wiertz, E. J., Jones, T. R., & Ploegh, H. L. (1997). The HCMV gene products US11 and US2 differ in their ability to attack allelic forms of murine major histocompatibility complex (MHC) class I heavy chains. *Journal of Experimental Medicine, 185*, 363-366.

McLaughlin-Taylor, E., Pande, H., Forman, S. J., Tanamachi, B., Li, C. R., Zaia, J. A., Greenberg, P. D., & Riddell, S. R. (1994). Identification of the major late human cytomegalovirus matrix protein pp65 as a target antigen for CD8+ virus-specific cytotoxic T lymphocytes. *Journal of Medical Virology, 43*(1), 103-110.

Mitchell, D. K., Holmes, S. J., Burke, R. L., Sekulovich, R., Tripathi, M., Doyle, M., & Duliege, A. M. (1997, March 5-9). *Immunogenicity of a recombinant human cytomegalovirus (CMV) gB vaccine in toddlers* [Abstract 50]. Sixth International Cytomegalovirus Workshop, Perdido Beach, AL.

Nankervis, G. A., Kumar, M. L., Cox, F. E., & Gold, E. (1984). A prospective study of maternal cytomegalovirus infection and its effect on the fetus. *American Journal of Obstetrics and Gynecology, 149*, 435-440.

Pande, H., Campo, K., Tanamachi, B., Forman, S. J., & Zaia, J. A. (1995). Direct DNA immunization of mice with plasmid DNA encoding the tegument protein pp65 (ppUL83) of human cytomegalovirus induces high levels of circulating antibody to the encoded protein. *Scandinavian Journal of Infectious Diseases. Supplementum, 99*, 117-120.

Plotkin, S. A., Starr, S. E., Friedman, H. M., Gonczol, E., & Weibel, W. E. (1989). Protective effects of Towne cytomegalovirus vaccine against low-passage cytomegalovirus administered as a challenge. *Journal of Infectious Diseases, 159*, 860-865.

Porath, A., McNutt, R. A., Smiley, L. M., & Weigle, K. A. (1990). Effectiveness and cost benefit of a proposed live cytomegalovirus vaccine in the prevention of congenital disease. *Reviews of Infectious Diseases, 12*, 31-40.

Rasmussen, L., Matkin, C., Spaete, R., Pachl, C., & Merigan, T. C. (1991). Antibody response to human cytomegalovirus glycoproteins gB and gH after natural infection in humans. *Journal of Infectious Diseases, 164*(5), 835-842.

Sedmak, D. D., Guglielmo, A. M., Knight, D. A., Birmingham, D. J., Huang, E. H., & Waldman W. J. (1994). Cytomegalovirus inhibits major histocompatibility class II expression on infected endothelial cells. *American Journal of Pathology, 144*(4), 683-692.

Snydman, D. R., Werner, B. G., Heinze-Lacey, B., Berardi, V. P., Tilney, N. L., Kirkman, R. L., Milford, E. L., Cho, S. I., Bush, H. L., Jr., Levey, A. S., et al. (1987). Use of cytomegalovirus immune globulin to prevent cytomegalovirus disease in renal-transplant recipients. *New England Journal of Medicine, 317*(17), 1049-1054.

Soderberg Naucler, C., Fish, K., & Nelson, J. A. (1997, March 5-9). *Reactivation of infectious human cytomegalovirus from allogeneically stimulated T cells induced monocyte derived macrophages from asymptomatic seropositive individuals* [Abstract 41]. Sixth International Cytomegalovirus Workshop, Perdido Beach, AL.

Stagno, S., Pass, R. F., Cloud, G., Britt, W. J., Henderson, R. E., Walton, P. D., Veren, D. A., Page, F., & Alford, C. A. (1986). Primary cytomegalovirus infection in pregnancy. Incidence, transmission to fetus, and clinical outcome. *Journal of the American Medical Association, 256*(14), 1904-1908.

Urban, M., Klein, M., Britt, W. J., Hassfurther, E., & Mach, M. (1996). Glycoprotein H of human cytomegalovirus is a major antigen for the neutralizing humoral immune response. *Journal of General Virology, 77*(Pt. 7), 1537-1547.

van den Berg, A. P., Klompmaker, I. J., Haagsma, E. B., Scholten-Sampson, A., Bijleveld, C. M., Schirm, J., van der Giessen, M., Slooff, M. J., & The, T. H. (1991). Antigenemia in the diagnosis and monitoring of active cytomegalovirus infection after liver transplantation. *Journal of Infectious Diseases, 164*(2), 265-270.

van Zanten, J., Harmsen, M. C., van der Meer, P., van der Bij, W., van Son, W. J., van der Giessen, M., Prop, J., de Leij, J., & The, T. H. (1995). Proliferative T cell responses to four human cytomegalovirus-specific proteins in healthy subjects and solid organ transplant recipients. *Journal of Infectious Diseases, 172*(3), 879-882.

Walter, E. A., Greenberg, P. D., Gilbert, M. J., Finch, R. J., Watanabe, K. S., Thomas, E. D., & Riddell, S. R. (1995). Reconstitution of cellular immunity against cytomegalovirus in recipients of allogeneic bone marrow by transfer of T-cell clones from the donor. *New England Journal of Medicine, 333*(16), 1038-1044.

Wiertz, E. J., Jones, T. R., Sun, L., Bogyo, M., Geuze, J. H., & Ploegh, H. L. (1996). The human cytomegalovirus US11 gene product dislocates MHC class I heavy chains from the endoplasmic reticulum to the cytosol. *Cell, 84,* 769-779.

VARICELLA-ZOSTER VIRUS

Background

Primary infection with VZV is manifested as chickenpox (varicella) and results in a lifelong latent infection. Reactivation of the latent virus leads to shingles (zoster).

Varicella

Prior to the introduction of the live-attenuated vaccine, approximately 4 million cases of varicella occurred annually, primarily in young children, with more than 90 percent of the U.S. population becoming seropositive (1). Chickenpox was estimated to cost about $400 million each year, much of this representing the cost to parents of lost income from work (2). As the use of the vaccine expands, it will lead to changes in the epidemiology and costs of this childhood illness in the United States.

Varicella can be complicated by a variety of serious conditions, including skin infections that can progress to systemic infections, infections of the brain, and pneumonia (3). Complications of varicella have been responsible for approximately 9,300 hospitalizations and 100 deaths annually. The risk of these complications is highest in adults: While less than 5 percent of varicella cases occur in adults more than 20 years of age, 55 percent of the deaths occur in this age group (4).

Zoster

Zoster typically involves large areas of skin that ulcerate and require several weeks to heal. The skin eruption itself is very painful, and it is often followed by postherpetic neuralgia (PHN), a pain syndrome that may persist for many months or years and that can be very disabling. There is no established prophylaxis or therapy for PHN. The incidence and severity of zoster and its complications increase with age. The incidence among 50-year-olds appears to be between 2 and 4 cases per 1,000 persons per year, and it more than doubles by the age of 80 years. More than one-half of all cases occur in persons 60 years of age and older (5). PHN is the major complication of zoster in the immunocompetent host: Rare in individuals less than 40 years of age, PHN is estimated to occur in 25 to more than 50 percent of patients with zoster who are more than 59 years of age (6).

Current Status and Key Issues in Research and Development

Humoral and cellular immune responses are elicited early in primary VZV infections, and their relative contribution to protection from disease is not well understood. The impact of active humoral immunity appears to be limited, but preexisting antibody has been shown to provide some level of protection. Passively acquired maternal antibody affords some protection to infants, and postexposure administration of VZV immunoglobulin (VZIG) to immunocompromised children reduces disease severity (7). In children receiving the live-attenuated Oka vaccine, the incidence and severity of breakthrough infection are inversely correlated with antibody titer to VZV glycoproteins (8), and possibly with the level of T-cell responses as well (9). Conversely, it is clear that cellular responses play the primary role in preventing disease associated with reactivation of latent VZV. While decreases in humoral immunity are not associated with increased risk of zoster (10), the age-related decline in cell-mediated responses to VZV antigens is proportional to the age-related increase in the incidence and severity of zoster (11, 12, 13), suggesting that this loss is a causative factor.

The role of viral immune evasion mechanisms in VZV infection is not well defined. For example, VZV is similar to HSV in that its glycoprotein gE forms a complex with gI and can act as an Fc receptor, but it is not known whether the similarity to HSV extends to providing protection from virus-specific antibody (14). Efforts are currently underway to identify VZV genes that may be associated with evasion of MHC class I- and class II-mediated immune responses (15).

A live-attenuated varicella vaccine, Oka, was developed in Japan in the early 1970s (16). In the United States, this vaccine is produced by Merck & Co., Inc., (VarivaxÒ). It was licensed for use in healthy individuals by the FDA in 1995; and is now recommended for universal use in early childhood by the Centers for Disease Control and Prevention's (CDC's) Advisory Committee for Immunization Practices (17), the American Academy of Pediatrics (18), and the American Academy of Family Physicians. The use of VarivaxÒ in the United States has been increasing steadily. According to Merck & Co., Inc., more than 16 million doses of VarivaxÒ have been distributed, and the immunization rate for 1- to 2-year-olds is approaching 70 percent. All States have ordered the vaccine for use in their immunization programs, and 14 have passed school and/or daycare requirements for varicella vaccination. Postlicensure surveillance in daycare centers indicates that the vaccine is generally well tolerated, leads to a lower attack rate, and protects from severe disease (19, 20). Long-term monitoring of vaccines to date indicates that immunity persists, and to some extent is stronger, at 5 years postvaccination (21). Further studies will establish whether immunization will provide protection as durable as that from natural infection, or whether boosting will be required to maintain protection through adulthood. The expanding use of this vaccine will undoubtedly alter the epidemiology and costs of varicella in the United States, and it affords the opportunity to study in greater detail the correlates of protection against infection and disease, and the viral functions associated with virulence and attenuation.

It also remains to be demonstrated whether the VZV vaccine will be effective in other populations, such as in the elderly for prevention of zoster, or in immunosuppressed transplant patients. Initial studies of vaccination in the elderly have shown that VZV-specific, cell-mediated immunity can be boosted significantly (22, 23).

In addition to further studies on the live-attenuated virus, there are continuing efforts to evaluate alternate vaccines. Inactivated virus showed some efficacy in protecting bone marrow transplant recipients from shingles (24), although this strategy also has been associated with a poorer MHC class I-restricted cytotoxic response (22) and reduced protection from varicella (25) when compared to the live-attenuated vaccine. Other strategies being pursued include disabled virus and plasmid DNA.

Recent Accomplishments and Developments

The availability of a live-attenuated VZV vaccine that is safe, effective, and FDA licensed for the prevention of varicella presents an opportunity to determine whether the same vaccination strategy might be effective for preventing zoster in the elderly. In 1994, the Veterans Administration Cooperative Studies Program (VA-CSP) approved a protocol for a multicenter, double-blind, placebo-controlled phase III study to determine whether VarivaxÒ can decrease the incidence and/or severity of zoster and its complications in adults age 60 and older. The primary outcome measure for the study is total burden of zoster-associated pain during a first occurrence of herpes zoster. In 1998, the study was initiated as a collaborative effort among VA-CSP; Merck & Co., Inc.; and the National Institute of Allergy and Infectious Diseases (NIAID). A total of 21 sites are participating, with a recruitment goal of 37,200. With a 3-year followup period, the study is expected to last approximately 5 years.

Next Steps and Challenges Ahead

The development of a VZV vaccine incapable of becoming reactivated, or of a subunit vaccine, will require much more basic research. Studies of the antigenic components most important for developing an immune response in humans, and of novel methods for presenting viral antigens to cells of the immune system, are in progress. The results of the phase III study described above will determine whether live-attenuated VZV can help prevent shingles in the elderly. Other populations at risk for severe VZV disease—e.g., pediatric renal transplant recipients—

are also candidates for studies evaluating the safety and efficacy of the live-attenuated vaccine.

Cantab Pharmaceuticals, Plc., (Cambridge, United Kingdom) is collaborating with Kaketsuken (Japan) to explore the development of a disabled VZV vaccine for chickenpox and shingles. Vical, Inc., (San Diego, CA) has a collaboration with Pasteur Merieux Connaught (Swiftwater, PA) to explore a plasmid DNA vaccine.

References

1 Weller, T. H. (1997). Varicella-herpes zoster virus. In A. S. Evans & R. A. Kaslow (Eds.), *Viral infections of humans: Epidemiology and control* (pp. 865-892). New York: Plenum Press.

2 Lieu, T. A., Cochi, S. L., Black, S. B., et al. (1994). Cost-effectiveness of a routine varicella vaccination program for U.S. children. *Journal of the American Medical Association, 271,* 375-381.

3 Arvin, A. M. (1996). Varicella-zoster virus. In B. N. Fields, D. M. Knipe, & P. M. Howley (Eds.), *Fields virology* (3rd ed., pp. 2547-2585). Philadelphia: Lippincott-Raven.

4 Centers for Disease Control and Prevention. (1997, May 16). Varicella-related deaths among adults—United States, 1997. *Morbidity and Mortality Weekly Report, 46,* 409-412.

5 Hope-Simpson, R. E. (1965). The nature of herpes zoster: A long-term study and a new hypothesis. *Proceeding of the Royal Society of Medicine, 58,* 9-20.

6 Ragozzino, M. W., Melton, L. J., III, Kurland, L. T., et al. (1982). Population-based study of herpes zoster and its sequelae. *Medicine (Baltimore), 61,* 310-316.

7 Brunell, P. A., Ross, A., Miller, L. H., et al. (1969). Prevention of varicella by zoster immune globulin. *New England Journal of Medicine, 280,* 1191-1194.

8 White, C. J., Kuter, B. J., Ngai, A., et al. (1992). Modified cases of chickenpox after varicella vaccination: Correlation of protection with antibody response. *Pediatric Infectious Disease Journal, 11,* 19-23.

9 Bergen, R. E., Diaz, P. S., & Arvin, A. M. (1990). The immunogenicity of the Oka/Merck varicella vaccine in relation to infectious varicella-zoster virus and relative viral antigen content. *Journal of Infectious Diseases, 162,* 1049-1054.

10 Webster, A., Grint, P., Brenner, M. K., et al. (1989). Titration of IgG antibodies against varicella zoster virus before bone marrow transplantation is not predictive of future zoster. *Journal of Medical Virology, 27,* 117-119.

11 Arvin, A. M., Pollard, R. B., Rasmussen, L. E., et al. (1980). Cellular and humoral immunity in the pathogenesis of recurrent herpes viral infections in patients with lymphoma. *Journal of Clinical Investigation, 65,* 869-878.

12 Meyers, J. D., Flournoy, N., & Thomas, E. D. (1980). Cell-mediated immunity to varicella-zoster virus after allogeneic marrow transplant. *Journal of Infectious Diseases, 141,* 479-487.

13 Ruckdeschel, J. C., Schimpif, S. C., Smyth, A. C., et al. (1977). Herpes zoster and impaired cell-associated immunity to the varicella-zoster virus in patients with Hodgkin's disease. *American Journal of Medicine, 62,* 77-85.

14 Nagashunmugam, T., Lubinski, J., Wang, L., et al. (1998). *In vivo* immune evasion mediated by the herpes simplex virus type 1 immunoglobulin G Fc receptor. *Journal of Virology, 72,* 5351-5359.

15 Abendroth, A., & Arvin, A. (1999). Varicella-zoster virus immune evasion. *Immunological Reviews, 168,* 143-156.

16 Takahashi, M., Otsuka, I., Okuno, Y., et al. (1974). Live vaccine used to prevent the spread of varicella in children in hospital. *Lancet, 2,* 1288-1290.

17 Centers for Disease Control and Prevention. (1996). Prevention of varicella: Recommendations of the Advisory Committee on Immunization Practices (ACIP). *Morbidity and Mortality Weekly Report, 45*(RR-11), 1-36.

18 American Academy of Pediatrics. (1995). Recommendations for the use of live attenuated varicella vaccine. *Pediatrics, 95,* 791-796.

19 Izurieta, H. S., Strebel, P. M., & Blake, P. A. (1997). Postlicensure effectiveness of varicella vaccine during an outbreak in a child care center. *Journal of the American Medical Association, 278,* 1495-1499.

20 Buchholz, U., Moolenaar, R., Peterson, C., et al. (1999). Varicella outbreaks after vaccine licensure: Should they make you chicken? *Pediatrics, 104,* 561-563.

21 Zerboni, L., Nader, S., Aoki, K., et al. (1998). Analysis of the persistence of humoral and cellular immunity in children and adults immunized with varicella vaccine. *Journal of Infectious Diseases, 177,* 1701-1704.

22 Hayward, A. R., Buda, K., Jones, M., et al. (1996). Varicella zoster virus-specific cytotoxicity following secondary immunization with live or killed vaccine. *Viral Immunology, 9,* 241-245.

23 Berger, R., Trannoy, E., Hollander, G., et al. (1998). A dose-response study of a live attenuated varicella-zoster virus (Oka strain) vaccine administered to adults 55 years of age and older. *Journal of Infectious Diseases, 178*(Suppl. 1), S99-103.

24 Redman, R. L., Nader, S., Zerboni, L., et al. (1997). Early reconstitution of immunity and decreased severity of herpes zoster in bone marrow transplant recipients immunized with inactivated varicella vaccine. *Journal of Infectious Diseases, 176,* 578-585.

25 Vans, I., & Vesikari, T. (1996). Efficacy of high-titer live attenuated varicella vaccine in healthy young children. *Journal of Infectious Diseases, 174*(Suppl. 3), S330-S334.

Irwin, M., Costlow, C., Williams, H., et al. (1998). Cellular immunity to varicella-zoster virus in patients with major depression. *Journal of Infectious Diseases, 178*(Suppl. 1), S104-S108.

Lungu, O., Panagiotidis, C. A., Annunziato, P. W., et al. (1998). Aberrant intracellular localization of varicella-zoster virus regulatory proteins during latency. *Proceedings of the National Academy of Sciences of the Untied States of America, 95,* 7080-7085.

Mahalingam, R., Wellish, M., Cohrs, R., et al. (1996). Expression of protein encoded by varicella-zoster virus open reading frame 63 in latently infected human ganglionic neurons. *Proceedings of the National Academy of Sciences of the United States of America, 93,* 2122-2124.

Riddell, S. R., Watanabe, K. S., Goodrich, J. M., et al. (1992). Restoration of viral immunity in immunodeficient humans by the adoptive transfer of T cell clones. *Science, 257,* 238-241.

Sadzot-Delvaux, C., Arvin, A. M., & Rentier, B. (1998). Varicella-zoster virus 1E63, a virion component expressed during latency and acute infection, elicits humoral and cellular immunity. *Journal of Infectious Diseases, 178*(Suppl. 1), S43-S47.

EPSTEIN-BARR VIRUS

Background

Based on serology, approximately 90 percent of the adult U.S. population has been infected with EBV. Primary childhood infection is often asymptomatic (1). In most developed countries, 35 to 75 percent of the young adult population remains seronegative. In 25 to 70 percent of such seronegative young adults, EBV infection results in infectious mononucleosis (2). In limited geographical areas and populations, EBV is associated with nasopharyngeal carcinoma (NPC) and with Burkitt's lymphoma (BL) (3). NPC and BL appear to require environmental, genetic, or chemical cofactors. In immunocompromised individuals, including AIDS patients, EBV is associated with lymphoproliferative diseases and lymphomas. Recent evidence also suggests a possible association with Hodgkin's lymphoma, T-cell lymphomas, and some gastric carcinomas.

Current Status and Key Issues in Research and Development

The principal target of EBV-neutralizing antibodies is the major virus surface glycoprotein gp350/220. A range of cell-mediated responses to EBV infection also has been described and is likely to be important in controlling persistent infection. CTLs specific for the latent EBV nuclear antigens EBNA-3A, -3B, and -3C are predominant in a large portion of seropositive adults and children (4, 5).

Several vaccine candidates based on gp350/220 have been developed. For subunit vaccination, this large, heavily glycosylated protein has been prepared from mammalian cell lines (CHO or mouse C127). Primate studies demonstrate that subunit vaccination can elicit a specific antibody response that is at least partially protective, and suggest that the choice of adjuvant is likely to be important in achieving acceptable efficacy (6). A phase I clinical study demonstrated that the subunit vaccine is well tolerated in seropositive and seronegative persons and that an immune response is induced (7). Live recombinant vectors also have been used to express and deliver gp350/220. Immunization with vaccinia recombinants provides some protection in primates (8) and in EBV-negative infants (9). Clinical trials of a peptide vaccine bearing an EBNA-3A epitope are underway in Australia (10).

Recent Accomplishments and Developments

A phase I clinical trial conducted by SmithKline Beecham Biologicals in collaboration with MedImmune, Inc., has provided initial safety data on a subunit vaccine for EBV. The vaccine under development contains the gp350/220 surface glycoprotein combined with a proprietary adjuvant from SmithKline Beecham Biologicals. The trial was a randomized, double-blind study to evaluate safety and immunogenicity in 67 healthy young adults. The study showed that the vaccine tested was safe and well tolerated. Laboratory tests showed evidence of immune response in vaccine recipients.

Next Steps and Challenges Ahead

It is not known whether vaccination with gp350/220 alone will be adequate to protect against primary infection, and whether such a protective response would be effective against EBV-associated tumors where the expression of viral gene products is limited and different. Little has been reported on the use of antigens other than gp350/220 in candidate subunit or recombinant vaccines. Further work also is needed on defining the CTL specificities that a candidate vaccine should target. Following up on their successful phase I trial of a gp350/220 subunit, the next step for SmithKline Beecham Biologicals will be a larger phase II study. Results from the Australian phase I evaluation of peptide vaccination are pending.

References

1 Henle, G., & Henle, W. (1970). Observations on childhood infections with the Epstein-Barr virus. *Journal of Infectious Diseases, 21,* 303-310.

2 Niederman, J. A., & Evans, A. S. (1997). Epstein-Barr virus. In A. S. Evans & R. A. Kaslow (Eds.), *Viral infections of humans: Epidemiology and control* (pp. 253-283). New York: Plenum Press.

3 Rickinson, A. B., & Kieff, E. (1996). Epstein-Barr virus. In B. N. Fields, D. M. Knipe, & P. M. Howley (Eds.), *Fields virology* (3rd ed., pp. 2397-2446). Philadelphia: Lippincott-Raven.

4 Khanna, R., Burrows, S. R., Kurilla, M. G., et al. (1992, July 1). Localization of Epstein-Barr virus cytotoxic T cell epitopes using recombinant vaccinia: Implications for vaccine development. *Journal of Experimental Medicine, 176,* 169-176.

5 Tamaki, H., Beaulieu, B. L., Somasundaran, M., et al. (1995). Major histocompatibility complex class I-restricted cytotoxic T lymphocyte responses to Epstein-Barr virus in children. *Journal of Infectious Diseases, 172,* 739-746.

6 Finerty, S., Mackett, M., Arrand, J. R., et al. (1994). Immunization of cottontop tamarins and rabbits with a candidate vaccine against the Epstein-Barr virus based on the major viral envelope glycoprotein gp340 and alum. *Vaccine, 12,* 1180-1184.

7 Aviron. (1999, August 11). *Aviron announces results of phase I clinical trial for Epstein-Barr virus vaccine* [Press Release]. Mountain View, CA.

8 Mackett, M., Cox, C., Pepper, S. D., et al. (1996). Immunization of common marmosets with vaccinia virus expressing Epstein-Barr virus (EBV) gp340 and challenge with EBV. *Journal of Medical Virology, 50,* 263-271.

9 Gu, S. Y., Huang, T. M., Ruan, L., et al. (1995). First EBV vaccine trial in humans using recombinant vaccinia virus expressing the major membrane antigen. *Developments in Biological Standardization, 84,* 171-177.

10 Moss, D. J., Burrows, S. R., Suhrbier, A., et al. (1994). Potential antigenic targets on Epstein-Barr virus-associated tumours and the host response. *Ciba Foundation Symposium, 187,* 4-13.

Jordan Perspective: Varicella Vaccine

In 1952, Weller and Stoddard (1) reported the successful cultivation in human tissue of the virus that causes chickenpox in children, and shingles in adults. No useful animal model could be developed, but it was demonstrated that the virus of herpes zoster was the virus of varicella reactivated from its latent state. Thus, it was designated varicella-zoster virus (VZV). In 1974, 2 years before I came to the National Institutes of Health (NIH), Takahashi and his associates (2) reported that VZV isolated in human embryonic lung cells from the vesicles of a 3-year-old child named Oka and attenuated by serial passage in human and then guinea pig embryonic cells had been effective as a live vaccine. This attenuated virus became known as the Oka strain.

Sometime after 1977 (date not recorded), Dr. George Galasso and I attended a meeting in Atlanta, Georgia, along with Dr. Maurice Hilleman of Merck. We encouraged Dr. Hilleman to import the Oka strain rather than spend the time to develop an attenuated virus of his own. He did, so VZV is clearly cell associated, as is Oka. Merck initially had difficulty producing reproducible lots; fortunately, Dr. Hilleman and his staff persisted and we could report to the Department of Health and Human Services (DHHS) that the vaccine was ready for expanded clinical trials.

Fortunately, Dr. Larry Gelb, a grantee, had developed the first of several assays that could distinguish between vaccine and wild-type virus, allowing classification of any rash disease. A multicenter trial was coordinated by Dr. Ann Gershon, then at New York University, with support provided by the National Institute of Allergy and Infectious Diseases (NIAID). The target population was a unique group of children at high risk for severe illness and death from chickenpox—children with leukemia. They were most in need of protection, but it had become customary to avoid the use of live vaccines in immunocompromised children. Leukemic children had been successfully—and safely—immunized in Japan after suspension of chemotherapy from 1 week before to 1 week after vaccination. Review boards allowed U.S. studies to include children in remission from acute lymphoblastic leukemia for at least a year whose maintenance of chemotherapy was withheld for 1 week before and 1 week after vaccination (3). Adverse reactions resembling a mild case of chickenpox—rash and fever—occurred in this and subsequent studies more often in U.S. children than in Japanese children, but these reactions could be managed with oral acyclovir. The vaccine induced a good immune response and a high degree of protection.

Subsequent studies in healthy children sponsored by Merck (4) and in healthy adults funded by NIAID (5) confirmed the safety and effectiveness of the vaccine. The vaccine was licensed for general use in March 1995 and added to the recommended childhood immunization schedule shortly thereafter. Expanded use has shown it to be highly effective in clinical practice (6). Trials are now underway to evaluate the effectiveness of the vaccine for the prevention of herpes zoster and post-herpatic neuralgia in the elderly.

Time from growth of virus: 43 years.
Time from licensed vaccine introduced in Japan: 21 years.
Time from beginning U.S. trials: 15 years.

With a concluding comment, I would like to express my admiration for the dedication and excellent work of Dr. Ann Gershon and her assistant Sharon Steinberg. During these trials, they moved from New York University to Columbia University College of Physicians and Surgeons without missing a beat. Dr. Gershon has successfully competed for grant and/or contract funding from NIAID since 1979.

References

1 Weller, T. H., & Stoddard, M. B. (1952). Intranuclear inclusion bodies in cultures of human tissue associated with varicella vesicle fluid. *Journal of Immunology, 68,* 311-.

2 Takahashi, M., Otsuka, T., Okuno, Y., Asano, Y., & Yazaki, T. (1974). Live vaccine used to prevent the spread of varicella in children in hospital. *Lancet, 2,* 1288-1290.

3 Gershon, A. A., Steinberg, S., & Gelb, L. (1984). NIAID-Collaborative-Varicella-Vaccine Study-Group. Live attenuated varicella vaccine: Efficacy for children with leukemia in remission. *Journal of the American Medical Association, 252,* 355-362.

4 Weibel, R., Neff, B. J., Kuter, B. J., et al. (1984). Live attenuated varicella vaccine efficacy trial in healthy children. *New England Journal of Medicine, 310,* 1409-1415.

5 Gershon, A. A., & Steinberg, S. (1988). NIAID-Collaborative-Varicella-Vaccine-Study-Group. Immunization of healthy adults with live attenuated varicella vaccine. *Journal of Infectious Diseases, 158,* 132-137.

6 Vazguez, M. A., LaRussa, P. S., Gershon, A. A., Steinberg, S. P., et al. (2001). The effectiveness of the varicella vaccine in clinical practice. *New England Journal of Medicine, 344,* 955-960.

Human Immunodeficiency Virus (HIV) Disease

Human Immunodeficiency Virus (HIV) Disease

OVERVIEW

The goal of the National Institute of Allergy and Infectious Diseases' (NIAID's) HIV vaccine research program is to identify a safe and effective vaccine that prevents HIV infection. An HIV vaccine is the best hope for controlling the worldwide spread of HIV. Although there have been ambitious HIV prevention campaigns over the years, HIV/ acquired immunodeficiency syndrome (AIDS) continues to ravage many parts of the world. Worldwide, there are approximately 40 million people living with AIDS. In 2000 alone, there were an estimated 5 million new HIV infections, or about 14,000 new infections each day, and more than 95 percent of these new infections occurred in developing countries. Researchers have made enormous strides since the discovery of HIV 20 years ago, and now scientific advances are generating renewed optimism that a vaccine to prevent the spread of HIV is attainable.

Global summary of the HIV/AIDS epidemic, December 2001

Number of people living with HIV/AIDS	Total	40 million
	Adults	37.2 million
	Women	17.6 million
	Children under 15 years	2.7 million
People newly infected with HIV in 2001	Total	5 million
	Adults	4.3 million
	Women	1.8 million
	Children under 15 years	800 000
AIDS deaths in 2001	Total	3 million
	Adults	2.4 million
	Women	1.1 million
	Children under 15 years	580 000

The concept of what may constitute an effective vaccine has evolved over the years and has helped shape current thinking. While the goal is to find a vaccine that is 100 percent effective in preventing infection, it is highly likely that the initial vaccines against HIV may not protect everyone from becoming infected and/or may work by controlling infection. Researchers recognize that even a partially effective vaccine could have a significant impact on the worldwide spread of new infections due to the effect of "herd immunity." By decreasing the number of people susceptible to HIV infection and/or able to infect others, fewer people would be passing the virus on to others. If that chain of protection is high enough and continues long enough, new infections could be reduced dramatically or even eliminated. Nonetheless, because a vaccine may be only partially effective and could lead people to relax their practice of safe behaviors,

education and prevention must continue to play a role in reducing new infections.

Since HIV can be transmitted through systemic and mucosal routes of exposure, by cell-associated and cell-free virus, researchers also recognize that an efficacious vaccine may need to induce several types of immunity. This includes humoral immunity, which uses antibodies to defend against free virus, and cell-mediated immunity, which uses cytotoxic T lymphocytes (CTLs) to directly kill or control infected cells. While earlier vaccine research focused primarily on vaccines that elicited antibodies, it is now generally believed that a broader immune response is needed. As a result, vaccine concepts that would induce a strong cellular response by eliciting CTLs are now being tested. Furthermore, in addition to systemic immunity, mucosal immunity, which includes antibodies in mucosal secretions and cells in the lining of the reproductive tract and nearby lymph nodes, may also be required. Recent studies indicate that mucosal transmission is relatively inefficient in the absence of other sexually transmitted diseases, thereby suggesting that moderate immune responses may prevent infection by mucosal routes.

RECENT ADVANCES

The current optimism in HIV vaccine research is predicated on a number of important scientific advances. Fundamental research has elucidated the three-dimensional structure of the HIV envelope and of broadly neutralizing antibodies, which has helped reveal specific targets for HIV vaccines and highlight several defenses that the virus uses to evade attack. Researchers also have provided information on how the HIV envelope enters target cells; improved understanding of the specificity and role of antibodies and CTLs in HIV/simian immunodeficiency virus (SIV) infection; and identified potential new targets for HIV vaccines, such as the HIV regulatory proteins Rev and Tat.

There also have been important advances in vaccine technology, such as improved systems for vaccine delivery (e.g., codon-optimized DNA; novel viral and bacterial vectors; and cytokine adjuvants) as well as advances in laboratory techniques. These include the development of the enzyme-linked immunospot (ELISPOT) assay, which allows researchers to detect and count cells producing cytokines in response to specific HIV peptides; tetramer binding assays that detect T cells that recognize specific HIV peptides bound to major histocompatability complex (MHC) class I molecules; and easier assays to measure neutralization of primary HIV isolates. All of these new discoveries serve to further the development of HIV vaccines.

It should be noted, however, that vaccine development is a lengthy process. Each stage of clinical study can take several years. For example, vaccine candidates that are currently in the pipeline will be tested in phase I and phase II clinical trials for several years before being tested in a large phase III efficacy trial. Efficacy trials can then take another several years after the last patient is enrolled in order to assess any protective effect. So, while there is a great deal of optimism, it is tempered with the realities of clinical investigation.

PROGRESSION OF CLINICAL HIV RESEARCH

The HIV Vaccine Trials Network (HVTN), established by NIAID in 2000, represents an important resource for advancing clinical HIV vaccine research. This comprehensive global network is designed to foster the development of HIV vaccines through testing and evaluating candidate vaccines in clinical trials and has the capacity to conduct all phases of clinical research, from evaluating candidate vaccines for safety and the ability to stimulate immune responses, to testing vaccine efficacy. Spanning four continents, the network includes 25 clinical sites; an operations, and statistical and data management center; and a central laboratory. HVTN is built on the previous work and accomplishments of NIAID's AIDS Vaccine Evaluation Group (AVEG) and the HIV Network for Prevention Trials (HIVNET).

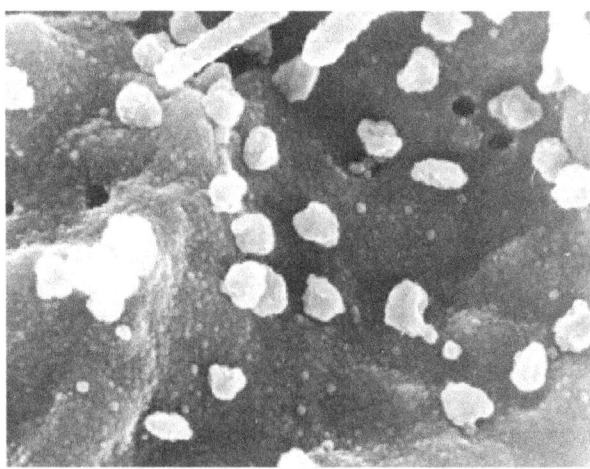

HIV bursting from CD4⁺ cells

To date, NIAID has supported more than 56 HIV vaccine trials, including 52 phase I trials and 4 phase II trials. A total of 29 candidate vaccines and 12 adjuvants have been tested with 1 or more of 10 routes or methods of administration. These trials have involved more than 3,700 international and U.S. volunteers.

Most of the initial HIV vaccine research (1987 to 1992) focused on the HIV envelope proteins (gp160 and gp120), peptides, induction of antibodies, and use of novel adjuvants. At least 13 different envelope candidates have been evaluated for safety and immunogenicity, and to date, all have been shown to be safe and effective at inducing neutralizing antibodies in nearly all of the volunteers tested. The initial emphasis on the HIV envelope protein was logical since envelope is the primary target for neutralizing antibodies in HIV-infected individuals. But the initial envelopes induced antibodies that were largely specific for clade B isolates, the subtype of HIV that is predominantly found in the United States and Europe. In order for a vaccine to be effective on a global scale, it will need to induce immune responses that are broadly reactive to the many different subtypes of HIV that circulate throughout the world.

There are several possible explanations as to why envelope proteins have induced limited immune responses. One theory is the degree to which the recombinant gp120 molecule resembles the envelope protein molecule on the surface of HIV. Because researchers have learned more about the actual structure of HIV and gp120, in particular, they are trying to create vaccines that more closely resemble the natural conformation of the HIV envelope on the virion surface. The envelope protein is a trimeric molecule—gp120 molecules bundled together in groups of three, held together with three transmembrane gp41 molecules. NIAID-supported researchers have identified ways to increase the stability of the gp120 protein trimer, which may help make it more potent and induce more broadly reactive antibodies.

Another theory is that the early envelope vaccines were based on laboratory strains of HIV (e.g., HIV isolates passaged repeatedly in cultured cell lines). Primary isolates of HIV, in contrast, have undergone minimal passage in fresh human peripheral mononuclear cells and are generally much less susceptible to neutralization by HIV antibodies.

In an effort to increase the breath of antibodies induced by envelope vaccines, the envelope candidates currently in a phase III trial are bivalent preparations comprised of two gp120s—one from a laboratory isolate and one from a primary isolate. Specifically, VaxGen, Inc., a company that manufacturers and tests preventive HIV vaccines, has developed two bivalent vaccines, AIDSVAX B/B and AIDSVAX B/E, which are currently in phase III trials (the former in North America and Europe, and the latter in Thailand). Results from the North America/Europe trial are expected at the end of 2002. Other groups also are designing polyvalent vaccines that include multiple envelopes.

Recognizing that an efficacious vaccine might need to induce a cellular (CTL) and antibody immune response, starting in 1992 researchers turned their attention to a combination or prime boost approach. In this approach, a recombinant vector vaccine (the prime) is followed by, or combined with, gp120 (the boost). Viral or bacterial vectors, as well as DNA vaccines, have been tested in combination with and without a subunit boost. A subunit is a synthetic structure component of HIV, such as an envelope or a core protein. NIAID has studied canarypox-HIV recombinant vaccines extensively alone and in combination with gp120 subunit boost. The canarypox-HIV vaccines are based on canarypox, which does not infect humans, and are genetically altered to contain selected HIV genes. For example, one canarypox vaccine, ALVAC vCP205, contains the *env* gene coding for the envelope protein gp120, the *gag* gene coding for the core protein p55, and the portion of the *pol* gene coding for the protease enzyme. The HIV genes in this vaccine come from clade B viruses, the predominant subtype of HIV found in the United States and Europe.

The combination approach has been shown to be safe and immunogenic in volunteers at low and high risk of HIV infection. Studies also have shown that this approach can stimulate cellular immunity, resulting in CTLs that can kill infected cells, as well as the production of HIV-neutralizing antibodies, which can stop HIV from infecting cells. Thus, the combination approach continues to hold promise because it stimulates production of HIV-neutralizing antibodies and cellular immunity.

Because the canarypox vaccine is the first candidate HIV vaccine shown to induce a CTL response against diverse HIV subtypes, HVTN conducted a phase I trial in 1999 in Uganda, a region in which clades A and D predominate. Although the vaccine was based on clade B, it elicited HIV-specific CTL responses in some volunteers that in the laboratory recognized several non-clade B strains. This study was extremely important because it demonstrated that a vaccine could induce cross-clade reactivity, and therefore may help protect against various subtypes of HIV. In addition, by successfully completing this trial, researchers showed that a vaccine trial could be conducted in Africa with high scientific and ethical standards, thus paving the way for additional international HIV vaccine trials in Africa.

Another NIAID-funded study found that among HIV-infected individuals in Uganda, the CTL response was as strong, if not stronger, to the clade B strain of HIV when compared to clade A. This study provides further justification for the evaluation of clade B-based vaccines in regions of the world where other subtypes are endemic.

At present, HVTN has two phase II trials underway to further evaluate the safety and immunogenecity of this combination vaccine approach. One trial, which is being conducted in the United States, is testing a canarypox vaccine (ALVAC 1452) in combination with a gp120 boost (AIDSVAX B/B). The second trial, which is being conducted in Haiti, Brazil, and Trinidad and Tobago, is also testing the use of ALVAC 1452, but in combination with a different gp120 product known as AIDSVAX MN. If specific immunogenicity criteria are met, the best available vaccine or combination of vaccines may enter an efficacy trial in early 2003.

Since 1997, researchers also have been exploring a range of other possible vaccines, including DNA vaccines (containing one or more HIV genes) with and without viral vectors, bivalent

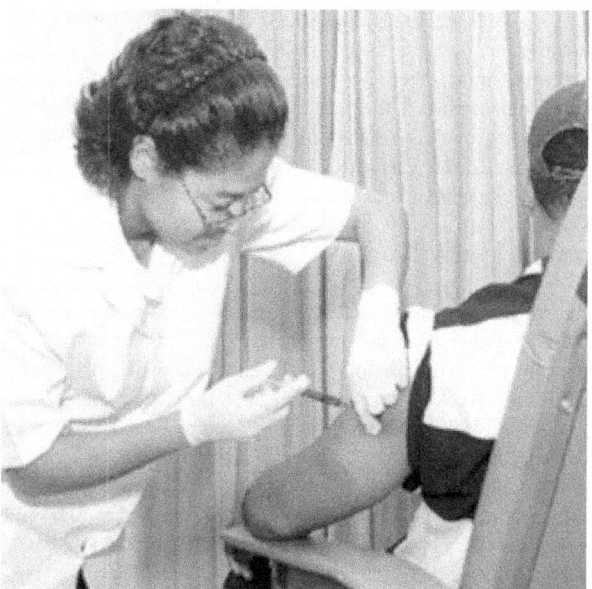

Start of ALVAC 1452 Study in Trinidad

envelope, Salmonella vectors, novel peptides (protein fragments), and p24. Studies demonstrated that the first DNA candidates were safe, but did not induce strong immune responses. New technologies for DNA vaccines, such as codon-optimized and particle-formulated DNA vaccine candidates, are being developed and are expected to enhance their performance. The frequency and strength of neutralizing antibodies and CTLs induced by peptides based on the viral envelope or internal proteins have also been disappointing, although new peptide-based approaches are under development. For example, scientists at NIAID recently tested in animals a vaccine using peptides expressed on the surface of phages, which infect bacteria. The phages were engineered to produce millions of random peptides, and upon screening, a few were found to react with HIV antibodies. Four out of five monkeys vaccinated with these phage-expressing peptides produced antibodies, and of those four, none got sick after being injected with virulent HIV. Additional research will be conducted to explore further the effectiveness of this approach.

PRECLINICAL DEVELOPMENTS

Animal models are extremely valuable in evaluating candidate HIV vaccines and continue to provide information that advances the field of HIV vaccine research. Since HIV does not infect monkeys, researchers have modified SIV, the related monkey virus. By taking parts of the HIV envelope and parts of the inner core of SIV, researchers have engineered simian-human immunodeficiency viruses (SHIVs), which mimic HIV infection and can cause AIDS-like illness in macaque monkeys. The chimeric viruses allow researchers to study the responses of the immune system to the vaccines, and the ability of these responses to stop or control the virus.

The goal of NIAID's preclinical HIV vaccine research effort is to identify the most promising vaccine candidates and ensure their entry into human trials. At present, there are more promising candidate vaccines in the preclinical pipeline than ever before. Specifically, NIAID is supporting the preclinical development of more than a dozen candidates through the HIV Vaccine Design and Development Teams, a program that brings together the skills and expertise of private industry and academic research centers, as well as through other mechanisms.

Recently, there have been promising studies in which some of these candidate vaccines were shown to protect rhesus macaques from disease following challenge with a highly pathogenic virus weeks to several months after the last immunization. In one study, NIAID-funded scientists combined two vaccines designed against SHIV. The first vaccine was a DNA vaccine containing genes for SIV and HIV proteins. When this DNA was injected into the monkeys, an immune response against SHIV was triggered. The immune response was then boosted with a second vaccine that added several of the same SHIV/HIV genes to a virus called modified vaccinia ankara (MVA), an attenuated strain of vaccinia that cannot replicate in humans. While immunized animals became infected, they controlled their infection, and in some cases, virus levels in the blood fell below detectable levels, and CD4+ T-cell levels remained stable. Since the vaccines induced strong immune responses that controlled virus replication and disease in the SHIV model in rhesus macaques, researchers will now seek to determine the safety and immunogenicity of this approach in human volunteers.

In other recent preclinical studies, researchers discovered that an HIV protein, Tat, might provide an effective way for fighting off infection. One study in monkeys found that killer T cells targeted to the Tat protein were able to contain SIV temporarily during the natural course of early infection. The Tat-specific killer T cells appeared to eliminate the original strain of SIV 4 weeks after the rhesus macaques were exposed to HIV. However, the monkeys still had some SIV that apparently resulted from small genetic changes from the infecting strain, which enabled the virus to escape immune attack. Other recent research involving Tat found that Tat and Rev, another regulatory protein, were frequent targets of HIV-specific CTLs. These studies provide important information on immune events in early SIV and HIV infection and represent a plausible new approach for vaccine design.

In addition to these promising studies, efforts are underway to molecularly engineer novel forms of HIV envelope proteins. To date, vaccines with recombinant envelope protein (gp120) have induced neutralizing antibodies, but only against the virus from which the protein was derived and closely related strains. Some researchers believe this is because the recombinant gp120 molecule does not resemble the molecule as it appears on the surface of the virus, while others believe that loops of the protein sequence protect the critical receptor-binding region of the gp120. To address this, NIAID-supported researchers engineered a molecule that in animals induced antibody responses that neutralize a broader range of laboratory-adapted strains and several primary isolates of HIV. Given the importance of inducing broadly reactive antibodies, this construct is now being developed further, and plans are underway to test it in clinical trials.

Adjuvants also have been shown to play an important role and may enhance immune-stimulating properties of a vaccine. One recent study with QS21, a saponin adjuvant, found that although it was not well tolerated, the adjuvant enabled recipients to receive a lower dose of gp120 and still achieve the same level of immune response as those who received a higher dose of gp120. Future research efforts will continue to explore the use of adjuvants, including cytokines, as well as other novel approaches, such as the use of alphavirus replicons (nonreplicating alphaviruses engineered to carry genes encoding HIV proteins), fowlpox, adenovirus, and novel peptides.

CHALLENGES

Despite the progress that has been made to date and the hope that has been generated, a number of critically important obstacles remain. In order to develop an effective HIV vaccine, researchers still need to improve upon current vaccine designs so that they will induce broadly reactive long-lasting neutralizing antibodies and CTL responses. The lack of validated immune correlates of protection limits confidence that any vaccine will prove efficacious, and it is hoped that once a candidate vaccine is shown to have some protection in humans, researchers will be better able to understand the type, magnitude, breadth, and/or location of the immune responses associated with that protection. In addition, the issue of clade or subtype diversity must be addressed in order for an HIV vaccine or vaccines to be effective on a global scale.

Researchers also need to explore the various types of outcomes possible from an effective or partially effective HIV vaccine and assess the value from an individual and a public health perspective. Vaccine recipients may be completely protected from HIV infection (sterilizing immunity) or may be able to remain healthy should they become infected after being vaccinated (controlled infection). If an HIV vaccine were not able to prevent infection, it is hoped that it would at least be able to keep the level of virus in the blood low enough in the vaccine recipient so that the recipient remains healthy and is not able to infect others. The greatest public health value of a vaccine will be in its ability to prevent transmission.

The ability to produce sufficient quantities of clinical grade vaccines, and the limitation of animal models represent other challenges to HIV vaccine research. The ability to conduct preventive HIV vaccine efficacy trials in the United States and in developing countries also poses substantial challenges. Because thousands of people would be required for an efficacy trial and because there is a relatively low incidence of HIV infection in industrialized countries, even among higher risk groups, an efficacy trial that enrolls all risk groups will require a large international collaborative effort. In developing countries, there are concerns regarding exploitation and unequal partnerships, access to a vaccine if it is proven efficacious, a lack of infrastructure (clinical, laboratories, supplies, equipment), and the need for increased training. Additionally, some populations that are at higher risk of HIV infection (such as high-risk women and injection drug users) are often harder to recruit and retain in a clinical trial. There is also a general mistrust and misunderstanding of vaccine research that creates barriers to HIV vaccine trial recruitment in some populations.

To help ensure adequate recruitment and retention in HIV vaccine efficacy trials, NIAID has continued its practice of including community representatives in all aspects of its HIV vaccine trial program. Among these efforts, community advisory boards at all NIAID-sponsored vaccine trial sites is a key element. In addition, in 2001, the National HIV Vaccine Communications Steering Group was established to stimulate and enhance the national dialogue concerning HIV preventive vaccines and to create a supportive environment for future vaccine studies. The group represents the diversity of communities affected by the AIDS pandemic and includes nationally recognized leaders in fields such as communications, the media, social marketing, community education and organizing, healthcare, advocacy, public policy, and HIV prevention.

CONCLUSION

Despite the ongoing challenges, new scientific and technological knowledge continues to advance the field of HIV vaccine research. There are promising data from animal model studies; a greater diversity of vaccine approaches being tested; and more products in the pipeline than ever before, including a large number of non-clade B products. Specifically, the NIH Dale and Betty Bumpers VRC and NIAID's HIV Vaccine Design and Development Teams are moving strong HIV vaccine candidates from the laboratory into human testing. The VRC recently initiated a phase I clinical trial of an HIV DNA to determine if the vaccine is safe and elicits an immune response. The HIV Vaccine Design and Development Teams program is developing a number of HIV DNA vaccines. Data from HVTN's two ongoing phase II trials will be available within the next year, possibly leading to an efficacy trial of the combination prime-boost vaccine concept with others to follow. As a result, there is greater optimism than ever before that the goal of identifying a safe and effective HIV vaccine is attainable.

Sources

HIV vaccine research always has been an integral part of NIAID's research portfolio, with the goal of identifying a safe and efficacious vaccine to prevent HIV infection and/or disease. In the last 7 years, in particular, the program has received an influx of funds that have enabled it to grow exponentially. From 1996 to 2001, funding for HIV vaccine research at the National Institutes of Health (NIH) increased from just more than $100 million to more than $356 million (estimated). These funds have enabled NIAID to establish a comprehensive and vibrant set of programs that support all stages of the vaccine development pipeline, including:

Dale and Betty Bumpers Vaccine Research Center (VRC) — Intramural vaccine research with a primary focus on the development of HIV vaccines

Innovation Grant Program — Investigator-initiated HIV vaccine research involving high-risk/high-impact studies at the earliest stages of concept genesis and evaluation

HIV Research and Design Program — Grants to support concept testing in animal models, development of potential vaccine candidates, studies of immune correlates, and animal model development

Integrated Preclinical/Clinical AIDS Vaccine Development Program — Grants that target research at the preclinical/clinical interface

HIV Vaccine Design and Development Teams — Consortia of scientists from industry and/or academia who have identified promising vaccine concepts and work under milestone-driven contracts

Vaccine Development Resources — Contracts for the manufacture and testing of vaccine candidates

Simian Vaccine Evaluation Units — Testing of promising SIV and HIV candidates in nonhuman primates

HVTN — Global research network with the capacity to conduct all phases of clinical trials, from evaluating candidate vaccines for safety and the ability to stimulate immune responses, to testing vaccine efficacy

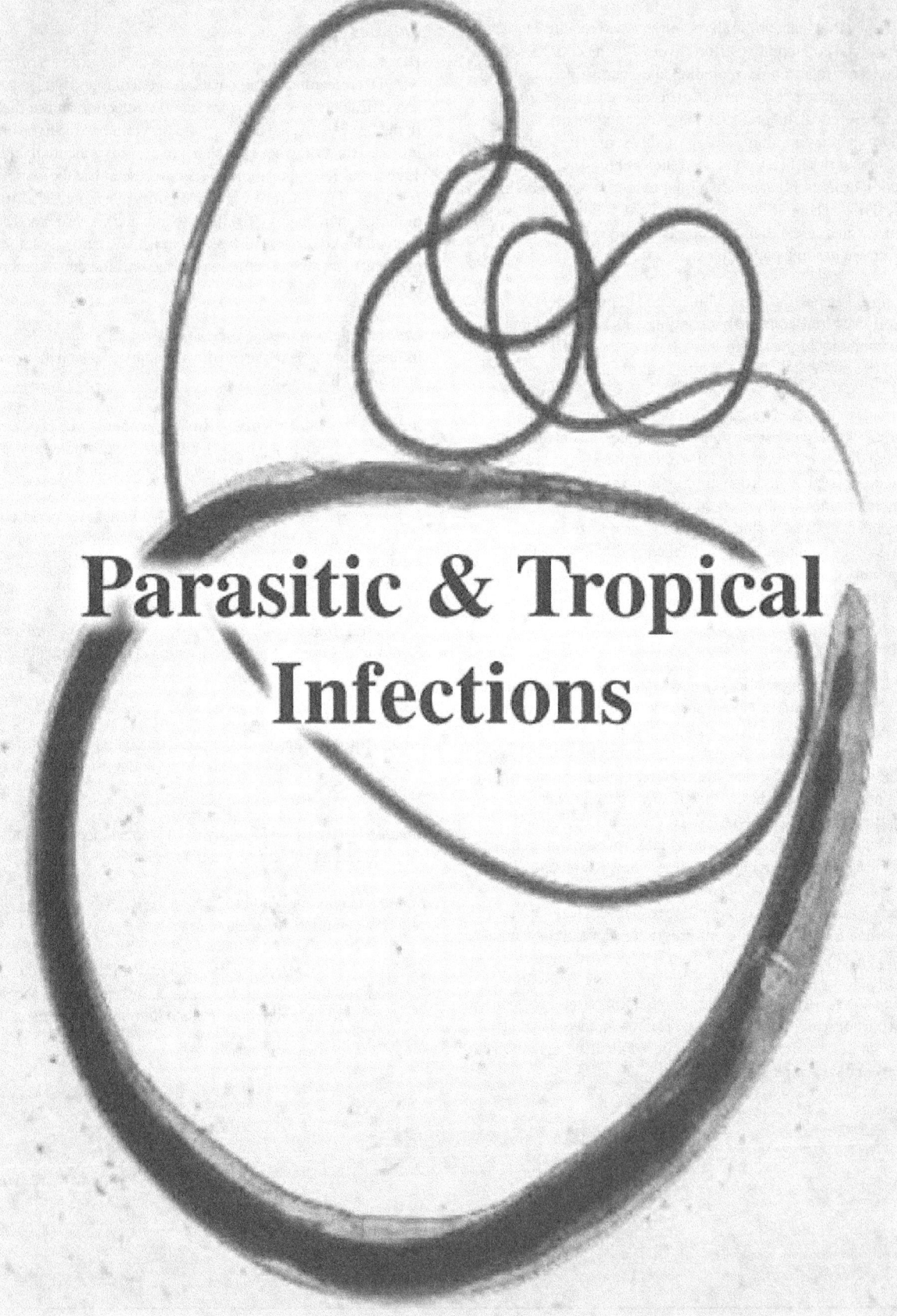

Parasitic & Tropical Infections

Parasitic and Tropical Infections

OVERVIEW

Parasitic diseases continue to plague billions of people in the modern world, killing millions annually and inflicting debilitating injuries, such as blindness and disfiguration, on additional millions. The World Health Organization (WHO) estimates that 1 person in every 10 is infected with a major tropical disease, and approximately one person in four harbors parasitic worms. These infections exact an enormous toll on world health and the global economy, particularly in less developed countries, where the diseases are often cited as a major impediment to economic progress. Despite efforts at control, some parasitic diseases are actually becoming more widespread because of drug resistance and changing water and land management policies that have brought humans in closer contact with parasite vectors.

Parasites remain a public health concern in the United States and other developed countries. Many parasites affecting humans are widely distributed in this country, but infections remain subclinical because of good nutrition and hygiene practices. In immunologically immature or immunosuppressed populations, however, parasitic infections represent a significant cause of morbidity and mortality. Moreover, symptomatic parasitic infections are becoming more widely observed in the United States as a consequence of the increased number of Americans traveling abroad, and of the increased number of immigrants from endemic areas. Recently, isolated endemic foci of some exotic parasitic infections (e.g., malaria and leishmaniasis) have been reported in the United States.

Despite the considerable global burden caused by protozoan and helminthic parasites, development of vaccines against these organisms has been arduous. In large part, the challenges of developing these vaccines derive from the fundamental biology of these organisms, which often have complex life cycles with developmental stages that are immunologically and biochemically distinct. These organisms are biologically much more complex than other microbes for which vaccines have been successfully developed. The genome of *Plasmodium falciparum*, for example, comprises 30 megabases; whereas the genomes of smallpox, polio, and *Haemophilus influenzae* type b are all 20 to 30 times smaller. Although radiation-attenuated parasites have provided useful insights into mechanisms of immunity in a variety of experimental settings, it has been impractical to develop vaccines based on attenuated versions of these organisms. Furthermore, these organisms often have sophisticated mechanisms to evade or undermine protective host immune responses, thus allowing them to establish chronic infections. Identifying protective immune responses as well as targets of protective immunity—thereby establishing surrogate markers and predictors of vaccine efficacy—has proven challenging even prior to setting out to design candidate vaccines.

As was noted by Dr. Jordan in his report some 20 years ago, the advent of molecular biology and recombinant DNA technologies, as well as molecular immunologic tools such as monoclonal antibodies, has been a tremendous boost to efforts to develop vaccines against protozoan and helminthic diseases. Subsequently, the development of recombinant viral and bacterial vectors capable of expressing cloned genes from protozoan or helminthic parasites has allowed the creation of novel hybrid vaccines. Even more recently, the availability of nucleic acid plasmids capable of expressing such genes in host tissue has created a whole new vaccine technology that is now being explored for its applicability to vaccines for parasitic infections.

These techniques have been applied to further understanding of the host-parasite relationship and to facilitate the identification and validation of antigens for inclusion in candidate vaccines. More than 40 antigens, for example, are currently considered as possible candidates for inclusion in or development as malaria vaccines. While one of the great advances of the last 20 years is the ability to sequence entire genomes of complex organisms like protozoan and helminthic parasites, the identification of the entire set of genes of an organism inevitably poses the daunting challenge of selecting among them to identify, validate, and ultimately create new vaccines. The recently completed *P. falciparum* genome, for example, has lead to the identification of 5,000 to 6,000 open reading frames within the genome. Included among

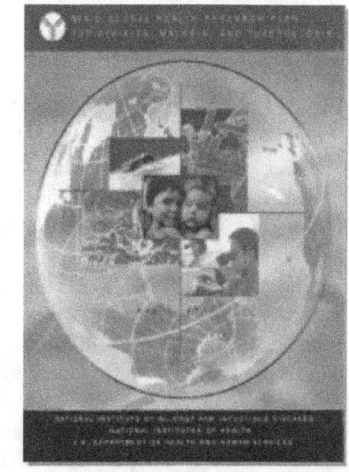

Global Health Plan Report Cover

these are two new gene families, rifins and stevors, which are now being investigated for their potential roles in vaccine development.

In addition to these scientific and technical advances, another important and encouraging change in recent years has been the growth of the number of groups supporting research on parasitic diseases and vaccine development. National Institute of Allergy and Infectious Diseases (NIAID)-supported programs, for example, have expanded, especially in the last decade [for example, NIAID's global health plans (http://www.niaid.nih.gov/dmid/global) and research to accelerate malaria vaccine development (http://www.niaid.nih.gov/dmid/malaria/malvacdv/toc.htm)].

New initiatives also have been launched in the public and private sectors. These include new entities such as the Malaria Vaccine Initiative (MVI) at the Program for Appropriate Technology in Health (PATH) [http://www.malariavaccine.org], and the Hookworm Vaccine Initiative (HVI) at the Albert B. Sabin Vaccine Institute (http://www.sabin.org/hookworm.htm), both of which are supported by the Bill & Melinda Gates Foundation; the European Malaria Vaccine Initiative (EMVI) [http://www.emvi.org]; the African Malaria Network (AMANET), formerly the African Malaria Vaccine Testing Network (http://www.amvtn.org); the Global Alliance for Vaccines and Immunization (GAVI) [http://www.vaccinealliance.org]; the Initiative on Public-Private Partnerships for Health; and the Initiative for Vaccine Research. Many of these organizations are already working in partnership with existing programs, such as those at the U.S. Agency for International Development (USAID), U.S. Department of Defense (DOD), WHO/Special Programme for Research and Training in Tropical Diseases (TDR), and elsewhere, to accelerate the development of vaccines against parasitic diseases.

LEPROSY

Leprosy, a chronic infectious disease caused by *Mycobacterium leprae*, has been a scourge of mankind since ancient times. It primarily affects the skin, peripheral nerves, mucosa of the upper respiratory tract, and eyes, often causing substantial disfigurement and disability if untreated.

M. leprae is an acid-fast, rod-shaped bacillus related to the bacterium that causes tuberculosis (*Mycobacterium tuberculosis*). Research on this bacterium has been markedly hampered by a continuing inability to culture it *in vitro*, and by its extremely slow doubling time (the slowest known for any prokaryote—approximately 13 days). The bacilli can be propagated in the foot pads of nude mice, but the only established animal model of disseminated disease is the nine-banded armadillo, which poses significant technical challenges of its own.

In the United States, there are an estimated 6,500 persons with leprosy, including those currently undergoing and those off treatment; 112 new cases were reported in 1998. WHO, which has led a global leprosy elimination program based on case detection and delivery of effective multidrug therapy (MDT), estimates that in 1997 there were 768,619 registered cases worldwide, with approximately 800,000 new cases detected. These figures represent a dramatic decrease in the prevalence of leprosy over the past few years; however, the number of new cases detected annually has been stable during this same period, and recently even appears to be on the increase. The reasons for this discrepancy between the remarkable effect of MDT on prevalence and the lack of noticeable impact on new cases detected are not clear, but the possibility of previously unknown reservoirs—either environmental or in the form of subclinical human infection—must be considered. India, Indonesia, and Myanmar currently account for approximately 70 percent of the world's

leprosy cases. Other "hot spots" for this disease continue to exist in Africa, Brazil, Colombia, and parts of Central and Eastern Europe. Leprosy is still considered endemic in 55 countries.

Dapsone was discovered to be effective against leprosy in the 1940s, but dapsone-resistant *M. leprae* gradually emerged, requiring the recent development of MDT for leprosy. Patients with leprosy are classified based on clinical manifestations and skin smear results into paucibacillary (PB) and multibacillary (MB) cases. Standard MDT consists of rifampicin, clofazimine, and dapsone given in a 6-month regimen for PB disease, and in a 2-year regimen for MB leprosy. A United Nations Development Programme (UNDP), World Bank, and WHO multicenter trial recently demonstrated that patients with PB disease with a single skin lesion could be cured with a single dose of rifampicin, ofloxacin, and minocycline. WHO also has indicated that it may be possible to adequately treat MB disease with a 12-month rather than 24-month course of standard MDT. These new regimens represent significant practical advances in the effort to control leprosy.

Major priorities in leprosy research are: Developing improved diagnostics (especially a sensitive and specific skin test); furthering understanding of the basic pathogenesis and epidemiology of the disease (it is not even clear how the disease is transmitted or whether there is a significant nonhuman reservoir); developing alternative treatments; and developing an effective vaccine.

Currently, there are only a handful of candidates in the leprosy vaccine development pipeline. One of these is the antituberculosis vaccine Bacillus de Calmette-Guerin (BCG), which has been demonstrated to be effective in preventing leprosy in some settings, but its use remains controversial. The Karonga Prevention Trial Group published the results of a double-blind, randomized, controlled trial of single BCG, repeat BCG, or combined BCG and killed-*M. leprae* vaccine in the prevention of leprosy and tuberculosis in Malawi. This study demonstrated that a second dose of BCG afforded an additional 50-percent protection against leprosy compared with a single BCG vaccination. In this trial, the addition of killed *M. leprae* did not improve the protection afforded by a primary BCG vaccination. A previous study by the Karonga Prevention Trial Group in the same part of Malawi demonstrated that a single BCG vaccination afforded approximately 50-percent protection against leprosy, but none against tuberculosis. A paper by M. D. Gupte and colleagues in the *Indian Journal of Leprosy* reported on a large leprosy vaccine trial comparing four vaccine candidates to placebo: BCG, BCG plus killed *M. leprae, M.w.,* and ICRC. The exact nature of the ICRC vaccine has not been made public, but it is reportedly based on a gamma-irradiated non-*M. leprae* mycobacterium. The study enrolled 171,400 subjects and, during a 5-year follow-up, found overall protective efficacies against leprosy of 65.5 percent for the ICRC vaccine, 64 percent for BCG plus *M. leprae,* 34.1 percent for BCG, and 25.7 percent for *M.w.* These exciting data suggest further analysis and testing of the ICRC and BCG plus killed *M. leprae* vaccines are warranted.

Another approach being pursued in leprosy vaccine development is the identification of major protective antigens and their use as the basis of subunit or recombinant BCG or vaccinia virus vector vaccines. As an example of such studies, one such protein, the 35-kilodalton (kD) protein of *M. leprae*, was identified as a major target of the human immune response to this pathogen. The 35-kD protein was expressed in the relatively fast-growing *Mycobacterium smegmatis* and shown to resemble the native antigen in forming multimeric complexes and in being recognized by monoclonal antibodies and sera from patients with leprosy. The *M. smegmatis*-derived recombinant antigen was recognized by almost all these patients via a T-cell proliferative or immunoglobulin (Ig) G antibody response, but not by most patients with tuberculosis. These findings suggest that the *M. leprae* 35-kD protein is a major and relatively specific target of the human immune response to *M. leprae*, and that it holds promise as a component of a potential antileprosy subunit, recombinant, or DNA vaccine.

Live atypical mycobacteria, including *M.w.* and *Mycobacterium habana*, are being investigated for their ability to elicit a cross-protective immune response, as are recombinant BCGs expressing other *M. leprae* antigen(s). Clinical testing of all these candidates would be vastly improved by the identification of correlates of human protective immunity.

Sequencing of the *M. leprae* genome is complete and should provide a significant boost to leprosy research in general, and vaccine development in particular—even more so than for many other microbial pathogens because of the extraordinary challenges involved in investigating this noncultivatable bacterium.

Sources

Gupte, M. D., et al. (1998). Comparative leprosy vaccine trial in South India. *Indian Journal of Leprosy, 70,* 369-388.

Karonga Prevention Trial Group. (1996). Randomised controlled trial of single BCG, repeated BCG, or combined BCG and killed *Mycobacterium leprae* vaccine for prevention of leprosy and tuberculosis in Malawi. *Lancet, 348,* 17-24.

Triccas, J. A., Roche, P. W., Winter, N., et al. (1996). A 35-kilodalton protein is a major target of the human immune response to *Mycobacterium leprae. Infection and Immunity, 64,* 5171-5177.

MALARIA

Malaria is a major health problem in the world's tropical areas, where it is responsible for high rates of morbidity and mortality, especially in children and pregnant women. The annual incidence of malaria is estimated to be approximately 300 to 500

million cases, resulting in greater than 1 million deaths each year. Because the control of malaria is difficult and has been further inhibited by the selection of drug-resistant parasites and insecticide-resistant mosquito vectors, the development of a malaria vaccine has been given high priority. Much work is now being done to determine the immunologic response to infection and to elucidate the protective antigens or epitopes that can be used in the construction of a synthetic or recombinant malaria vaccine. Such vaccines would target the infective sporozoite stage, the replicating liver or blood stages, or the sexual stages that are infective for the mosquito vector. Over the past few years, an increasing number of malaria vaccines have been tested in clinical trials.

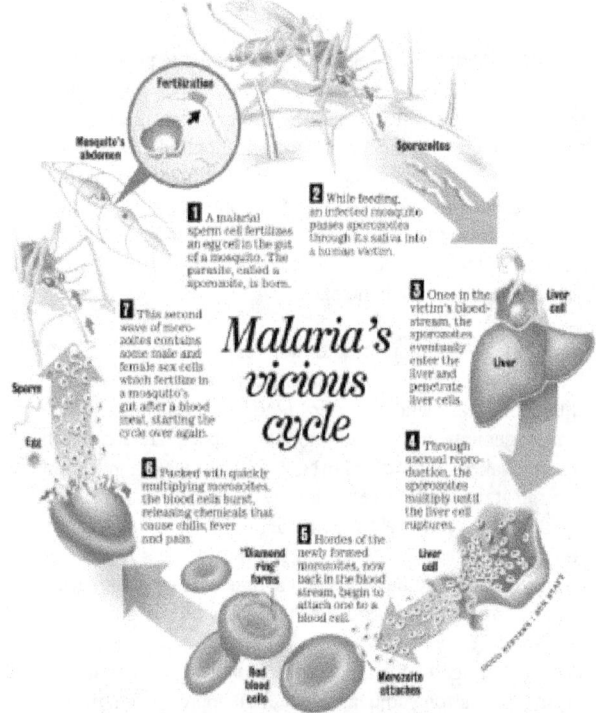

Vaccines Against Pre-Erythrocytic Stages of Malaria Parasites

Trials done in the 1970s with irradiated sporozoites resulted in good protection in volunteers challenged with infectious parasites. Several years later, an additional study was undertaken to take advantage of improved immunological techniques for the identification of immune correlates of resistance. Four of five vaccinated volunteers were protected, as measured by the absence of, or the delayed onset of, parasitemia following challenge infection. Protected individuals developed antibodies to sporozoites, including the repeat region of the circumsporozoite (CS) protein, as well as to antigens expressed by liver-stage parasites. T-cell proliferation, cytotoxicity, and cytokine production also have been observed in response to recombinant CS protein.

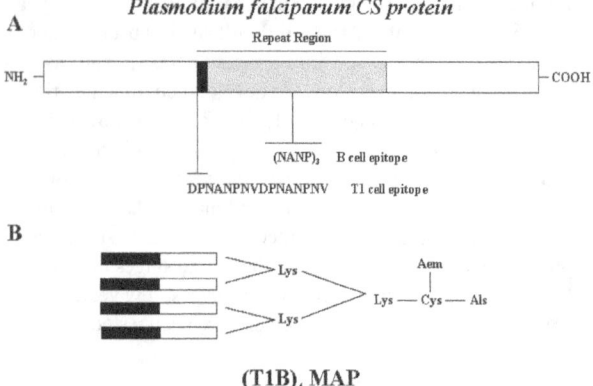

A

Plasmodium falciparum CS protein

Repeat Region

NH₂ — [ ] — COOH

(NANP)₃   B cell epitope

DPNANPNVDPNANPNV   T1 cell epitope

B

> Lys
> Lys
                    Aem
         Lys — Cys — Als
> Lys

(T1B)₄ MAP

In studies in animal models, CS-based synthetic peptide and recombinant vaccines conferred protection when given with strong adjuvants. Early trials with CS-based vaccines demonstrated enough immunogenicity to warrant challenge studies. When such studies were carried out with adjuvants approved for human use, however, the degree of protection was disappointing. These results were interpreted to mean that better immunogenicity could be achieved if more powerful adjuvants were available for use in humans.

During the 1990s, many studies were carried out with various candidate malaria vaccine formulations that included different adjuvants. These studies either failed to demonstrate adequate immunogenicity or failed to demonstrate adequate protection against challenge infection. In early 1997, however, investigators working at the Walter Reed Army Institute of Research (WRAIR) reported that a candidate vaccine (RTS,S), based on recombinant fusion proteins of the CS protein and the hepatitis B surface antigen, could provide protection against challenge infection with a homologous parasite when the vaccine was formulated with an appropriate novel adjuvant. These results were encouraging and validated the importance of incorporating into vaccine formulations strong adjuvants that elicit appropriate immune responses. Unfortunately, subsequent studies indicated that the protection conferred against experimental challenge by this vaccine alone is not long lived. An additional study has been carried out in The Gambia that demonstrated that under conditions of natural exposure to malaria, the candidate vaccine could elicit protection as defined as a delay in time to first infection in semi-immune adult men. Such protective immunity did not appear to be restricted to homologous parasites, but again was short lived. Overall vaccine efficacy was 34 percent, but was higher (71 percent) in the first 9 weeks of follow-up than in the last 6 weeks. Volunteers who received a fourth dose the next year, prior to the onset of the malaria season, again exhibited statistically significant protection (47 percent) over a 9-week follow-up period. Additional studies are now underway to improve the formulation and address other means by which the immunity provided might be enhanced. Of interest, an initial study to assess the combination of RTS,S and another recombinant protein corresponding to the pre-erythrocytic antigen

thrombospondin-related adhesion protein/sporozoite surface protein 2 (TRAP/SSP2) resulted in an apparent loss of protective efficacy compared to RTS,S alone. These results suggest that interactions among constituent antigens in vaccines may actually be detrimental rather than beneficial, and thus serve as a cautionary note.

Building on the increased awareness of the importance of strong adjuvants, some investigators have returned to the concept of immunizing with long synthetic peptides formulated with stronger adjuvants. Investigators at the University of Lausanne in Switzerland carried out a phase I clinical trial of an approximately 100 amino acid long synthetic peptide corresponding to the C-terminal portion of the CS protein, formulated with a strong adjuvant (Montanide ISA 720). Subsequent analyses showed that the vaccine was safe and well tolerated and elicited antibody and cellular immune responses, including antigen-specific production of an important cytokine, interferon gamma (IFNg).

An alternative approach that appears promising is to identify specific regions of the CS protein that stimulate immune responses and then incorporate several copies of those regions into a synthetic structure called a multiple antigenic peptide (MAP). MAPs based on CS protein structures have been shown to elicit high antibody titers in animal models and are capable of boosting preexisting malaria-specific immune responses. One potential problem associated with evaluation of synthetic peptide-based vaccines such as MAPs is that genetic factors may limit immune responses to the vaccine. This is particularly important because the candidate vaccine might be rejected as nonimmunogenic if the responsive individuals are not adequately represented in the initial immunogenicity study. To address this issue, collaborating scientists from New York University, the University of Maryland, USAID, and NIAID developed an innovative design for a recent phase I clinical trial of a CS-based MAP vaccine. Volunteers for this clinical trial were prescreened for presumed immune response genes to ensure that an adequate number of responder individuals was included. In this trial, only the pre-identified responder individuals mounted significant immune responses.

To address the limitations imposed on such epitope-based vaccines by the genetic restriction elements, investigators from New York University and their collaborators took a novel approach. Peptide epitopes were first synthesized to yield homogeneous products, and these peptide products were then linked to a small core peptide via oxime bonds. These multiple epitope constructs were shown to be immunogenic in mice. To overcome the genetic restriction, investigators created a construct that also incorporated a "universal" T-cell epitope (i.e., one that was not subject to narrow genetic restriction). This construct was subsequently shown to elicit robust immune responses in mice and in humans with diverse genetic backgrounds. Most recently, the B- and T-cell epitopes studied in the MAP trials have been incorporated into a recombinant viral-like particle based on a molecularly engineered version of the hepatitis B core antigen. This particle functions as a particularly immunogenic platform, and the engineered CS-HBc particle elicits robust immune responses to *P. falciparum* sporozoite antigens. Clinical trials with this construct are now in the planning stage.

Attention also has been directed to the nonrepeat domains of the CS polypeptide. A genetically conserved region within these domains has been implicated in parasite attachment to liver cells. Although shown to be safe and immunogenic in a clinical trial, a vaccine based on a genetically engineered CS-derived polypeptide in which the central repeat region was excised failed to confer protection against experimental challenge in the immunized volunteers.

While malaria vaccine efforts in the past have focused primarily on the humoral aspects of immunity, increasing attention is being directed to the important role played by T cells. In addition to enhancing antibody responses and conferring immunological memory, T cells also mediate cytotoxic immunity and induce the production of cytokines, such as IFNg. CS-responsive T-cell clones have been established from cells of vaccinees immunized with attenuated parasites; they may prove to be useful in future studies on the development of immune responsiveness. Epitopes of CS polypeptides recognized by helper T cells, as well as by cytotoxic T cells, have been identified and are being incorporated into recombinant vaccine candidates for further testing. To identify new candidate vaccine components, investigators employed a new approach called reverse immunogenetics. Using this technique, they have identified a peptide component of a liver-stage parasite protein (*LSA-1*) that is efficiently recognized by cytotoxic T cells from individuals who are resistant to severe malaria. Other liver-stage antigens (e.g., *LSA-3*) are also being evaluated in preclinical and clinical studies for their potential as candidate malaria vaccines.

Pre-erythrocytic antigens also have been incorporated into multicomponent vaccines (see below). In the case of DNA vaccines, a construct incorporating the gene for the CS antigen was evaluated as a "proof of concept" in a clinical study carried out by the U.S. Navy Malaria Program and its collaborators. The construct elicited cell-mediated immune responses in study volunteers, but did not elicit antibody responses and did not confer protection against experimental challenge.

Investigators are expressing pre-erythrocytic stage antigens in a variety of viral and bacterial vectors and evaluating their potential either as vaccines by themselves or as part of a heterologous prime-boost strategy (i.e., one type of vaccine is used to prime; and a second, different type is used to boost the immune response).

Vaccines Against Asexual Blood Stages of Malaria Parasites

Until recently, obtaining conformationally correct, immunogenic recombinant proteins based on candidate asexual blood-stage

vaccines has hampered progress. However, scientists have now established a number of approaches to produce such recombinant proteins. These include expression of recombinant proteins in a number of systems, including *Escherichia coli*, *Salmonella* spp., baculovirus, *Saccharomyces cerevisiae*, *Pichia pastoris*, Drosophila cells, and transgenic mammalian cells. In addition, crystallographic data are providing insights into the structure of the 19-kD C-terminal fragment of merozoite surface protein 1 (MSP1).

A number of blood-stage vaccine candidates are in development. In studies in Aotus monkeys, recombinant protein candidates based on the 42-kD and 19-kD C-terminal fragments of MSP1 have elicited protection. A phase I clinical trial of the candidate based on the 19-kD fragment of MSP1 was carried out at Baylor College of Medicine and demonstrated that the vaccine as formulated was poorly immunogenic and had unacceptable side effects. Additional work will be required before further development and clinical evaluation.

In collaboration with GlaxoSmithKline and USAID, investigators at WRAIR recently expressed the 42-kD C-terminal fragment of the major MSP1 in *E. coli*. Based on reactivity with a panel of monoclonal antibodies, the antigen appears to be conformationally correct. The antigen was subsequently formulated with the same adjuvant used in the RTS,S studies (see above). In clinical trials carried out in the United States, this vaccine appeared to be safe and immunogenic, although the addition of the MSP1 42-kD antigen to RTS,S did not appear to enhance protective efficacy against experimental challenge. A clinical trial of the recombinant MSP1 42-kD fragment for assessment of safety and immunogenicity in malaria-endemic populations has been initiated in Kenya.

Under a cooperative research and development agreement, NIAID and Genzyme Transgenics Corporation evaluated the feasibility of producing genetically engineered animals capable of secreting a recombinant version of the MSP1 42-kD C-terminal fragment in the animals' milk. Because *Plasmodium* species do not carry out substantial N- or O-linked glycosylation, site-specific mutations were introduced into the native sequence to prevent glycosylation in the transgenic animals. When glycosylated and nonglycosylated versions of these recombinant proteins were compared in a head-to-head study in Aotus monkeys, only the nonglycosylated version elicited protective immunity. Taken in collaboration with studies of the same recombinant protein expressed from a baculovirus construct in insect cells, these results suggest that the extent of glycosylation in some expression systems may alter or obscure the immunogenicity of protective epitopes. A recombinant version of the ectodomain of apical merozoite antigen 1 (AMA1) in which the glycosylation sites were also mutagenized also has been shown to elicit protective immunity in Aotus monkey studies.

Other antigens that are being produced in recombinant protein expression systems include the 175-kD erythrocyte binding antigen (EBA175) of *P. falciparum,* and its paralog in *Plasmodium vivax*, the Duffy binding antigen (DBA). Preclinical studies have been conducted already for these antigens, and it may be expected that once formulated as candidate vaccines, they will move into clinical trials in the future.

In addition to the studies with vaccines based on recombinant proteins, two clinical trials have been carried out recently with vaccines based on long synthetic peptide versions of MSP3, and the glutamine-rich protein (GLURP). Results of these studies are expected in the near future.

Vaccines Against Sexual Stages of Malaria Parasites and Mosquito Vector Components (Transmission-Blocking Vaccines)

Antigens of the sexual stages of the malaria parasite that can induce transmission-blocking activity also have been identified. Investigators at the NIAID Malaria Vaccine Development Unit (MVDU) have expressed in yeast a recombinant protein corresponding to a 25-kD molecule found in *P. falciparum* (Pfs25). Immunization with this molecule elicits transmission-blocking antibodies in animals; from these studies, however, it is clear that attaining and maintaining a high titer of transmission-blocking antibody is likely to

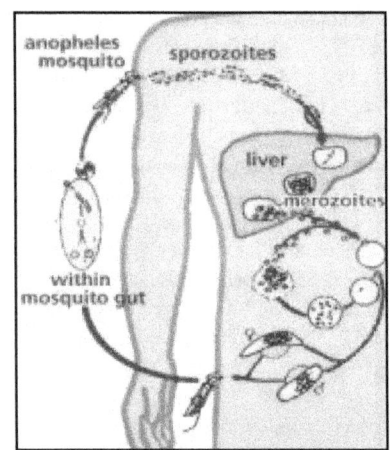

Plasmodium life cycle

be important for efficacy. Phase I clinical testing of this vaccine candidate formulated with alum has been conducted, and preliminary results indicate that improved formulation will be required. Experiments are underway to improve the preclinical profile and immunogenicity. A recombinant antigen corresponding to a similar 25-kD antigen found in *P. vivax* has also been produced by recombinant DNA technology by MVDU and shown to elicit transmission-blocking activity in monkeys. A phase I clinical trial is planned for late 2002.

Multicomponent Vaccines

Multicomponent vaccines directed against different antigens and different stages of the parasite life cycle may offer an advantage over single-component vaccines because they may provide multiple levels of protection. Such vaccines also may reduce the spread of vaccine-resistant strains, which can arise when the parasite changes a surface protein to avoid detection by the immune system.

Almost 10 years ago, a blood-stage vaccine (SPf66) developed in Colombia was reported to delay or suppress the onset of disease during trials in that country. In a randomized, double-blind trial conducted in Colombia, the vaccine was reported to have an overall efficacy of 40 percent. Two other clinical trials in South America reported similar results. These studies, however, were carried out in areas of low or seasonal malaria transmission, and thus the utility of this vaccine in areas of high transmission and in other geographic locations was questioned. To address these issues, randomized, double-blind, controlled clinical trials were carried out in Tanzania, The Gambia, and Thailand. In the Tanzanian study, the estimated efficacy of SPf66 was 30 percent, but with wide variability. In the Gambian and Thai studies, however, no significant efficacy was demonstrated. A later study in Brazil also did not demonstrate any efficacy of SPf66.

A combination vaccine consisting of recombinant proteins corresponding to fragments of three blood-stage antigens [MSP1, MSP2, and ring-infected erythrocyte surface antigen (RESA)] also has been in development by Australian investigators and their collaborators, and has undergone clinical evaluation. In phase I studies, the vaccine components were shown to be safe and immunogenic. Subsequently, the vaccine underwent field testing in Papua, New Guinea. In this study in children 5 to 9 years old, a statistically significant 62-percent reduction in parasite density was seen in vaccinees compared to controls. Vaccine-elicited immune responses also appeared to select against the specific form of MSP2 targeted by the vaccine. However, there was no difference in the number of clinical episodes between the vaccine and control groups.

An alternative approach to peptide or protein-based combination vaccines has been to use recombinant attenuated viruses because they can incorporate multiple exogenous genes and express the foreign malaria antigens. Vaccinia virus has been used extensively as a smallpox vaccine and has demonstrated a good safety profile in large numbers of individuals. However, disseminated vaccinosis has been a problem in immunocompromised individuals, suggesting that a malaria vaccine based on a recombinant vaccinia virus might not have an appropriate safety profile for use in areas where human immunodeficiency virus (HIV) infection has a high prevalence. This concern is being addressed by the development of attenuated, replication-defective viruses that could be used as a basis for a recombinant vaccine. However, as the virus is attenuated, it becomes less immunogenic; a balance has to be met between safety and vaccine efficacy. An attenuated vaccinia vectored 7-antigen vaccine (NYVAC-Pf7) has been tested in phase I and II trials, but resulted in poor antibody production and no protection.

Another exciting approach that is being developed for malaria as well as for a number of other infectious diseases is a DNA-based vaccine. Such vaccines have the advantage that they may elicit humoral and cellular arms of the immune response and that they may simplify evaluation of vaccines involving multiple different antigens. Thus, they may find utility at several stages in the vaccine identification and development process. However, because DNA vaccines are so new, experience with them is limited. The issues of safety, immunogenicity, and efficacy, especially in the long term, still need to be addressed. A phase I trial of a CS-based DNA vaccine was conducted at the Naval Medical Research Institute. The vaccine failed to induce antibody responses, but did induce cytotoxic T cells. Studies are now underway to elucidate means to enhance the immunogenicity of this candidate vaccine. A number of laboratories have reported that in experimental systems, giving a primary immunization with a DNA-based vaccine followed by a boosting immunization with a recombinant virus-based or recombinant protein malaria vaccine, enhances the immune response. In addition, multivalent DNA vaccines are also under development.

It is clear that before an ideal vaccine can be developed, more information is needed on the immune response to malaria and the factors involved in protection, including the use of immunogenicity-enhancing adjuvants and carrier proteins. Under its research plan for malaria vaccine development (http://www niaid nih.gov/dmid/malaria/malvacdv/toc htm) and its Global Health Research Plan for HIV/AIDS, Malaria, and Tuberculosis, NIAID has stimulated research in this area with recent initiatives and support activities. Novel vaccine targets, delivery systems, and alternative strategies to prime and boost protective immune responses differentially are being investigated. A resource for the collection of malaria research and reference reagents, named the Malaria Research and Reference Reagent Resource Center, has been established at the American Type Culture Collection to provide a central source of quality-controlled, malaria-related reagents and information to the interna

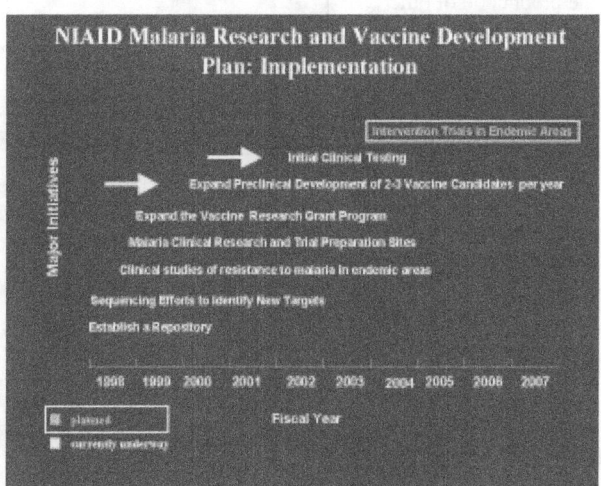

tional malaria research community. As part of a consortium, NIAID, along with the collaborators Wellcome Trust, Burroughs Wellcome Fund, DOD, National Human Genome Research Institute, and Stanford University, is supporting large-scale sequencing of genomes of Plasmodium parasites. Such efforts are ex

pected to result in the identification of new targets for potential vaccines and drugs. The assembled sequence of the *Anopheles gambiae* genome is available through two sites, National Center for Biotechnology Information (NCBI) and European Bioinformatics Institute (EBI). These data are provided on an interim basis since analysis by Celera Genomics and its partners in the Anopheles Genome Sequencing Consortium is ongoing. In 2001, NIAID awarded a grant to Celera Genomics to sequence the *A. gambiae* genome as part of an international consortium of *A. gambiae* researchers and genome sequencing centers. Finally, efforts are also in progress to expand capabilities to produce candidate malaria vaccines and to accelerate their evaluation domestically and internationally.

SCHISTOSOMIASIS

Schistosomiasis is another parasitic disease with a major human health impact. It is estimated that 200 million people worldwide are infected with this helminth, and approximately 600 million people live under conditions in which they are directly exposed to infection. Schistosomiasis is primarily a chronic disease associated with significant morbidity and loss of productivity; nevertheless, the mortality rate is estimated in the hundreds of thousands.

Recent research on schistosomiasis has focused on the identification of candidate vaccine antigens. Several of these candidates have been shown to provide partial protection in a mouse model of infection with the human parasite *Schistosoma mansoni*, a form found in South America and Africa. Many antigens are molecules associated with the invasive larval stage of the parasite; these antigens were initially distinguished by their reactivity with protective monoclonal or polyclonal antibodies. They include the enzymes glutathione-S-transferase (GST) and triose phosphate isomerase (TPI), as well as a 38-kD antigen with prominent carbohydrate epitopes that are shared between the larval and egg stages.

Another promising candidate, calpain, was recently identified based on the ability of a T-cell clone to transfer protection against challenge infection in mice. Several other antigens also have demonstrated partial protective activity. *Schistosome paramyosin*, a muscle protein, has been shown to induce a protective, cell-mediated immune response based on the production of IFNg-activated macrophage effector cells. Several vaccine candidates are being tested for efficacy against *S. mansoni* in baboons. One, a 28-kD GST of *S. mansoni*, has been shown to reduce worm burden or egg excretion in baboons and cattle. A myosin-like antigen also has shown efficacy against *S. mansoni* in mice and baboons. MAPs, based on selected regions of TPI and a 23-kD antigen, also have shown promise as candidate vaccines against *S. mansoni* in mice.

Additional investigations on mechanisms to enhance the level of protective immunity achieved with purified native or recombinant-derived antigens are underway; these studies include evaluations of the benefit of combining antigens or of varying the method used to present antigen to cells of the immune system. DNA-based vaccines also are being explored to identify promising routes of administration, combinations of vaccines, and protective immune effector mechanisms. Studies carried out in Egypt, Brazil, and Kenya have identified antigen-specific immunologic correlates of resistance to reinfection in populations at risk.

A candidate vaccine based on *Schistosoma haematobium* GST has been evaluated in phase I and II clinical trials. The vaccine appeared to be safe and well tolerated, and elicited high titers of IgG3 and IgA, as well as T helper (Th) 2 cytokine responses.

In certain settings, animal reservoirs may constitute a significant source of infectious parasites, and it has been proposed that immunizing the reservoir hosts may block transmission. Results obtained in water buffalo immunized with paramyosin and GST from *Schistosoma japonicum* are promising in this regard.

OTHER PARASITIC DISEASES

Candidate vaccine antigens have been identified for other parasitic diseases, including leishmaniasis, toxoplasmosis, amoebiasis, filariasis, onchocerciasis, hookworm, and taeniasis. Leishmaniasis is caused by several species of protozoan parasites found in most areas of the world, but particularly in the tropics. In its severest forms, this disease can cause serious disfigurement as well as death, and WHO estimates worldwide prevalence to be approximately 12 million cases. Several WHO-supported efficacy trials of vaccines based on a combination of whole, killed Leishmania parasites and BCG have been carried out recently. In one published clinical trial evaluating efficacy against anthroponotic cutaneous leishmaniasis in Iran, no difference was found between the vaccine and the control groups; a subgroup analysis, however, suggested that the vaccine might have a protective effect in boys. This apparent protective effect in boys was unanticipated and may be a chance finding. A second trial in Iran that evaluated protection against zoonotic cutaneous leishmaniasis found no efficacy, but only a single dose of vaccine was given. A subsequent study in Sudan that evaluated two doses of vaccine plus BCG, compared to BCG alone, found no evidence of protective efficacy against visceral leishmaniasis. An alternative approach involving the development of attenuated Leishmania vaccines based on gene replacement in *Leishmania major* is in early stages of preclinical investigation.

Two Leishmania surface antigens serve as ligands for the attachment of the parasite to host macrophages, thereby enabling infection to be initiated. They are gp63, a glycoprotein with protease activity, and a glycoconjugate known as lipophosphoglycan. When tested as candidate vaccines, both antigens have been shown to induce protection in a mouse model of leishmaniasis. In addition, a 46-kD promastigote antigen, derived from *Leishmania amazonensis*, has been shown to protect mice when administered as the native molecule admixed with adjuvant or as a recombinant vaccinia construct. Expres-

sion cloning has been used to identify a novel parasite antigen known as Leishmania-activated C kinase (LACK) that appears to be related to a family of enzyme receptors. When administered with interleukin (IL)-12, this antigen also has been shown to confer protection against leishmaniasis in susceptible mice. P4, a protein expressed in the intracellular forms of Leishmania parasites, has been demonstrated to immunize mice against infection. Protection correlates with establishment of an IFNg response. In subsequent studies, P4 also was shown to elicit IFNg production in peripheral blood lymphocytes obtained from patients with American cutaneous leishmaniasis. P4 is now being further characterized and has been shown recently to have nuclease activity, suggesting a possible function for this molecule in intracellular survival of Leishmania parasites.

NIAID-supported investigators have demonstrated that T-lymphocyte-dependent host responses to the Leishmania parasites determine whether the disease is progressive or self-limited in experimental animal models. More specifically, when a Th1 lymphocyte response (characterized by the production of cytokines, such as IL-2 or IFNg) is dominant, the disease is self-limited, whereas when a Th2 lymphocyte response (characterized by the production of other cytokines, such as IL-4 and IL-5) is dominant, the disease is progressive.

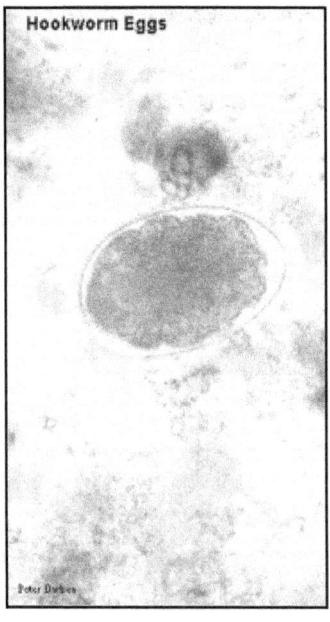

Hookworm Eggs

NIAID-supported investigators demonstrated that incorporation of the cytokine IL-12, a specific stimulator of Th1 responses, into an experimental vaccine against leishmaniasis resulted in complete protection of susceptible mice against progressive disease. Neither IL-12 alone nor the experimental vaccine without IL-12 conferred protection. Other NIAID-supported investigators have extended these findings by demonstrating that immunostimulatory oligodeoxynucleotides given as adjuvants, or a recombinant Leishmania antigen, LeIF, are also capable of eliciting IL-12 and Th1 responses and conferring protection.

DNA immunization is also being used to identify and validate candidate vaccine antigens for leishmaniasis. In mice, protection against *L. major* has been demonstrated following immunization with DNA constructs encoding gp63 and LACK antigens. A combination vaccine for leishmaniasis, comprising three antigens of *L. major* expressed as recombinant proteins in *E. coli*, is also under investigation and is expected to enter clinical trials in the near future.

In recent years, it has been appreciated that the sandflies that transmit Leishmania parasites also contribute to the pathogenesis directly. In particular, it has been observed that the sandfly saliva present when the insect takes a blood meal and transmits the parasite comprises substances that modulate blood and immune responses. NIAID-supported investigators recently identified a 15-kD protein in sandfly saliva that, when given as a vaccine, conferred protection against infection. The mechanism of protection appears to be host cell-mediated responses to the 15-kD protein that are elicited when the sandfly takes a blood meal.

Toxoplasmosis is primarily a disease of the central nervous system that affects individuals with immature or compromised immune systems. It usually is associated with neurological problems in the developing fetus; however, more recently it has been identified as a major opportunistic infection in acquired immunodeficiency syndrome (AIDS) patients. The possibility of effective vaccination against this protozoan parasite was suggested by experiments showing that mice immunized with a temperature-sensitive mutant of *Toxoplasma gondii* were resistant to further infection with a potentially lethal strain. In addition, a major surface antigen of *T. gondii*, called p30, has now been cloned. This antigen has been shown to stimulate cytotoxic T lymphocytes with parasiticidal activity *in vitro*. Purified native p30 recently has been demonstrated to protect mice against parasite challenge *in vivo*.

Amoebiasis, caused by invasion of the intestinal wall and gut-associated organs by the protozoan parasite *Entamoeba histolytica*, has been estimated to result in more than 100,000 deaths per year; the prevalence of infection may be as high as 50 percent in some developing countries. Recent studies have identified a galactose-inhibitable amoebic lectin involved in adherence of the parasite to the colonic mucosa. Gerbils immunized with this lectin showed a significant reduction in development of liver abscesses following infection, suggesting that this molecule might form the basis of a potential vaccine against amoebiasis. Investigators are working to identify the regions of the lectin that elicit protective immunity and to develop genetically engineered and recombinant subunit vaccines based on these regions. In addition, investigators are working to identify new antigens and delivery systems, especially those that would target mucosal immunity.

Lymphatic filariasis is endemic in many tropical and subtropical countries, where it is estimated to afflict approximately 90 million people. In its chronic form, this infection causes inflammation and blockage of the lymphatic system, resulting in the condition known as elephantiasis. Immunization with several *Brugia malayi* antigens has been demonstrated to facilitate the clearance of bloodstream forms (microfilariae) of the parasite in animal models. One such antigen is paramyosin, a 60-kD antigen. In addition, filarial collagen has been shown to partially inhibit the development of infective larvae into adult worms.

Onchocerca volvulus, a filarial parasite, is the causative agent of African river blindness. There has been considerable progress in the identification, characterization, and cloning of antigens of *O. volvulus*. A number of these antigens have exhibited promise as vaccines in animal models.

Hookworms are a leading cause of anemia and protein malnutrition globally. Considerable progress has been made in recent years to accelerate development of hookworm vaccines. With support from NIAID and HVI at the Albert B. Sabin Vaccine Institute, investigators of hookworm at George Washington University have identified and cloned a number of potential vaccine candidates. Recombinant expression systems for production of these candidates are now being examined. Studies are also underway to increase understanding of the immunological protective mechanisms.

Finally, considerable progress has been made in recent years in the development of vaccines against parasites of veterinary importance, including *Taenia ovis*, *Echinococcus granulosis*, *Boophilus microphilus*, *Fasciola hepatica*, *Haemonchus contortus*, *Ostertagia* spp., and *Trichostrongylus* spp. The results support the biological feasibility of developing vaccines against these and related infectious agents. Furthermore, in some cases it may be possible either to modify veterinary vaccines for future use in humans, or to disrupt the transmission of these parasites to humans by immunizing animal hosts.

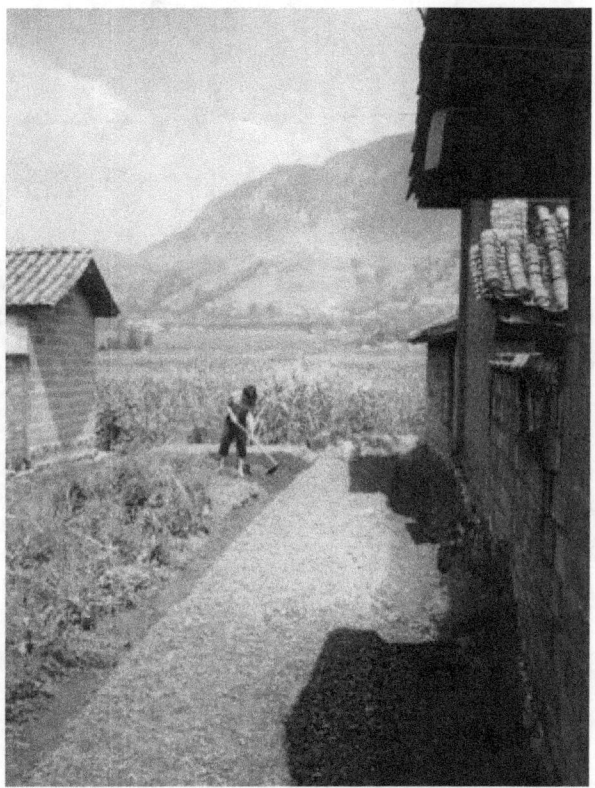

China ICTRD site which conducts research for parasitic infections.

Respiratory Infections

Respiratory Infections

OVERVIEW

Infections of the respiratory tract continue to be the leading cause of acute illness worldwide. Upper respiratory infections (URIs) such as the common cold, strep throat, sinusitis, and otitis media are very common, especially in children, but seldom have serious or life-threatening complications. Lower respiratory infections (LRIs) include more serious illnesses such as influenza, bronchitis, pertussis (whooping cough), pneumonia, and tuberculosis and are the leading contributor to the more than 4 million deaths caused each year by respiratory infections. According to the *1999 World Health Report*, acute LRIs and tuberculosis are among the top 10 leading causes of death from an infectious disease worldwide. In the United States, pneumonia and influenza are the sixth leading cause of death and are responsible for 3.7 percent of all deaths. The populations at greatest risk for developing a fatal respiratory infection include the very young, the elderly, and the immunocompromised. In developing countries, most of the deaths caused by respiratory infections occur in children younger than 5 years of age, and the World Health Organization (WHO) estimates that 30 percent of these deaths are attributable to pneumonia. The most common etiological agents of pneumonia are *Streptococcus pneumoniae*, *Haemophilus influenzae*, and respiratory syncytial virus. In the elderly, influenza-related pneumonia remains a leading cause of infectious disease-related deaths. Nosocomial or hospital-acquired pneumonia is a major infection-control problem. Pneumonia is the second most common type of nosocomial infection, accounting for approximately 15 percent of all nosocomial infections, with associated mortality rates of 20 to 50 percent. Nosocomial pneumonia can prolong hospital stays by 4 to 9 days, resulting in additional costs of approximately $1.2 billion annually in the United States.

Although generally considered less severe than LRIs, URIs have a major effect on global health. The common cold accounts for approximately 20 percent of all acute illness in the United States, with associated direct costs estimated at more than $500 million annually. Otitis media, which can be caused by a variety of etiologic agents, including nontypeable *H. influenzae*, *S. pneumoniae*, and *Moraxella catarrhalis*, is responsible for substantial morbidity and can have long-term effects on speech and language development in children.

According to the 1995 National Health Interview Survey conducted in the United States, there were more than 223 million acute cases of respiratory infections, with half requiring medical attention. Acute respiratory infections accounted for an estimated 640 million restricted activity days, 152 million bed days, and 134 million days of work lost among employed persons older than 18 years of age.

In addition, respiratory infections were responsible for millions of visits to hospital emergency rooms, outpatient departments, and doctors' offices.

Adequate clinical management of infections depends primarily on the rapid and accurate identification of the causative agent and is essential to avoid the indiscriminate use of antibiotics, which ultimately favors the development of antimicrobial resistance. Treatment of infections caused by antibiotic-resistant pathogens often requires the use of more expensive and potentially more toxic drugs and usually results in longer hospital stays. The difficulty in identifying the causative agent, the rapid global emergence of antibiotic-resistant organisms, and the increased incidence of atypical pathogens as the cause of respiratory infections have complicated the management of LRIs. The burden of respiratory infections is not only the loss of lives, but also the substantial effect they have on health resources.

A major goal of the National Institute of Allergy and Infectious Diseases (NIAID) Respiratory Diseases Branch is to stimulate and support research that may lead to more effective and accepted prophylactic and therapeutic approaches for preventing and controlling respiratory infections. Areas of interest include developing and licensing vaccines and therapeutic agents for respiratory pathogens; stimulating basic research on the pathogenesis, immunity, and structural biology of respiratory pathogens; developing more accurate and more rapid diagnostic tools; and understanding the long-term health effects of acute respiratory infections in various populations.

BORDETELLA PERTUSSIS

Even in the age of vaccine availability, *Bordetella pertussis*, or whooping cough, continues to be a major cause of childhood morbidity and mortality. An estimated 50 million cases and 300,000 deaths occur every year worldwide; case fatality rates in developing countries may be as high as 4 percent in infants. In the United States, an estimated 6,755 cases were reported for 2000.

During the past 20 years, there have been significant developments in the field of pertussis. The most notable is the recent availability of the acellular pertussis vaccine for use in infants and toddlers. Since the late 1940s, the incidence of pertussis has decreased dramatically in most developed countries as a result of widespread immunization. Initial vaccine formulations, which are still in use, consist of killed, but otherwise intact, *B. pertussis* cells. Concerns regarding documented and perceived adverse side effects accompanying whole cell vaccination prompted the development of acellular vaccines based on a subset of highly purified components of the organism. Several acellular vaccines are now licensed for use in the United States, beginning at 6 weeks of age. This followed a series of seven phase III clinical trials in Europe and North Africa that were completed in 1995. These efficacy studies all demonstrated levels of protection for most of the acellular pertussis vaccines that were equivalent to the whole cell vaccine. Vaccines containing three or more antigens were, generally, more efficacious than vaccines containing only one or two antigens. Furthermore, all the acellular vaccines demonstrated fewer adverse events for local and systemic reactions compared to the whole cell products following a primary immunization. Interestingly, this was not the case in children receiving a booster dose of an acellular vaccine between the ages of 4 and 6 years. In comparison to a fourth dose of an acellular vaccine administered at 18 to 24 months of age, the rate of local reactions increased following the fifth dose, while systemic reactions remained similarly low or decreased. Furthermore, when evaluating the safety and immunogenicity of various acellular vaccines among 4 to 6 year olds, children who had previously received four doses of either an acellular vaccine or whole cell vaccine showed local reactions that were significantly more frequent after five consecutive doses of the acellular vaccine than after an acellular vaccine following four previous doses of a whole vaccine.

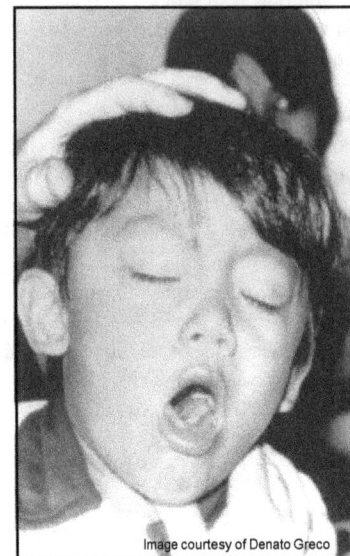

Image courtesy of Denato Greco

Child with Bordetekka pertussis

The first acellular vaccine, manufactured by Wyeth-Lederle, was licensed for use in infants and children in the United States in 1996. Since then, several other acellular products have been licensed, including products manufactured by Aventis Pasteur and GlaxoSmithKline. All of the licensed vaccines in the United States contain chemically or genetically inactivated pertussis toxin. The acellular vaccines also contain additional surface proteins either in the form of filamentous hemagglutinin, pertactin, or fimbriae.

Widespread vaccination of infants and children has resulted in several interesting changes in the epidemiology of *B. pertussis*. Although the frequency of the disease has declined overall, the organism continues to pose a problem, as observed by a change in the clinical spectrum and age-related incidence of the disease. In the prevaccine era, 85 percent of the cases of disease in the United States occurred in children 1 to 9 years of age. By the

DIP Vaccines: Chronology

1906	Organism is isolated and grown in artificial media (Bordet-Gengou)
1912-14	Vaccine made from killed whole cell *B. purchases* first introduced into children
1930's	Hendrick refines and uses whole cell vaccine in children
1942	Hendrick combines improved killed vaccine with Diphtheria and Tetanus Toxoids (DIP)
1947	DIP vaccine first recommended for routine administration in UPS.
1965	Many states in UPS. pass school-entry laws requiring DIP immunization
1974-77	Questions about the safety of whole cell vaccines in Great Britain and Japan. Vaccine uptake falls; cases increase dramatically
1979	Sweden discontinues use of whole cell vaccines due to safety issues and lack of efficacy
1981	The British National Childhood Encephalopathy Study is published suggesting rare association with acute necrologic reactions. Japan initiates routine immunization of two year-olds with several cellular vaccines
1986	National Childhood Vaccine Injury Act is passed by the UPS. Congress
1991-92	Several major efficacy studies begin in Europe and Africa
1993	Institute of Medicine publishes findings on the nature, frequency and circumstances of adverse events following purchases
1994-95	Seven efficacy trials for evaluating eight cellular vaccines completed

Courtesy of Carole Heilman and David Klein

1990s, only 41 percent of all cases occurred in infants, while 27 percent occurred in persons 10 years of age or older. Disease in infancy is due to exposure before sufficient levels of protection can be achieved through vaccination. In contrast, postchildhood disease results from the waning of vaccine-induced and natural immunity, resulting in repeat infections throughout life and the opportunity for transmission to susceptible infants. Although pertussis is rarely considered or diagnosed in older children or adults, it appears to be epidemiologically significant since it provides a reservoir for infection of unprotected individuals. Ultimately, the successful control of pertussis in the community may require routine immunization of adolescents and adults.

One area of concern that has developed in recent years is the adaptation or mutation of the *B. pertussis* organism to vaccination, thereby promoting resistance to the vaccines used to immunize the population. According to Dutch researchers, the organism appears to be disguising itself from the immune system by changing certain antigenic features on its surface. This has resulted in an increased incidence of disease in the Netherlands, United States, and elsewhere. Comparing old and new strains of pertussis over time has shown that at least two surface proteins, important in the development of protection against disease, have changed sufficiently to allow for an increase in the incidence of disease due to a reduced level of protection against the more recently isolated strains of the organism. The major surface variants have all been associated with altered forms (based on DNA fingerprinting) of either pertussis toxin or pertactin, two important virulence factors. Interestingly, fewer vaccine-type pertactin variants have been observed among vaccinated individuals compared to unvaccinated, which suggests the need for continued vaccination, especially with the newer acellular vaccines.

In recent years, an increasing proportion of pertussis cases has been documented in adolescents and adults. In adolescents and adults, the spectrum of disease is quite wide and may manifest itself as either a mild respiratory infection all the way to a paroxysmal cough with apnea. Pertussis is thought to be the cause of 12 percent to 26 percent of cases of cough illness in adults. Overall, the information about pertussis disease in the adult and adolescent patient is minimal compared to what is known about the disease in children. However, it is clear that adults and adolescents can transmit the disease to infants, and thus may represent the primary reservoir for the continued cycling of this disease in a community. Even though pertussis is preventable in all age groups, it is rarely considered or diagnosed in older children or adults. Natural and vaccine-induced protection from pertussis wanes as children age, resulting in repeat infections throughout life and an increased opportunity for transmission of this disease from infected adolescents and adults to susceptible infants.

A clinical trial was recently completed in 2,784 subjects 15 to 65 years of age to define the incidence (number of new cases per a given number of individuals per year), clinical spectrum, and epidemiology of pertussis infection and disease in adolescents and adults, as well as to define the safety, immunogenicity, and efficacy of an acellular pertussis vaccine designed for use in older individuals. The acellular vaccine was shown to be safe. A total of 3,171 cough illnesses lasting longer than 5 days occurred among the study cohorts, yielding a yearly incidence of 65 cough illnesses per 100 persons per year. Half had no cough illnesses, and 25 percent had more than two episodes. Confirmed pertussis occurred in two vaccinees and nine controls, yielding an efficacy of 78 percent. This means the vaccine works approximately as well in this group of adolescents and adults as it does in young children. The incidence of pertussis was approximately 4 cases per 1,000 subjects per year. This incidence represents an estimated 800,000 cases per year of pertussis among older individuals in the United States; such illnesses are often long lasting and not benign. Extensive experience in children suggests that an acellular pertussis vaccine given to adolescents and adults in the form of a diphtheria and tetanus toxoids and acellular pertussis (DTaP) vaccine combined booster would be safe and effective in reducing the burden of disease in this population, in addition to reducing transmission to infants. Other target groups [e.g., those with asthma or cystic fibrosis (CF), or immunocompromised individuals] would benefit as well. In addition, immunizing adolescents and adults should not involve significantly higher costs than the current diphtheria/tetanus immunization boosters that adolescents and adults receive.

Suggested Reading

Carbonetti, N. H., Tuskan, R. G., & Lewis, G. K. (2001). Stimulation of HIV gp120-specific CTL responses *in vitro* and *in vivo* using a detoxified pertussis toxin vector. *AIDS Research and Human Retroviruses, 17,* 819-827.

Heininger, U., et al. (2000, November 12-14). *Reactogenicity data following fourth and fifth doses of the Wyeth-Lederle Takeda acellular pertussis component vaccine – The Erlangen Trial.* Abstract presented at the Acellular Pertussis Vaccine Conference, Bethesda, MD.

Mooi, F. R., et al. (1998). Polymorphism in the *Bordetella pertussis* virulence factors P69/pertactin and pertussis toxin in the Netherlands: Temporal trends and evidence for vaccine-driven evolution. *Infection and Immunity, 66,* 670-675.

Strebel, P., et al. (2001). Population-based incidence of pertussis among adolescents and adults, Minnesota, 1995-1996. *Journal of Infectious Diseases, 183,* 1353-1359.

Ward, J. I., et al., & APERT Study Group. (2001, April 28-30). *Adult efficacy trial using an acellular pertussis vaccine.* Abstract presented at the meeting of the Society for Pediatric Research, Baltimore, MD.

CHLAMYDIA PNEUMONIAE

Background

Chlamydia pneumoniae (CP) is recognized as an important cause of acute respiratory tract infections, including pharyngitis, sinusitis, and bronchitis; in addition, severe systemic infections, while uncommon, do occur. It is a common cause of pneumonia, accounting for approximately 10 percent of all cases of pneumonia and 5 percent of all cases of bronchitis in the United States. Infection is usually asymptomatic, especially in young age groups. Most children become infected between the ages of 5 and 14 years. However, the disease is more severe and has the highest incidence in the elderly; case fatalities of 6 to 23 percent have been reported in this population. Transmission of the disease is person to person via respiratory droplets. Although CP has been isolated from the nasopharynx of healthy individuals, the rate of asymptomatic carriage in the normal population is unknown. Epidemics of pneumonia caused by CP have been documented in a number of geographic locations (mostly in northern Europe). In addition, CP has been implicated as a causative agent in chronic obstructive pulmonary disease (COPD) and has been associated with the exacerbation of asthma. Studies indicate that approximately 40 to 60 percent of the adult population worldwide has antibodies to CP, suggesting that the infection is universal.

Clinical disease manifestations associated with CP extend beyond respiratory illnesses. For example, there has been a recent association of CP with cardiovascular disease. Initially, this association was made on the basis of elevated immunoglobulin (Ig) G and IgA antibodies and increased chlamydial lipopolysaccharide (LPS)-containing immune complexes in 50 to 60 percent of patients with coronary heart disease or acute myocardial infarction, compared to 7 to 12 percent in control patients. Subsequent to these studies, several other investigators in the United States and other countries have reported similar findings in patients with coronary heart disease and have come to similar conclusions. Recent studies indicate that CP can be identified in postmortem brain samples of patients with Alzheimer's disease, and in the cerebral spinal fluid of patients with multiple sclerosis. CP also has been associated with Guillain-Barré syndrome and endocarditis. Infections caused by CP can result occasionally in shock and multiorgan dysfunction syndrome and have been associated with acute pulmonary exacerbation in some patients with CF. CP has been isolated from immunosuppressed patients, such as those with acquired immunodeficiency syndrome (AIDS); however, its role as an opportunistic pathogen is unclear. Thus, infections attributed to or associated with CP have a substantial impact on the public health in the United States and worldwide. Although conventional antibiotic therapy has been shown to be effective against CP, recurrent infections have been shown to occur following treatment. Consequently, alternative strategies such as vaccine development should be considered.

As a group, Chlamydia cause important infections in animals and humans. Chlamydia are distinguished from other bacteria by having a unique life cycle with an orderly alternation of dimorphic forms that are functionally and morphologically distinct. The infectious form, known as the elementary body (EB), is specialized for invasion into susceptible host cells. Following endocytosis, the EB differentiates into a larger form called the reticulate body (RB). Once inside the cells, the organism resides inside membrane-bound vesicles and can modify the inclusion membrane, resulting in evasion of lysosomal fusion and immune detection. Chlamydia grow only intracellularly and require and use substrate and energy pools of the host cells for growth, and as such have been termed energy parasites. A special property of Chlamydia is their ability to persist in cells, and this property may result in latent or chronic infections. The chronic state may be related to the ability of the organisms to develop into morphologically aberrant forms that do not divide or differentiate into EBs; this state may favor the development of immune-mediated diseases and the avoidance of host defense strategies. Studies show that these aberrant forms can be induced experimentally by the administration of cytokines, such as interferon gamma, and are characterized by the absence of typical inclusions, low-grade infectivity, and altered expression of key membrane surface proteins. There is a lack of understanding about the mechanisms by which Chlamydia cause disease, and very little information is available on factors associated with virulence. The organisms possess two major surface proteins: Outer membrane protein (OMP) 1 and LPS. Chlamydial LPS has a low endotoxic activity when compared to the LPS of enterobacteria; however, the role of LPS or the OMPs in pathogenesis has not been defined. Studies indicate that the aberrant form has an altered expression of the OMP. Chlamydia do not have a peptidoglycan layer, but do have penicillin-binding proteins on their cell walls. In addition, they express a number of heat shock proteins (HSPs).

Certain characteristics, such as DNA homology, distinguish CP from two other closely related organisms, *Chlamydia trachomatis* and *Chlamydia psittaci*. Thus far, CP has been found to have one immunotype, TWAR (derived from the first two strains, TW-183 and AR-39). However, more recent studies indicate that CP strains are antigenically different from each other, suggesting that more than one serovar of CP exist. The organism forms dense round inclusions in tissue culture cells that are more similar to *C. psittaci* than to *C. trachomatis*. In addition, CP has a characteristic pear-shaped EB that is surrounded by a periplasmic space. Ultrastructural studies of the entry of CP organisms into HeLa cells show that the mode of attachment and endocytosis of CP are different from those of *C. trachomatis* and *C. psittaci*.

Current Status of Research and Development

Very little research has been done on the development of vaccines against diseases caused by CP. At present, most studies are focused on methods of diagnosis, the immunobiology of CP, and the response of the host to infections caused by CP. Recent advances in isolation techniques have improved tremendously the capacity to detect the organism in clinical specimens. Monoclonal antibodies specific for CP are now commercially available for culture confirmation, and several CP-specific primers have been used in polymerase chain reaction (PCR) detection of organisms. However, efforts are being made to develop a more sensitive multiplex PCR system.

Several studies have been conducted over the years to examine the mechanisms involved in abnormal immune reactions associated with CP. For example, genes encoding HSPs associated with immunopathology and those associated with protective responses have been identified in CP. Among these, HSP60, recognized by using sera from individuals infected with CP, is expressed at high levels during periods of stress and is particularly high in the aberrant form of the organisms; for example, high levels are expressed during chronic, persistent chlamydial infections. In a study designed to examine the significance of HSPs in the development of atherosclerosis, it was shown that chlamydial HSP60 can induce a variety of proinflammatory cytokines as well as increase the expression of cellular adhesion molecules on immune and vascular cells. In addition, at the molecular level, HSP60 induced the activation of nuclear factor kappa B (NFkB), which may contribute to the gene expression of these molecules. In another study, it was shown that a peptide from heart muscle that has homology with CP OMP can induce an autoimmune inflammatory heart disease, suggesting that CP may be linked to heart disease by antigenic mimicry of heart muscle protein.

There is a tremendous gap in understanding the host immune responses to infections caused by CP. Cell-mediated immune responses can be demonstrated in individuals infected with CP by blast transformation assays using peripheral blood mononuclear cells and have been demonstrated in experimental studies using CP EB antigens. CP infections also induce serum IgM, IgA, and IgG antibody responses. However, the role of cell-mediated or humoral immunity in recovery from infections caused by CP remains to be determined. Studies indicate that immunity to CP may be dependent on the expression of interferon gamma, a characteristic product of T helper 1 (Th1) T cells. Recently, a number of species-specific, potentially immunogenic antigens have been characterized. Two of these, an OMP2 and a HSP, have epitope configurations consistent with the capacity to induce a T-cell proliferative response.

Considerable research has been directed at understanding the association of CP with coronary heart disease. Indeed, morphological as well as microbiological evidence indicating the presence of CP in atheromatous plaques has been obtained using electron microscope studies, immunocytochemical staining, and PCR testing of coronary, carotid, and aortic atheroma. In most studies, it is clear that the organisms are more commonly found in diseased than in normal tissue. However, the role of CP infection in the progression to atherosclerosis is unclear. Other studies have focused on elucidating the mechanisms of pathogenesis. The results of these studies suggest that the initial events may be the colonization of CP in alveolar macrophages. Indeed,

macrophages or monocytes are likely to play a key role in the infection, serving as a vehicle for dissemination and responsible for the inflammatory response to infection through the elaboration of a variety of inflammatory mediators. Studies show that CP can grow in blood monocytes, monocyte cell lines, and a variety of vascular cells. CP also can induce the expression of cytokines, including tumor necrosis factor-alpha (TNF-a), interleukin (IL)-6, IL-1 beta, and interferon gamma, as well as increase the expression of cellular adhesion molecules. In addition to the release of cytokines from macrophages, activated T cells produce cytokines that cause infiltration of monocytes and lymphocytes from the blood. However, it is not clear how these events lead to the development of atherosclerosis.

It is still not clear whether CP actually causes atherosclerosis or is merely a bystander in the process. Studies in animals show that CP is capable of initiating and accelerating the development of atherosclerosis. For example, a combination of CP infection and small amounts of cholesterol supplementation enhanced the development of atherosclerosis in rabbits; however, antibiotic treatment of rabbits significantly reduced the development of atherosclerotic lesions. Three prospective human studies, conducted to examine whether cardiovascular diseases are amenable to antibiotic treatment, have now been reported. These studies indicate that cardiovascular events are reduced following treatment. However, in light of other studies showing conflicting results, the future of antibiotic therapy is uncertain. Several other treatment trials are underway.

There are currently no licensed vaccines for CP. Recent advances in immunological techniques and molecular genetics now make the development of such a vaccine feasible. Little is known about the microbial components of CP that may serve as vaccine targets. Studies show that the major outer membrane protein (MOMP) of *C. trachomatis* induces the activation of T cells that are protective against *C. trachomatis* infections. There have been conflicting reports, on the other hand, regarding the immunogenicity of the MOMP of CP. Some studies indicate that this antigen is poorly immunogenic, whereas other studies show a moderate to high level of immunogenicity. Clearly, this area of research needs to be investigated further using purified CP MOMP. Recently, two novel genes encoding CP OMPs have been identified and found to be immunogenic in mice. A major impediment in the development and application of a vaccine against CP is poor understanding of the host defense mechanisms against this organism. Animal experiments show that a Th1-type immune response to infection promotes protection, whereas animals that are susceptible to infection manifest a Th2-type immune response.

There are three experimental animals available for CP infections: Mouse, rabbit, and monkey. Mice have been shown to be the most susceptible to intravenous, subcutaneous, or intracerebral infection. These experimental animal models can be used to examine potential vaccine candidates. For example, although CP is primarily a respiratory pathogen, it is conceivable that vaccine administration may prevent systemic spread to other organs. In an effort to understand latent infection caused by CP, it has been reported that CP lung infection in mice can be reactivated by treatment with cortisone; however, the underlying mechanisms remain to be clarified.

Recent Accomplishments and Developments

Although CP is a well-known causative agent of respiratory infections, it also has been associated with cardiovascular and neurologic disease (including multiple sclerosis, stroke, and Alzheimer's disease). There is now considerable interest in understanding the mechanisms involved in the process of atherogenesis; there are studies in progress to determine how CP organisms colonize and destroy the walls of blood vessels. The earliest lesions seen consist of foam cells (mainly lipid-laden macrophages) and T lymphocytes intermixed with smooth muscle cells. Previous studies using electron microscopy have identified CP within foam cells. In a recent study, it was shown that CP LPS, a major bacterial cell wall component, could induce foam cell formation, suggesting that CP contributes directly to atherogenesis. In another recent study, it was observed that chlamydial HSP60 induced cellular oxidation of low-density lipoprotein; this finding offers a mechanism whereby CP may promote the development of atherosclerosis. In addition, a number of treatment trials are ongoing based on the concept that the administration of antimicrobial agents may decrease the risk of cardiovascular disease.

Future Steps and Challenges

Efforts should be made to obtain more accurate and more rapid diagnostic methods to ensure timely detection of CP. Studies should be done with more sensitive assays to obtain a better understanding of the epidemiology of diseases caused by CP. Important risk groups should be defined because immunization recommendations will depend on who is at risk. Studies should be conducted to obtain information on the cell biology and molecular genetics of the organism, characterize CP-specific proteins, and identify microbial components that may serve as vaccine targets. Molecular mechanisms associated with attachment and invasion should be defined, and the host defense mechanisms, strategies for immune evasion, as well as the underlying mechanisms of protection should be elucidated. Major efforts should be made to develop vaccines against infections caused by CP. It is also necessary to develop appropriate animal models that could be useful in investigating chronic or latent CP infections. Specifically, basic research studies should be conducted to determine which factors contribute to the development of atherosclerosis, as well as other cardiovascular and neurological diseases. Further, experiments should be done to evaluate the impact of antibiotic treatment on CP-associated coronary heart disease, as well as the impact of such treatment on the mortality associated with CP infections.

Sources

Bachmaier, K., Neu, N., de la Maza, L. M., Pal, S., Hessel, A., & Penninger, M. (1999). Chlamydia infections and heart disease linked through antigenic mimicry. *Science, 283,* 1335-1339.

Huang, J., Wang, M. D., Lenz, S., Gao, D., & Kaltenboeck, B. (1999). IL-12 administered during *Chlamydia psittaci* lung infection in mice confers immediate and long-term protection and reduces macrophage inflammatory protein-2 level and neutrophil infiltration in lung tissue. *Journal of Immunology, 162,* 2217-2226.

Jackson, L. A., Campbell, L. A., Schmidt, R. A., Kuo, C., Cappuccio, A. L., Lee, M. J., & Grayston, J. T. (1997). Specificity of detection of *Chlamydia pneumoniae* in cardiovascular atheroma: Evaluation of the innocent bystander hypothesis. *American Journal of Pathology, 50,* 1785-1790.

Kalayoglu, M. V., Hoerneman, B., LaVerda, D., Morrison, S. G., Morrison, R. P., & Byrne, G. I. (1999). Cellular oxidation of low-density lipoprotein by *Chlamydia pneumoniae. Journal of Infectious Diseases, 180,* 780-790.

Knudsen, K., Madsen, A. S., Mygind, P., Christiansen, G., & Birkelund, S. (1999). Identification of two novel genes encoding 97- to 99-kilodalton outer membrane proteins of *Chlamydia pneumoniae. Infection and Immunity, 67,* 375-383.

Kol, A., Bourcier, T., Lichtman, A. H., & Libby, P. (1999). Chlamydial and human heat shock protein 60s activate human vascular endothelium, smooth muscle cells, and macrophages. *Journal of Clinical Investigation, 103,* 571-577.

Muhlestein, J. B. (1998). Bacterial infections and atherosclerosis. *Journal of Investigative Medicine, 46,* 396-402.

Ross, R. (1999). Atherosclerosis—An inflammatory disease. *New England Journal of Medicine, 340,* 115-126.

GROUP A STREPTOCOCCI

Group A streptococci (GAS) cause a broad spectrum of disease that ranges from uncomplicated pharyngitis and skin infections to life-threatening invasive illness that includes pneumonia, bacteremia, necrotizing fasciitis, streptococcal toxic shock syndrome (STSS), and nonsuppurative sequelae consisting of acute rheumatic fever (ARF) and glomerulonephritis. Streptococcal pharyngitis has been and continues to be one of the most common childhood illnesses throughout the world. Skin infections caused by GAS are a particular problem in tropical and subtropical climates and summer months of temperate or northern climates. Outbreaks of necrotizing fasciitis and STSS with significant rates of morbidity and mortality among otherwise healthy individuals were first reported in the 1980s in the United States, Europe, and Japan and have continued into the 21st century.

Although the incidence of ARF has varied in the United States—decreasing in the 1970s, reappearing in the 1980s, and being limited to Utah and occasional outbreaks in the 1990s—this disease continues to be a serious public health problem in developing countries. Recurrent infections with GAS following ARF result in rheumatic fever and rheumatic heart disease (RF/RHD), requiring costly resources for medical and surgical treatment. RF/RHD is the major cause of heart disease in children around the world. Postinfectious glomerulonephritis is the most common form of glomerulonephritis in children, and GAS are the most frequent infectious etiology. The frequency and severity of poststreptococcal glomerulonephritis seem to be diminishing in the United States, and epidemics have been rare since 1965. However, sporadic outbreaks of poststreptococcal glomerulonephritis continue to be reported in developing countries and close communities with poor hygiene. The high burden of disease from streptococcal infections emphasizes the need for a safe and efficacious vaccine.

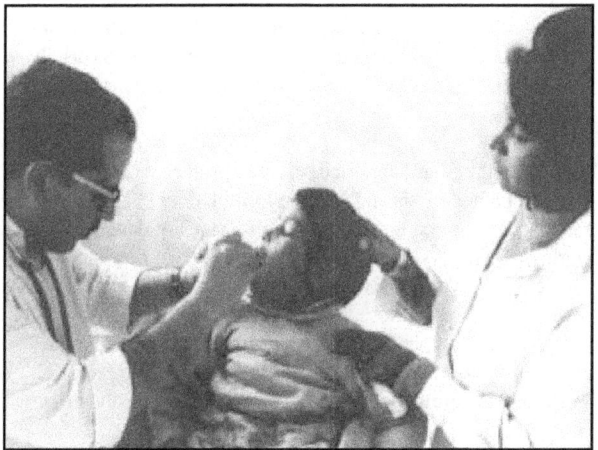

Confirmation of Group A Streptococci

A GAS vaccine has been a high priority at NIAID (see Appendix A, table of priority vaccines from first *Jordan Report*). The most significant obstacle to the development of a GAS vaccine has been circumventing an autoimmune response. The basis of this concern is the immunological cross-reactivity that has been demonstrated between the streptococcal epitopes and host tissues, including heart, kidney, articular cartilage, and basal ganglia of brain. The role of cross-reactive antibodies in the pathogenesis of GAS disease, especially ARF, has not been elucidated yet. Because humans are the only host for GAS, the development of animal models has been a challenge that has hindered progress. Human clinical trials to evaluate GAS vaccine candidates were impacted for more than 20 years following the report of ARF in volunteers receiving an M protein-based GAS vaccine in 1976. During that time, the use of biotechnology and advances in streptococcal research resulted in new vaccine candidates that are in various stages of development. The most significant scientific advance that has allowed progress in vaccine development was the identification of M protein protective

epitopes and M protein human tissue cross-reactive epitopes, providing a basis for inclusion or exclusion of epitopes to design safe vaccines. State-of-the-art biotechnology methods were used to dissect and manipulate streptococcal DNA and proteins for the elucidation and characterization of epitopes and provide tools to prepare vaccines for preclinical testing. Twenty years ago, efforts related to GAS vaccines were focused on M protein serotype specific protection. Recently, vaccine development has extended to the evaluation of surface molecules common among GAS to design vaccines that would evoke broadly protective immune responses after immunization.

Type-specific sequences of the M protein have been used to develop GAS vaccines because immunity to GAS is mediated predominantly by opsonic serotype-specific antibodies to the M protein. A multivalent approach is necessary because antibodies to a specific M protein serotype are only protective for that homologous serotype, and there are more than a hundred different M serotypes. Epidemiologic studies will guide the selection of M serotypes to be included in a GAS vaccine. A prototype hexavalent GAS vaccine was developed that in preclinical testing did not produce human tissue cross-reactive antibodies in an animal model. The hexavalent vaccine consists of a recombinant protein adjuvanted with alum. It is currently being evaluated for safety in an open label, phase I, dose escalation clinical trial at the Center for Vaccine Development, a NIAID-supported Vaccine and Evaluation Treatment Unit. The vaccine was administered parenterally and was found to be well tolerated in volunteers in the first and second cohorts; testing in a third cohort was initiated in early 2002. A newer formulation consisting of 26 serotypes, StreptAvaxä, is being evaluated in Canada by ID Biomedical Corporation. By selecting the highest frequency of serotypes, it is expected that the collection of peptides in this formulation should create antibodies to more than 90 percent of GAS serotypes currently found in North America.

Conserved sequences of M protein also have been used for developing a GAS vaccine. This approach is based on several studies demonstrating that adults have antibodies to peptides in the conserved region, a reflection of continuous exposure to GAS. Epitopes from the conserved region of the M protein that do not cross-react with human tissue have been evaluated for use in several vaccine candidates. One strategy uses a live vector delivery system, the oral commensal *Streptococcus gordonii*, which has been genetically manipulated to express a conserved M protein epitope from *Streptococcus pyogenes*. The vaccine is designed to evoke a GAS-specific mucosal immune response following administration via an intranasal/oral route, colonization, and expression of the conserved M protein epitope on the surface of *S. gordonii*. Because of the novel delivery system, clinical trials to test the reactogenicity, colonization, and eradication of the *S. gordonii* vector were necessary. Phase I clinical trials to evaluate safety have been conducted at the Center for Vaccine Development. The live *S. gordonii* vector was well tolerated. All volunteers were colonized for at least 1 day, and the vector was eliminated either spontaneously or with antibiotics.

Several M protein strategies are being used for the development of a GAS vaccine designed for the Australian Aboriginal population. The approaches involve an epitope of the conserved region of the M protein, either alone or in combination with M serotype epitopes. Earlier work was focused on identifying a minimum, helical, nonhost-cross-reactive epitope from the conserved region of the M protein. This epitope was placed in a non-M protein peptide sequence designed to maintain helical folding and antigenicity. Because this conserved region of the M protein is identical in only 70 percent of GAS isolates, common M serotypes were identified in communities with endemic GAS. Recently, seven serotype peptides were linked to the hybrid peptide with the conserved epitope to create a heteropolymer. This construct demonstrated excellent immunogenicity and protection in mice.

Twenty years ago, vaccine efforts were focused on M protein-based vaccines. Although this work has continued, recent efforts have involved other GAS proteins as vaccine candidates. Each has been shown to induce nonserotype-specific immunity. Animal studies involving these vaccine candidates were described in the *Jordan Report 2000*. A brief summary of promising GAS vaccine candidates under development follows.

C5a peptidase (SCPA) has an important role in the virulence of GAS. Antibodies to SCPA have been detected in adults, but are lacking in young children, reflecting exposure to GAS. Vaccine efforts are focused on preventing nasopharyngeal colonization, thereby reducing the incidence of streptococcal pharyngitis and more serious complications. Previous studies with intranasal administration of highly pure SCPA demonstrated protection to intranasal challenge with heterologous serotypes of GAS. Recent studies demonstrated an immune response in mice following vaccination with a recombinant truncated form of SCPA that was administered with adjuvant (monophosphoryl lipid A and alum).

S. pyogenes exotoxins (SPE) belong to a large family of proteins secreted by GAS. SPE A and SPE C are being developed as vaccine candidates because of their association with invasive GAS diseases, e.g. STSS. Vaccine toxoids have been constructed for SPE A and SPE C that are nontoxic and protective when used as vaccines against experimental STSS in rabbits. Although these toxoids are likely to have a significant effect on reducing the incidence of STSS and scarlet fever, they may or may not have protective effects against other invasive streptococcal diseases. SPE B contributes to streptococcal virulence and also is being developed as a vaccine candidate. Recent studies support the role of SPE B in the production of cutaneous and invasive disease. Studies in animals demonstrated that antibodies to SPE B enhance survival of mice challenged with highly virulent GAS.

Another streptococcal protein that is being developed as a GAS vaccine candidate is fibronectin-binding protein I (SfbI). This is a multifunctional protein that mediates bacterial attachment to host cells and allows GAS to evade phagocytosis by polymorphonuclear leukocytes. This protein is highly conserved, located on the bacterial surface, expressed by a large number of clinical isolates from different serotypes, and lacks cross-reactivity with host tissues. Several formulations of SfbI are being explored. The intranasal route of administration has been used to demonstrate protection against homologous or heterologous lethal challenge with GAS. It is currently being used to evaluate immune responses after intranasal administration with SfbI derivatives. Another approach under investigation is the constitutive expression of SfbI and SfbII in an attenuated *Salmonella typhimurium aroA* live oral delivery system. It is interesting to note that this system demonstrated protective immunity in studies in the late 1980s when it was used for the expression of cloned streptococcal M protein.

The potential for GAS carbohydrate to protect against GAS infections has been under investigation. Most human sera contain antibodies to GAS carbohydrate, and acquisition of antibodies appears to be age related. Animal studies using passive and active immunization have demonstrated that GAS carbohydrate antibodies protect against lethal challenge. GAS carbohydrate antibodies raised in animals were not cross-reactive with human tissues.

NIAID funding has supported research projects related to streptococcal pathogenesis and vaccine formulations. Vaccine candidates have emerged that are in various stages of development. During the past 5 years, clinical trials have been conducted at the Center for Vaccine Evaluation to evaluate GAS vaccines and vaccine approaches. Research efforts will continue to be supported with an emphasis on GAS virulence determinants, immune response to GAS, and pathogenesis of GAS infections. The future is optimistic for the development of safe and effective GAS vaccines.

Sources

Brandt, E. T., Sriprakash, K. S., Hobb, R. I., et al. (2000). New multi-determinant strategy for a group A streptococcal vaccine designed for the Australian Aboriginal population. *Nature Medicine, 6,* 455-459.

Cleary, P., Stafslien, D., Carlson, B., et al. (1999, October). A streptococcal C5a peptidase vaccine induces protection to intranasal challenge with heterologous serotypes of group A streptococci. Abstract from the XIV International Lancefield Meeting on Streptococci and Streptococcal Diseases, New Zealand.

Dale, J. (2000). Multivalent group A streptococcal vaccine designed to optimize the immunogenicity of six tandem M protein fragments. *Vaccine, 17,* 193-200.

McCormick, J. K., Yarwood, J. M., & Schlievert, P. (2001). Toxic shock syndrome and bacterial superantigens: An update. *Annual Review of Microbiology, 55,* 77-104.

Poirier, T. P., Kehoe, M. A., & Beachey, E. H. (1988). Protective immunity evoked by oral administration of attenuated *aroA Salmonella typhimurium* expressing cloned streptococcal M protein. *Journal of Experimental Medicine, 168*, 25-32.

Sabharwal, H., Blake, J., Michon, F., & Zabriskie, J. (1999, October). Immunization with group A streptococcal carbohydrate protects against group A streptococcal infections in mice. Abstract from the XIV International Lancefield Meeting on Streptococci and Streptococcal Diseases, New Zealand.

Schulze, K., Medina, E., Talay, S. R., et al. (2001). Characterization of the domain of fibronectin-binding protein I of *Streptococcus pyogenes* responsible for elicitation of a protective immune response. *Infection and Immunity, 69*, 622-625.

Towers, R., Gillen, C., McArthur, J., et al. (1999, October). Constitutive expression of the *Streptococcus pyogenes* fibronectin binding proteins SfbI and SfbII in an attenuated *Salmonella typhimurium aroA* oral vaccine delivery system. Abstract from the XIV International Lancefield Meeting on Streptococci and Streptococcal Diseases, New Zealand.

GROUP B STREPTOCOCCI

In the 1970s, Group B streptococci (GBS) emerged as the most important infectious cause of neonatal morbidity and mortality and pregnancy-related morbidity. Two syndromes in infants had been recognized: Early onset disease (primarily sepsis, pneumonia, and bacteremia within the first 7 days of life), and late onset disease (primarily meningitis between 7 and 90 days of age). GBS are vertically transferred from a colonized mother during delivery and can cause invasive disease. Neonatal disease prevention strategies in the United States have focused on the identification of vaginal and rectal colonization in pregnant women, and the use of antibiotics during labor and delivery in those women who are colonized. Although there has been a decrease in the incidence of early onset neonatal infections (65 percent) and invasive GBS infections in pregnant girls and women (21 percent), the incidence of late onset GBS disease in infants has not changed. While this strategy is effective, it is an interim solution. It has not been able to eliminate GBS disease and encourages the widespread use of antibiotics, with related concerns that include emergence of drug resistance in GBS. Recent data indicate that 15 percent of GBS isolates are resistant to clindamycin, and 21 percent to erythromycin.

Active immunization of women during the third trimester of pregnancy to induce antibodies and passively protect their newborns has great potential for the prevention of maternal and infant disease. GBS vaccines produced under a NIAID-supported contract have been found to be safe and induce high levels of functional antibodies in women of childbearing age. Recently, a phase I clinical trial in healthy, low-risk, third trimester pregnant women was completed. The vaccine was well tolerated and all deliveries resulted in a normal neonatal outcome.

The main obstacle in developing a GBS vaccine for neonates from invasive GBS disease is a litigation concern related to liability of vaccine manufacturers. The feasibility of maternal immunization has been demonstrated. Worldwide immunization of pregnant women for the prevention of infection in the infant is used routinely for neonatal tetanus, a major cause of infant mortality. However, safety data related to neonatal outcomes other than tetanus have not been collected. The risk involved in maternal immunization needs to be better defined. The current use of inactivated influenza vaccine in pregnant women in the United States provides an opportunity to design studies to collect safety data to demonstrate the safety of this approach.

Recent data report an increase in the incidence of invasive GBS disease in nonpregnant adults. The majority of these cases occur in adults with significant underlying conditions, such as diabetes, neurological impairment, breast cancer, and cirrhosis. Common clinical manifestations of GBS disease in adults include skin and soft tissue infections, bone and joint infections, and pneumonia. Meningitis and endocarditis are less common but, when present, are associated with serious morbidity and mortality. The case fatality rate is higher in adults than in neonates, and adults over the age of 65 are at the highest risk of dying from invasive GBS disease. These adults are an at-risk population that may benefit from a GBS vaccine, but the protective role of vaccine-induced antibodies is unknown. A challenge for GBS vaccine development is to better understand innate and adaptive responses of the immune system in relation to GBS pathogenesis in these populations.

The development of a GBS vaccine has been supported by NIAID since 1976. The primary focus of vaccine development has been GBS capsular polysaccharides (CPS). GBS serotypes are identified on the basis of the CPS structure, and antibodies generated against the CPS confer protective serotype-specific immunity to GBS infection. The first *Jordan Report* noted that GBS vaccines were being evaluated for antigenicity in human clinical trials. Phase I studies were in progress with vaccines that consisted of GBS CPS types III, II, and Ia. Although these vaccines were safe, they were not very immunogenic. Conjugate vaccines became the focus of improving immunogenicity, with early studies optimizing parameters such as the CPS component, GBS and nonproteins as carrier molecules, and amount of cross-linking of CPS to a protein carrier. NIAID contracts have supported these vaccine design studies, as well as the production of GBS glycoconjugate vaccines for serotypes Ia, Ib, II, III, and V. Starting in 1993, phase I and phase II trials have been conducted with conjugated GBS vaccines. Approximately 120 volunteers received uncoupled CPS, and 662 volunteers received CPS-protein conjugates. A summary follows:

- Conjugated vaccines were compared to unconjugated CPS vaccines to evaluate reactogenicity and immunogenicity and to determine optimal dose. Each CPS was individually conjugated to tetanus toxoid (TT), and a second type V conjugate was prepared with the mutant diphtheria toxoid cross-reactive material 197 (CRM$_{197}$). The vaccines were well tolerated and the CPS-TT vaccines were more immunogenic than uncoupled homologous CPS (CRM conjugate was not compared to uncoupled GBS type V CPS). Functional antibody of vaccine-induced antibodies was demonstrated in an *in vitro* opsonophagocytosis assay.

- Most clinical trials involved monovalent vaccine preparations, with the exception of a bivalent study in which a GBS III-TT and GBS II-TT were administered together. The magnitude of the immune response with the bivalent vaccine was comparable to that observed in the monovalent vaccine recipients.

- A single injection of vaccine was administered in the clinical trials, with the exception of one study in which volunteers received a GBS III-TT booster 21 months after the first dose. A booster response was only observed in a group that had undetectable GBS III CPS-specific IgG before the first dose of GBS III-TT conjugate vaccine.

- The effect of an alum adjuvant on immunogenicity was tested. Adsorption of a GBS III-TT to alum did not improve the immune response to the type III CPS antigen in a study in which unadsorbed and adsorbed GBS III-TT vaccine were administered to volunteers.

- A randomized, double-blind, placebo-controlled, phase I clinical trial was completed in which a GBS III-TT was administered to healthy, low-risk, third trimester pregnant women. The vaccine was well tolerated, healthy babies were delivered by all vaccine recipients, and vaccine-induced type III CPS-specific IgG was shown to be efficiently transported to the infant and functionally active through 2 months of age. These data suggest that a GBS CPS conjugate vaccine has the potential to prevent early onset and late onset infant GBS disease and invasive disease in pregnant women.

Although these data demonstrate progress in GBS vaccine development, there are several challenges that relate to CPS conjugate vaccines. The first involves the multiplicity of serotypes. GBS serotypes Ia, Ib, II, III, and V are the predominant serotypes that have been isolated from neonates, young infants, pregnant women, and adults with invasive GBS disease in the United States. Because antibodies against GBS CPS are serotype specific, a multivalent vaccine will need to be developed to provide broad protection. Parameters that will need to be optimized for a multivalent vaccine include the number and amount of the protein carriers in the CPS formulation. The second relates to use of a GBS vaccine for maternal immunization, in that a correlate of immunity needs to be determined for GBS serotype. The success of using antibiotics for prevention of neonatal sepsis has reduced the number of cases of GBS neonatal sepsis in the United States, resulting in problems for conducting efficacy trials of GBS vaccines and presenting the need for antibody levels that correlate with protection. Although some data

are currently available, information for all serotypes causing invasive GBS disease is required.

An alternative strategy for prevention of GBS disease is to develop a vaccine based on a GBS surface protein. Some advantages of this approach are that these proteins are immunogenic and do not need to be conjugated to other molecules. Recombinant DNA techniques can be used to produce large amounts of antigens for vaccine preparation. For example, investigations with a and b subunits of the C protein, Rib protein, type V a-like and Rib proteins, and surface immunogenic protein (Sip) have demonstrated that these proteins are capable of eliciting antibodies in mice and protect against lethal bacterial challenges. In addition to their use as immunogens, surface proteins have been used as carriers for CPS antigens. As compared to GBS CPS vaccines conjugated with TT, these conjugates have the advantage of enhancing the immunogenicity of the polysaccharide component of the vaccine and eliciting additional antibodies protective against GBS infections. Examples of surface proteins that have been conjugated to CPS antigens and are being pursued as vaccine candidates include GBS C5a peptidase and a C protein. Studies with anti-C5a peptidase antibodies demonstrated opsonic activity, suggesting that inclusion of C5a peptidase in a polysaccharide vaccine can produce another level of protection that is serotype independent.

Additional formulations of GBS vaccines is another area of active research. A study with a bivalent vaccine composed of purified Rib and a proteins mixed with alum demonstrated that this approach resulted in an antibody response in mice to the two proteins and protected against lethal infection with GBS (serotypes Ia, Ib, II, and III). In another study, a GBS CPS type III conjugated with recombinant cholera toxin B subunit administered intranasally improved the mucosal as well as systemic immune response to GBS in a mouse model.

There has been a lot of progress in the development of GBS vaccines during the last 20 years. Better CPS-conjugate vaccines have emerged and the use of GBS proteins, as immunogens or conjugated with CPS, holds great promise. Additional research is needed to expand serological findings to define protective levels of GBS antibodies and define immune defects in adults that result in invasive disease. NIAID has funded basic research and clinical trials in the past and will continue to support these activities using grants, contracts, and a network of resources for clinical trials.

Sources

Areschoug, T., Stalhammar-Carlemalm, M., Larsson, C., & Lindahl, G. (1999). Group B streptococcal surface proteins as targets for protective antibodies: Identification of two novel proteins in strains of serotype V. *Infection and Immunity, 67*, 6350-6357.

Baker, C. J., Paoletti, L. C., Rench, M. A., et al. (2000). Use of capsular polysaccharide-tetanus toxoid conjugate vaccine for type II group B *Streptococcus* in healthy women. *Journal of Infectious Diseases, 182,* 129-138.

Baker, C. J., Paoletti, L. C., Wessels, M. R., et al. (1999). Safety and immunogenicity of capsular polysaccharide-tetanus toxoid conjugate vaccines for group B streptococcal types Ia and Ib. *Journal of Infectious Diseases, 179,* 142-150.

Baker, C. J., Rench, M. A., & McInnes, P. (2001). Safety and immunogenicity of group B streptococcal type III capsular polysaccharide-tetanus toxoid conjugate vaccine in pregnant women. *Clinical Infectious Diseases, 33,* 1151.

Brodeur, B. R., Boyer, M., Charlebois, I., et al. (2000). Identification of group B streptococcal Sip protein, which elicits cross-protective immunity. *Infection and Immunity, 68,* 5610-5618.

Cheng, Q., Carlson, B., Pillai, S., et al. (2001). Antibody against surface-bound C5a peptidase is opsonic and initiates macrophage killing of group B streptococci. *Infection and Immunity, 69,* 2302-2308.

Farley, M. M. (2001). Group B streptococcal disease in nonpregnant adults. *Clinical Infectious Diseases, 33,* 556-561.

Gravekamp, C., Kasper, D. L., Paoletti, L. C., & Madoff, L. C. (1999). Alpha C protein as a carrier for type III capsular polysaccharide and as a protective protein in group B streptococcal vaccines. *Infection and Immunity, 67,* 2491-2496.

Kasper, D. L., Paoletti, L. C., Wessels, M. R., et al. (1996). Immune response to type III group B streptococcal polysaccharide-tetanus toxoid conjugate vaccine. *Journal of Clinical Investigation, 98,* 2308-2314.

Larsson, C., Stalhammar-Carlemalm, M., & Lindahl, G. (1999). Protection against experimental infection with group B streptococcus by immunization with a bivalent protein vaccine. *Vaccine, 17,* 454-458.

Lin, K. Y., Philips, J. B., III, Azimi, P. H., et al. (2001). Level of maternal antibody required to protect neonates against early onset disease caused by group B streptococcus type Ia: A multicenter, seroepidemiology study. *Journal of Infectious Diseases, 184,* 1022-1028.

Shen, X., Lagergard, T., Yang, Y., et al. (2001). Preparation and preclinical evaluation of experimental group B streptococcus type III polysaccharide-cholera toxin B subunit conjugate vaccine for intranasal immunization. *Vaccine, 19,* 850-861.

HAEMOPHILUS INFLUENZAE TYPE B

The incidence of invasive disease due to *Haemophilus influenzae* type b (Hib) has significantly decreased since the conjugate polysaccharide vaccines were introduced. Unfortu-

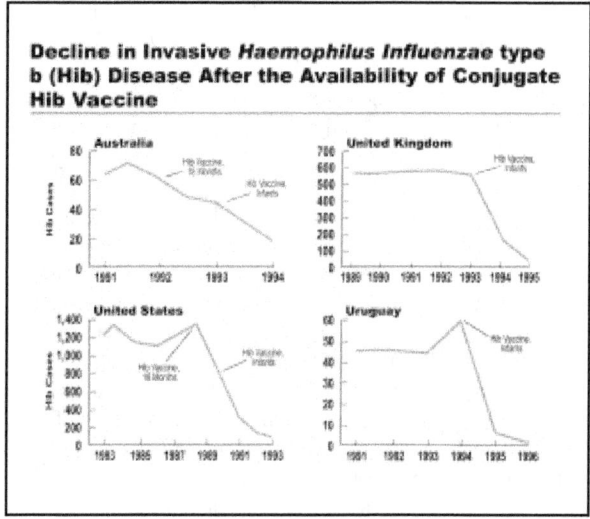

Decline in Invasive *Haemophilus Influenzae* type b (Hib) Disease After the Availability of Conjugate Hib Vaccine

nately, the introduction of each new vaccine has added to the overall number of shots that burden children during their first 2 years of life. Thus, pediatricians and vaccine manufacturers have been pursuing the introduction of complex combinations of vaccines that include, in one form or another, DTaP, Hib, hepatitis B virus (HBV), and inactivated poliovirus (IPV).

The combination of DTaP-Hib was licensed in Germany in 1996. A postlicensing trial was designed to determine whether lower antibody titers induced by this formulation were clinically significant. Earlier studies had shown that the Hib mean antibody concentration (GMC) is lower for the Hib combination than when it is given alone. Even though the GMC achieved with the combination is lower, it is still significantly above the theoretical level of protection of 0.15 ug/ml. The postlicensing trial included evaluation of a number of invasive Hib disease cases as well as surveys of microbiology laboratories determining the prevalence of Hib isolated from children.

Following the adoption of the combination vaccine in Germany, the number of cases of invasive Hib disease has continued to decrease up to the present time. The efficacy of the combination vaccine after three doses has been calculated to be 98.8 percent. During the study period, there were 91 cases of invasive disease due to *H. influenzae*, of which 41 were serotype b. Compliance with the vaccine schedule was only 74 percent, and most cases of invasive Hib disease occurred in nonimmunized children. This suggests that invasive Hib disease cases are not due to vaccine failure, but most likely due to the failure to vaccinate. The data also imply that combination vaccines such as DTaP-Hib are clinically effective despite inducing an antibody response that is lower than the response observed with Hib vaccine alone. Therefore, while preserving immunogenicity, administration of combination vaccines should increase vaccine uptake by minimizing the number of injections given to children.

Research in this field continues to define the genetics and function of the human antibody repertoire of the Hib capsular polysaccharide (Hib PS). Using the Hib PS as a model, efforts have been made to delineate the rules governing the expression of antipolysaccharide antibody specificities in humans and elucidate the structural determinants of protective immunity to this encapsulated bacteria. Studies have demonstrated the importance of avidity in determining protective efficacy of antibodies to Hib, and recently this observation has been extended to the pneumococcal system. Several molecular mechanisms also have been identified that can account for variation in anti-PS antibody avidity. These mechanisms include differential variable (V) region gene utilization, subtle alterations in V region sequence acquired during the process of antibody gene assembly, and extent of somatic hypermutation. Molecular analysis of the infant Hib PS repertoire has shown that infant antibodies contain amino acid polymorphisms not previously observed in adult antibodies. This structural variation among infant antibodies provides a molecular explanation for the differential functional efficacy of antibodies elicited in infants by Hib PS protein conjugate vaccines. Researchers have shown that closely related germline V gene homologs are not equivalent in their potential to form high affinity anti-Hib PS antibodies; therefore, inherited differences in the V repertoire can affect, in principle, the ability to generate protective polysaccharide immunity. Recent efforts involve studying the development of the Hib PS antibody repertoire from fetal life to old age. The results indicate that certain V region genes encoding Hib PS antibodies are assembled as early as the beginning of the second trimester. This pattern of V gene usage in the Hib PS repertoire is maintained throughout adult life and into advanced age. Additional studies have examined the extent of somatic hypermutation in the Hib PS antibody repertoires. The majority of infant Hib PS antibodies utilizing the recently recognized heavy and light chain genes associated with the Hib serum antibody repertoire show no evidence of somatic mutation, i.e., they are in the germline configuration. In contrast, the canonical H and L chains in elderly subjects appear to have acquired a significant mutational load. This finding suggests that the generation of immunological memory to Hib PS is accompanied by hypermutation. The impact this mutation has on antibody function is not yet known, but based on previous serological studies, it has been predicted that this mutation does not adversely affect antibody protective efficacy. This knowledge will help in understanding the cellular and molecular bases of protective immunity and may allow for the design of more effective vaccines against encapsulated bacterial pathogens.

Sources

Lucas, A. H., & Granoff, D. M. (2001). Imperfect memory and the development of *Haemophilus influenzae* type b disease. *Pediatric Infectious Disease Journal, 20*, 235-39.

Lucas, A. H., Granoff, D. M., Mandrell, R. E., Connolly, C. C., Shan, A. S., & Powers, D. C. (1997). Oligoclonality of serum immunoglobulin G antibody responses to *Streptococcus pneumoniae* capsular polysaccharide serotypes 6B, 14 and 23F. *Infection and Immunity, 65*, 5103-5109.

Lucas, A. H., Moulton, K. D., & Reason, D. C. (1998). Role of kII-A2 L chain CDR-3 junctional residues in human antibody binding to the *Haemophilus influenzae* type b polysaccharide. *Journal of Immunology, 161*, 3776-3780.

Lucas, A. H., & Reason, D. C. (1998). Aging and the immune response to the *Haemophilus influenzae* type b capsular polysaccharide: Retention of the dominant idiotype and antibody function in elderly individuals. *Infection and Immunity, 66*, 1752-1754.

Lucas, A. H., & Reason D. C. (1999). Polysaccharide vaccines as probes of antibody repertoires in man. *Immunological Reviews, 171*, 89-104.

Reason, D. C., Wagner, T. C., Tang, V. R., Moulton, K. D., & Lucas, A. H. (1998). Polysaccharide binding potential of the human A2/A18 kappa light chain homologues. *Infection and Immunity, 67*, 994-997.

Usinger, W. R., & Lucas, A. H. (1999). Avidity as a determinant of the protective efficacy of human antibodies to pneumococcal capsular polysaccharides. *Infection and Immunity, 67*, 2366-2370.

NONTYPEABLE *HAEMOPHILUS INFLUENZAE*

Nontypeable *H. influenzae* is a bacterium that frequently causes recurrent infections of the respiratory tract in humans, and whose environmental reservoir is the nasopharynx. From this point of origin, pathogenic varieties of this organism can make their way to the lungs, middle ear, bloodstream, and tissues surrounding the central nervous system causing such diseases as pneumonia, otitis media, and meningitis. If identified in a timely fashion, infection by this organism may be treated with antibiotic therapy. In addition, vaccines are available as a safeguard against Hib, one of the most prevalent pathogenic subtypes of *H. influenzae*.

Although the introduction of Hib conjugated polysaccharide vaccines significantly decreased the prevalence of invasive Hib disease, pediatric infections due to nontypeable *H. influenzae* are still highly prevalent. The organism is an important human pathogen in several settings and is most often associated with otitis media, sinusitis, and bronchitis. Nontypeable *H. influenzae* is consistently a major cause of otitis media in infants and children and is responsible for approximately one-quarter to one-third of all episodes. This amounts to approximately 5 million episodes of acute otitis media annually in the United States. Otitis media represents an enormous national health problem from the standpoints of human suffering and cost. This is most evident in the tremendous morbidity associated with hearing loss and delays in speech and language development in children. Approximately 80 percent of children will have had at least one episode of otitis media by the age of 3. Otitis media is the most common reason for visits to pediatricians, and the annual cost of medical care for this disease nationally is estimated to be $2 to $5 billion. Serologic studies and studies of the effect of antibiotics indicate that nontypeable *H. influenzae* also is an important cause of LRIs in patients (adults) with COPD. COPD is the fourth leading cause of death in the United States and in the world, with infections being the major contributing factor. Recent studies have implicated *H. influenzae* as a common cause of bacterial pneumonia in patients with AIDS. Carefully performed studies in Papua New Guinea, Hong Kong, Pakistan, and Gambia have demonstrated the importance of nontypeable *H. influenzae* as a common cause of LRIs in children, accounting for a significant fraction of the more than 5 million deaths in this population annually. Neonatal sepsis caused by nontypeable *H. influenzae* has been recognized with increasing frequency during the past decade. The infection is associated with a 50 percent mortality overall and a 90 percent mortality among premature infants. Little is known about the pathogenesis of this infection. Based on this huge amount of morbidity and mortality associated with nontypeable *H. influenzae*, children and adults would benefit greatly from a vaccine to prevent infections due to this organism.

All strains of *H. influenzae* have in common the fact that they require the iron-containing compound known as heme for growth. *H. influenzae* cannot make its own heme, so it has to acquire heme from its human host to grow in the body and cause an infection. The human body contains large amounts of heme, but all of this heme is bound to the hemoglobin protein in red blood cells or bound to other proteins. To grow and cause an infection in the body, *H. influenzae* has evolved specific mechanisms that allow this bacterial pathogen to steal heme from these human proteins and use it for its own purposes.

The inhibition of the ability of *H. influenzae* to steal heme from its human host may kill *H. influenzae* or otherwise prevent it from growing in the human body and causing disease. Testing of the ability of heme proteins to induce the synthesis of antibodies protective against nontypeable *H. influenzae* in an animal model is in progress.

A major problem among children is the reoccurrence of middle ear infections by what appears to be the same *H. influenzae* organisms. It is, therefore, the most common cause of recurrent otitis media and is implicated in a substantial proportion of otitis media with effusion. NIAID-supported research has revealed the mechanism of recurrent infections in this setting. Studies of the OMPs have revealed that the surface characteristics of the bacterium allow for these recurrent infections. When a child gets an episode of otitis media, the immune system makes antibodies to one specific region of one specific molecule (loop 5 of the OMP P2). This was proven by immunizing animals and rigorously studying their immune response. These studies revealed that the bacterium induces the host to make an immune response to a

specific portion of the protein. This portion of the P2 porin protein shows extreme heterogeneity among strains. Therefore, the immune response made by the child is effective at clearing the bacterium from the middle ear, but is only effective for that particular strain that caused the infection. Consequently, the child remains susceptible to other strains of *H. influenzae,* which have different protein sequences in the loop 5 region. This observation has important implications in the design of vaccines to prevent nontypeable *H. influenzae* infections. Additional work has identified another molecule (P6) that does not show sequence differences among strains. This P6 OMP has many unique characteristics, suggesting that it will be an effective vaccine antigen. Early clinical trials have demonstrated the safety and immunogenicity of P6.

Many investigators have concluded that the successful vaccine for nontypeable *H. influenzae* will most likely include more than one antigen. Therefore, several other *H. influenzae* surface proteins also have been identified as strong vaccine candidates. A recombinant form of a novel *H. influenzae* OMP designated Hin47 has been clinically developed by Aventis through a technology license agreement with Antex Biologics, Inc. The vaccine, which relies on an adhesin-receptor technology and is combined with an adjuvant, has undergone phase I testing in adults to determine its safety and immunogenicity. The ultimate intent is to develop an effective vaccine that will prevent otitis media and its complications in the pediatric population.

Another highly conserved protein associated with Hib and nontypeable *H. influenzae* strains is a 42-kDa membrane lipoprotein referred to as protein D. GlaxoSmithKline has been studying this nonacylated form of lipoprotein D as a potential carrier for their Hib and pneumococcal conjugate vaccines, as well as a vaccine for nonencapsulated strains of *H. influenzae*. Preclinical studies in rats have demonstrated high titers of bactericidal antibody against homologous and heterologous *H. influenzae* strains following hyperimmunization. Clinical testing of protein D as a carrier has shown the vaccine to be safe and immunogenic.

Lipooligosaccharide (LOS) has been shown to be a major surface antigen of nontypeable *H. influenzae*, capable of eliciting bactericidal and opsonic antibodies in animals. When prepared as a detoxified protein conjugate [i.e., LOS linked to TT or other high molecular weight (HMW) *H. influenzae* proteins], IgG anti-LOS antibody levels rose significantly in mice and rabbits to the homologous LOS following two or three injections administered subcutaneously or intramuscularly. These results were enhanced by the addition of monophosphoryl lipid A plus trehalose dimycolate.

Two additional HMW proteins that have been identified are referred to as HMW1 and HMW2. Both proteins are encoded by genes that are 80 percent identical and found in 70 to 75 percent of nontypeable *H. influenzae* strains. HMW1 and HMW2 also are effective adhesions that facilitate the binding of bacteria to the host cell wall. HMW1 is thought to be more important for binding than HMW2. The ability of HMW1 and HMW2 to protect against nontypeable *H. influenzae* infection was tested in chinchillas. After administration of the vaccine, the animals' middle ears were inoculated with nontypeable *H. influenzae*. All animals in the placebo group developed otitis media. Although only 50 percent of vaccinated chinchillas were fully protected against disease, bacterial counts in the middle ear were fiftyfold lower in immunized animals. In addition, by using intravenous Ig, it has been demonstrated *in vitro* that human antibodies have good activity against this protein. Although 25 percent of nontypeable *H. influenzae* do not express either HMW1 or HMW2, they express another critical adhesin called *H. influenzae* adhesin (hia), which is likely to be immunogenic. These findings suggest that frequently expressed nontypeable *H. influenzae* adhesins represent potential candidate vaccines.

Suggested Reading

Barenkamp, S. J. (2000). *Development of a vaccine for nontypeable Haemophilus influenzae for the prevention of otitis media*. Abstract 1139 presented at the 40th Interscience Conference on Antimicrobial Agents and Chemotherapy, Toronto, Canada, 535.

Cope, L. D., Hrkal, Z., & Hansen, E. J. (2000). Detection of phase variation in expression of proteins involved in hemoglobin and hemoglobin:haptoglobin binding by nontypeable *Haemophilus influenzae*. *Infection and Immunity, 68,* 4092-4101.

Faden, H. J., et al. (1989). Otitis media in children. The systemic immune response to nontypeable *Haemophilus influenzae*. *Journal of Infectious Diseases, 160,* 999-1004.

Grass, S., & St. Geme, J. W., III. (2000). Maturation and secretion of the non-typeable *Haemophilus influenzae* HMW1 adhesin: Roles of the N-terminal and C-terminal domains. *Molecular Microbiology, 36,* 55-67.

Klein, J. O. (1994). Otitis media. *Clinical Infectious Diseases, 19,* 823-833.

Maciver, I., et al. (1996). Identification of an outer membrane protein involved in the utilization of haemoglobin:haptoglobin complexes by nontypeable *Haemophilus influenzae*. *Infection and Immunity, 64,* 3703-3712.

Murphy, T. F., & Sethi, S. (1992). Bacterial infection in chronic obstructive pulmonary disease. *American Review of Respiratory Diseases, 146,* 1067-1083.

Ren, Z., Jin, H., Morton, D. J., & Stull, T. L. (1998). HgpB, a gene encoding a second *Haemophilus influenzae* hemoglobin- and hemoglobin-haptoglobin-binding protein. *Infection and Immunity, 66,* 4733-4741.

Yi, K., & Murphy, T. F. (1997). Importance of an immunodominant surface-exposed loop on outer membrane protein P2 of nontypeable *Haemophilus influenzae*. *Infection and Immunity, 65,* 150-155.

INFLUENZA

Among viruses, influenza is notable in its ability to produce annual epidemics in all age groups worldwide. Recorded as pneumonia and influenza (P&I) morbidity and mortality, an average of 20,000 P&I-related deaths occur each year in the United States, with higher rates occurring during years with more severe outbreaks.

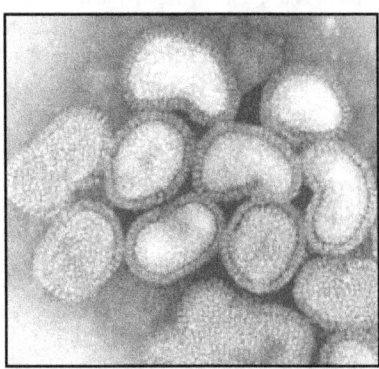

Despite prior vaccination or infection, the population's susceptibility to infection is renewed annually due to the accumulation of point mutations in the two major surface glycoproteins of the virus. Over time, the accumulation of these subtle mutations results in

Influenza vinons

the antigenic drift of the virus, often leaving current influenza vaccines outdated and unable to provide protection against the drifted virus. While antigenic drift is the basis for the annual review and frequent update of the content of influenza vaccines, a second form of antigenic variation occurs in influenza with little or no predictability. Due to the segmented nature of the influenza virus genome, these viruses also can acquire a gene for an entirely new glycoprotein from an avian or other animal influenza virus. This sudden emergence of an influenza virus with a completely new glycoprotein subtype in the human population is referred to as an antigenic shift, and if the virus also can spread efficiently from person to person, a worldwide epidemic known as a pandemic can result. Since 1889, at least five pandemics have occurred, with the most catastrophic being the Spanish influenza of 1918, which resulted in more than 20 million deaths worldwide.

Influenza viruses were first isolated in the early 1930s. The earliest vaccines against influenza were whole virus vaccines that were produced by growing the virus in embryonated chicken eggs and inactivating it with formalin. Starting in the 1940s, the U.S. military conducted clinical trials in healthy adults and demonstrated that the vaccine was 70 to 90 percent effective in preventing influenza provided there was a good match between the viruses in the vaccine and those causing the epidemic. In 1945, licenses were issued to several companies in the United State for the production of influenza vaccines. While contemporary inactivated influenza vaccines are still produced in embryonated eggs, a series of improvements in manufacturing over the years has resulted in a more highly purified split product or subunit vaccine that is less reactogenic. Today, inactivated influenza vaccines continue to be the primary means of preventing annual influenza disease and influenza-related complications in all age groups. Recommendations for the use of influenza vaccines in the United States include individuals 50 years of age or older and individuals 6 months of age and older with chronic underlying disease that places them at increased risk for complications from influenza disease. Over the last 10 years, annual influenza vaccination rates in persons 65 years of age or older have steadily risen; however, the effectiveness of the current vaccine in preventing influenza illness in some elderly populations can be as low as 30 to 40 percent. The goal of the Influenza Program at NIAID is to stimulate and support basic and applied research that leads to more effective approaches to controlling influenza virus infections, with an emphasis on exploring new ways of improving the effectiveness of influenza vaccines in naive populations and those at high risk, especially the elderly.

Over the last 25 years, NIAID and/or the private sector supported a series of clinical studies to assist in the development of a live-attenuated influenza vaccine. Live-attenuated influenza vaccines may be an attractive alternative to the inactivated vaccine because they are thought to stimulate local, humoral, and cellular immunity, and are administered intranasally. One approach has built on the cold-adapted influenza virus that was initially described by Dr. Hunein Maassab in 1967 at the University of Michigan. The unique characteristic of these cold-adapted influenza viruses is their ability to grow at 25°C and inability to grow at temperatures greater than 38°C (temperature sensitivity). This characteristic allows the virus to undergo limited replication in the cooler nasopharynx, but not the warmer lower respiratory tract. The first clinical studies with a cold-adapted, live-attenuated virus vaccine were done in 1976. NIAID-supported studies over the next 19 years evaluated monovalent, bivalent, and trivalent preparations of the cold-adapted virus vaccine in more than 8,000 adults and children. The results of these studies demonstrated that the live-attenuated influenza vaccine was safe, well tolerated, and likely to be at least as effective as the inactivated vaccine.

In 1995, NIAID signed a Cooperative Research and Development Agreement (CRADA) with Aviron for the continued development of a trivalent formulation of the live-attenuated influenza vaccine delivered with a nasal spray-syringe delivery system (FluMist™). Over the past 7 years, NIAID and Aviron have collaborated on more than nine clinical studies to test the safety, immunogenicity, and efficacy of FluMist™ in various populations. In 1997, the results of a phase III placebo-controlled efficacy study conducted by the Division of Microbiology and Infectious Diseases' (DMID's) Vaccine and Treatment Evaluation Units (VTEUs) in more than 1,600 children indicated that FluMist™ influenza vaccine was approximately 93 percent efficacious in preventing culture-confirmed cases of influenza. During the second year of the trial, the 1997 to 1998 formulation of FluMist™ was 100 percent efficacious against culture-con-

firmed influenza for strains included in the vaccine, and 86 percent efficacious against a mismatched influenza strain. Follow-on studies were done in 1998 to evaluate the efficacy against influenza A/H1N1, and in 1999 to assess the safety of revaccination of prior FluMist™ recipients. The results of this series of studies have shown that live-attenuated FluMist™ vaccine is safe, immunogenic, and efficacious in preventing culture-confirmed influenza virus illness. In addition, NIAID's VTEUs have evaluated the safety and immunogenicity of FluMist™ in high-risk groups, including human immunodeficiency virus (HIV)-infected adult and pediatric populations. In 1998, the safety and immunogenicity of a single dose of FluMist™ was evaluated in 57 asymptomatic or mildly symptomatic HIV-infected adults. HIV- and non-HIV-infected recipients of FluMist™ had a higher incidence of rhinorrhea on Days 2 and 3 postvaccination compared with placebo recipients; however, the rates of other local and systemic reactions were similar in HIV-infected and non-HIV-infected FluMist™ recipients as well as in FluMist™ recipients and placebo recipients. A similar study was initiated in 1999 to evaluate the safety of FluMist™ in HIV-infected children 1 to 7 years of age with aysmptomatic or mild HIV disease compared to non-HIV-infected children of similar age. Twenty-four HIV-infected and 25 non-HIV-infected children participated in the study. The results of this study indicated that FluMist™ was generally safe and well tolerated by children with asymptomatic or mildly symptomatic HIV infection. HIV RNA measurements, CD4 counts, and CD4 percentage in the peripheral blood remained stable throughout the 5-month study period in HIV-infected participants, and no evidence of increased shedding of the live-attenuated influenza vaccine viruses was detected in HIV-infected children in this study compared to the non-HIV-infected children. Aviron submitted a Biologics License Application for FluMist™ to the Food and Drug Administration (FDA) in 2000. The FDA review of the application is ongoing.

Although influenza vaccines have been reliably produced in embryonated chicken eggs for more than 50 years, new production technologies that reduce dependence on eggs are being increasingly sought. Forging partnerships with industry to develop non-egg-based technologies is an important part of NIAID's commitment to influenza vaccine development. In 2000, NIAID launched a new initiative to encourage private-sector involvement through its Challenge Grant Program. This milestone-driven mechanism is aimed at providing matching funds to companies also willing to commit their own dollars and resources. Three awards were made to private-sector companies for the development of egg-free influenza vaccine technologies and for the production of vaccines against influenza viruses with high pandemic potential. Awards were made to Aventis Pasteur for the development and testing of a DNA-based technology that will allow the rapid production of influenza vaccine candidates; to Aviron for the development of a live-attenuated influenza vaccine aimed at protection from possible pandemic strains; and to Novavax, Inc., for the production of a vaccine made with recombinant influenza proteins. Increasingly, other private-sector companies also are reporting progress on the development of novel mammalian cell lines as an alternative to egg-grown influenza vaccines.

The NIAID Influenza Program continues to support independent investigators and partnering with the private sector to develop and evaluate strategies aimed at improving the effectiveness of influenza vaccines. Additional NIAID collaborations on the development of new vaccine strategies have included the support of preclinical and clinical studies on the use of a variety of novel adjuvants, alternative delivery systems, and recombinant protein vaccines, as well as the evaluation of different doses of the inactivated vaccine.

Sources

Arden, N. H., Patriarca, P. A., & Kendal, A. P. (1986). Experiences in the use and efficacy of inactivated influenza vaccine in nursing homes. In A. P. Kendal & P. A. Patriarca (Eds.), *Options for the control of influenza* (pp. 155-168). New York: Alan R. Liss, Inc.

Belshe, R. B., Gruber, W. C., Mendelman, P. M., Cho, I., Reisinger, K., Block, S. L., Wittes, J., Iacuzio, D., Piedra, P., Treanor, J., King, J., Kotloff, K., Bernstein, D. I., Hayden, F. G., Zangwill, K., Yan, L., & Wolff, M. (2000, February). Efficacy of vaccination with live attenuated, cold-adapted, trivalent, intranasal influenza virus vaccine against a variant (A/Sydney) not contained in the vaccine. *Journal of Pediatrics, 36*(2), 168-175.

Belshe, R. B., Mendelman, P. M., Treanor, J., King, J., Gruber, W. C., Piedra, P., Bernstein, D. I., Hayden, F. G., Kotloff, K., Zangwill, K., Iacuzio, D., & Wolff, M. (1998, May 14). The efficacy of live attenuated, cold-adapted, trivalent, intranasal influenza virus vaccine in children. *New England Journal of Medicine, 338*(20), 1405-1412.

Centers for Disease Control and Prevention. (2002). Prevention and control of influenza: Recommendations of the Advisory Committee on Immunization Practices (ACIP). *Morbidity and Mortality Weekly Report, 51*(RR-03), 1-31.

Edwards, K. M., Dupont, W. D., Westrich, M. K., Plummer, W. D., Palmer, P. S., & Wright, P. F. (1994). A randomized controlled trial of cold-adapted and inactivated vaccines for the prevention of influenza A disease. *Journal of Infectious Diseases, 169*, 68-76.

Kilbourne, E. D. (1987). *Influenza.* New York: Plenum Medical Book Company.

King, J. C., Jr., Fast, P. E., Zangwill, K. M., Weinberg, G. A., Wolff, M., Yan, L., Newman, F., Belshe, R. B., Kovacs, A., Deville, J. G., & Jelonek, M. (2001, December). Safety, vaccine virus shedding and immunogenicity of trivalent, cold-adapted, live attenuated influenza vaccine administered to human immunodeficiency virus-infected and noninfected children. *Pediatric Infectious Disease Journal, 20*(12), 1124-1131.

King, J. C., Jr., Treanor, J., Fast, P. E., Wolff, M., Yan, L., Iacuzio, D., Readmond, B., O'Brien, D., Mallon, K., Highsmith, W. E., Lambert, J. S., & Belshe, R. B. (2000, February). Comparison of the safety, vaccine virus shedding, and immunogenicity of influenza virus vaccine, trivalent, types A and B, live cold-adapted, administered to human immunodeficiency virus (HIV)-infected and non-HIV-infected adults. *Journal of Infectious Diseases, 181*(2), 725-728.

Kistner, O., Barrett, P. N., Mundt, W., Reiter, M., Schober-Bendixen, S., & Dorner, F. (1998). Development of a mammalian cell (Vero) derived candidate influenza virus vaccine. *Vaccine, 16*, 960-968.

Maassab, H. F., Heilman, C. A., & Herlocher, M. L. (1990). Cold-adapted influenza viruses for use as live vaccines for man. In A. Mizrahi (Ed.), *Viral vaccines: Advances in biotechnological processes* (pp. 205-236). New York: Wiley-Liss Publishers.

National Institutes of Health, National Institute of Allergy and Infectious Diseases. (1997, July 14, Monday). *Nasal spray flu vaccine proves effective in children* [News Release].

Nichol, K. L., Margolis, K. L., Wuorwnma, J., & VonSternberg, T. (1994). The efficacy and cost effectiveness of vaccination against influenza among elderly persons living in the community. *New England Journal of Medicine, 331*(12), 778-784.

Patriarca, P. A., Weber, J. A., Parker, R. A., et al. (1985). Efficacy of influenza vaccine in nursing homes: Reduction in illness and complications during an influenza A (H3N2) epidemic. *Journal of the American Medical Association, 253*, 1136-1139.

Powers, D. C., Smith, G. E., Anderson, E. L., Kennedy, D. J., Hackett, C. S., Wilkinson, B. E., Volvovitz, F., Belshe, R. B., & Treanor, J. J. (1995). Influenza A virus vaccines containing purified recombinant H3 hemagglutinin are well tolerated and induce protective immune responses in healthy adults. *Journal of Infectious Diseases, 171*, 1595-1599.

MEASLES

Measles is still endemic in many countries and results in approximately 1 million deaths per year. However, the reported incidence of measles in the United States has been less than 1 case per million for the past few years (1997, 138 cases; 1998, 100 cases; 1999, 100 cases; 2000, 86 cases). Between 1981 and 1988, about 3,000 cases of measles occurred in the United States consistently each year. This rate was a reduction of more than 99 percent from the 400,000 to 700,000 annual cases reported before the introduction of a vaccine in 1963. However, in the early 1990s, a resurgence of measles occurred in the United States. From 1989 to 1991, there were 55,165 cases with 123 deaths reported. The major cause of the reemergence of measles in the United States was the failure to vaccinate children at the appropriate age rather than failure of vaccine efficacy. The United

States undertook a major effort to increase vaccine coverage, and in 2000, a total of 86 confirmed measles cases were reported, representing a record low number of measles cases. Of the 86 cases, 30 percent were imported, and 18 of the indigenous cases were linked to imported cases. In the past few years, there have been periods when there were no reports of indigenous cases, and transmission of the virus appears to have been interrupted.

Worldwide, measles reporting is incomplete, but the annual disease burden recently was estimated at 36.5 million measles cases and 1 million deaths. Measles remains a major health problem, accounting for 10 percent of global mortality from all causes among children younger than 5 years of age. There is substantial underreporting of measles cases, but the number of cases officially reported to WHO dropped from 1,330,589 in 1990 to 817,161 in 2000. The majority of these cases (520,120) were in the African region. Of the remaining cases, the European region accounted for 21,104; the Western Pacific region for 176,494; the Southeast Asia region for 61,975; the Eastern Mediterranean region for 34,971; and the American region for 2,515.

Measles vaccine coverage worldwide has gone from 12 percent in 1980 to 80 percent in 2000. The success of the polio eradication campaign and the success in reducing measles in the Americas have led to a global call for increased efforts to control measles worldwide. To accomplish this, measles control has incorporated lessons learned from the polio eradication campaign. For measles, this approach has been termed the "keep-up, catch-up, follow-up" program, and it has been extremely successful in many countries, particularly in South America. However, some countries have used other control strategies, and the U.S. experience with a two-dose immunization schedule demonstrates that maintenance of high levels of routine immunization also can lead to successful interruption of virus transmission.

Unfortunately, two recent experiences with measles have illustrated that many challenges remain for measles elimination programs. In 1997, despite a well-coordinated measles control program, measles reemerged in Brazil. By the middle of the year, the state of Sao Paulo reported more than 400 cases, after having virtually eliminated measles for the previous 6 years. In 1997 in Canada, despite a successful change from a one-dose to two-dose schedule and extensive catch-up campaigns, measles reemerged. An epidemic started after importation of measles into a university setting and spread within British Columbia and later to Alberta. These epidemics are being studied to understand their cause and to fine tune measles control strategies.

As a public health tool, the current vaccine has some deficiencies. It has a primary vaccine failure rate of about 5 percent; thus, susceptible individuals accumulate in the population. This failure rate is higher if the current vaccine is given to children younger than 12 months of age, when maternal antibody interferes with vaccine efficacy. In developing countries, where measles continues to claim more than 1 million lives each year, infants are at greatest risk for serious disease and complications

during the interval between loss of maternal antibody and receipt of vaccine, at 9 to 12 months of age. Because currently licensed vaccines have lower than desired efficacy in very young infants, research has been directed toward developing an effective vaccine that can be safely administered earlier in infancy. In addition, there is a potential need for an improved measles vaccine for future immunization schedules that will evolve to emphasize administration of vaccines at earlier ages in infancy and will make use of multiple combinations of vaccines.

To develop improved measles vaccines, research had concentrated on the selection of more potent measles vaccine strains or the development of high-titer vaccine formulations that might effectively immunize a higher percentage of vaccinees and might be given to infants at 6 months of age or younger. However, studies in some parts of the world had shown that high-titer vaccines might be associated with an increase in childhood mortality during a period of up to 2 years following immunization at 6 months of age. Although the reasons for this are not known, it was suggested that the immunosuppression that results from natural measles might occur with high-titer vaccines as well. Consequently, in 1992, WHO recommended that high-titer measles vaccines not be used.

Unfortunately, measles is a difficult virus to study because there are no satisfactory animal models. Within the past few years, basic and applied measles vaccine studies have been accelerated by complementary WHO and National Institutes of Health (NIH) funding for the development of a reliable measles monkey model. Considerable progress also has been made in applying basic molecular virology approaches to define the genetic, molecular, and antigenic characteristics of measles. After elucidation of the molecular structure of this virus, the major focus of research has been to express antigens (particularly antigenic sites on H, F, M, and N proteins) in a form suitable for use as a vaccine. A request for applications issued by NIAID in late 1992 stimulated measles research and resulted in the development of a number of new potential measles vaccine candidates, including immunostimulatory complexes (ISCOMs), nucleic acid vaccines, pox-vectored vaccines, viral subunit immunogens, and Bacillus de Calmette-Guerin (BCG)-vectored vaccines. In addition, this research program helped advance the development of the new primate model systems. These systems have been used to directly compare the immunogenicity of new potential vaccine candidates in nonimmune monkeys and in monkeys passively given measles antibody to mimic maternal antibody. Although data in primates are incomplete, it currently appears that ISCOMs, poxvirus vectored vaccines, and the nucleic acid vaccine have the greatest potential for inducing a protective immune response in the presence of maternal antibodies.

Primates also have been given standard vaccine, high-titer vaccine, and older killed vaccine (frozen old stocks and recreated 1960s-era products) in an attempt to use modern immunological tools to determine what caused the vaccine-related sequelae with inactivated vaccine in the 1960s and with live high-titer vaccine in the 1990s. It now appears that older killed vaccines induced an unbalanced immunological response that did not protect against wild-type measles.

Sources

Bell, A., King, A., Pielak, K., et al. (1997). Epidemiology of measles outbreak in British Columbia—February 1997. *Canada Communicable Disease Report, 23*(7), 49-51.

Buckland, R., & Wild, T. (1997). Is CD46 the cellular receptor for measles virus? *Virus Research, 48*(1), 1-9.

Case control study finds no link between measles vaccine and inflammatory bowel disease. (1997). *Communicable Disease Report. CDR Weekly, 7*(38), 339.

Centers for Disease Control and Prevention. (1997). Measles—United States, 1996, and the interruption of indigenous transmission. *Morbidity and Mortality Weekly Report, 46*(11), 242-246.

Centers for Disease Control and Prevention. (1997). Status report on the childhood immunization initiative: National, state, and urban area vaccination coverage levels among children aged 19-35 months—United States, 1996. *Journal of the American Medical Association, 278*(8), 622-623.

Centers for Disease Control and Prevention. (2002). Measles—United States, 2000. *Morbidity and Mortality Weekly Report, 51*(6), 120-123.

deQuadros, C., et al. (1996). Measles elimination in the Americas: Evolving strategies. *Journal of the American Medical Association, 275*(3), 224-229.

Etchart, N., et al. (1997). Class I-restricted CTL induction by mucosal immunization with naked DNA encoding measles virus haemagglutinin. *Journal of General Virology, 78*(Pt 7), 1577-1580.

Feeney, M., Ciegg, A., Winwood, P., et al. (1997). A case-control study of measles vaccination and inflammatory bowel disease. *Lancet, 350*(9080), 764-766.

Karp, C., et al. (1996). Mechanism of suppression of cell-mediated immunity by measles virus. *Science, 273*, 228-231.

Knudsen, K., et al. (1996). Child mortality following standard, medium, or high titer measles immunization in West Africa. *International Journal of Epidemiology, 25*(3), 665-673.

Reuman, P., Sawyer, M., Kuter, B., et al. (1997). Safety and immunogenicity of concurrent administration of measles-mumps-rubella-varicella vaccine and PedvaxHIB vaccines in healthy children twelve to eighteen months old. *Pediatric Infectious Disease Journal, 16*(7), 662-667.

World Health Organization. (2001). *Measles update*. Geneva, Switzerland: WHO Press.

World Health Organization Department of Vaccines and Biologicals. (2001). *WHO vaccine-preventable diseases: Monitoring system—2001 global summary*. www.who.int/vaccines-documents/.

Yang, K., et al. (1997). Early studies on DNA-based immunizations for measles virus. *Vaccine, 15*(8), 888-891.

MUMPS

Mumps vaccine was licensed in the United States in 1967. Since that time, the number of cases has dropped more than 99 percent to 338 in 2000. This drastic drop in cases occurred because of an increasingly inclusive vaccination policy at the State and Federal levels. The recent introduction of a second measles immunization using measles-mumps-rubella (MMR) vaccine has accelerated the reduction of mumps cases.

In contrast to the elimination of polio and measles, elimination of mumps has not been an important global health goal. However, a recent study indicates that elimination of mumps might not only eliminate the acute mumps illness, but might also eradicate endocardial fibroelastosis. The study screened for the presence of genome material of various viruses in autopsy tissue from 29 pediatric patients with endocardial fibroelastosis. This study included tissue samples from 1955 to 1992, and more than 70 percent of the heart tissue contained genetic material from the mumps virus. Only 1 of 65 matched controls contained any viral material, and that was from an enterovirus. Endocardial fibroelastosis was once relatively common, occurring in 1 of 5,000 births, but the cases have declined sharply. Interestingly, almost all the tissue samples before 1980 contained mumps viral material, whereas none after 1980 did.

Sources

Centers for Disease Control and Prevention. (2002). Summary of notifiable diseases—United States, 2000. *Morbidity and Mortality Weekly Report, 49*(53), 1-102.

Ni, J., et al. (1997). Viral infection of the myocardium in endocardial fibroelastosis: Molecular evidence for the role of mumps virus as an etiologic agent. *Circulation, 95*(1), 133-139.

Reuman, P., Sawyer, M., Kuter, B., et al. (1997). Safety and immunogenicity of concurrent administration of measles-mumps-rubella-varicella vaccine and PedvaxHIB vaccines in healthy children twelve to eighteen months old. *Pediatric Infectious Disease Journal, 16*(7), 662-667.

World Health Organization. (1996). *State of the world's vaccines and immunization*. Geneva, Switzerland: WHO Press.

RUBELLA

Worldwide, rubella remains a common benign febrile disease of childhood. The most serious effects of rubella—spontaneous abortions, miscarriages, stillbirths, and congenital rubella syndrome (CRS)—follow infection during early pregnancy. The currently licensed vaccine is highly effective, and its combined use with measles and mumps vaccines in childhood immunization programs has drastically reduced the number of cases of rubella in the United States. From 1969 to 1989, the number of cases of rubella reported annually dropped 99.6 percent. Although there was a slight reemergence of rubella cases between 1989 and 1992, from 1992 to 2000, an average of only 100 to 200 rubella cases occurred annually. Most recently, rubella has occurred in adults born in countries without rubella immunization programs. It is estimated that the average cost of a single case of CRS is more than $500,000. Sixty-seven cases of CRS were reported in the United States in 1970, the year the vaccine was licensed, and except for the reemergence of CRS in the early 1990s (33 cases in 1991), CRS cases have steadily declined, with only 9 cases reported in 2000.

It can be generally concluded that in the developing world, natural rubella infection occurs early in life and almost universally. In such a situation, unless the epidemiology of rubella changes, there is no pressing need to immunize against rubella. However, recently it came to the attention of WHO officials that many countries, on their own, have purchased MMR for their measles campaigns, and thus have already started to alter the natural circulation of rubella. Once this interference has occurred and "natural immunization" with rubella is not universal, rubella immunization programs must be continued aggressively. Consequently, rubella control and eradication have again been catapulted into the public health spotlight.

The epidemiology of rubella in the United States has changed from the 1980s in that since 1994, 84 percent of the cases occur in patients older than 15. Apparently, most cases occur among unvaccinated adults born in countries without immunization programs. Ninety-three percent of cases were indigenous to the United States; many imported cases came from countries that do not routinely provide rubella immunization (e.g., Mexico). From 1991 to 2000, the percentage of cases among Hispanics increased from 19 percent to 78 percent. Therefore, immunization programs now focus more efforts on adolescents and adults and on selected ethnic groups that have lower rates of immunization and have close contact with people coming from countries without comprehensive rubella immunization programs. Attempts to eliminate rubella from the United States would clearly benefit from improved global immunization programs.

Although the total number of cases of rubella is low and the number of cases of CRS is limited, the recent reemergence of natural rubella led to a campaign to increase vaccination coverage in all age groups in the United States. Consequently, many adult women were immunized against rubella, and a longstanding concern was again raised about possible vaccine-associated arthritic complications in these women. Early reports of naturally occurring rubella epidemics noted an increased incidence of arthropathy, predominantly in adult women. Like natural rubella, there are reports that the rubella vaccine causes transient joint symptoms in a significant proportion of women vaccinees. Joint complaints have been reported in up to 25 percent of previously seronegative vaccinees; these symptoms may last from 1 day to 3 weeks after immunization. Investigators in Canada had reported preliminary data indicating that a small percentage of adult female vaccinees develop a more severe and persistent arthropathy. One suggestion was that these complications might increase with the age of the vaccinee or the presence of low or incomplete rubella immunity. The causal relationship of rubella vaccination to the acute type of arthritis was highlighted in a recent Institute of Medicine report on vaccine safety, but its relationship to chronic arthritis remains unclear. Two large studies of immunized populations suggested that long-term arthritic complications are not commonly associated with rubella immunization. More basic research studies have shown that for rubella virus to replicate, it must bind to host cellular proteins. These cellular proteins are under investigation as to their potential role as autoantigens and their potential contribution to arthropathy.

Basic research on rubella is now proceeding at a reduced level of funding, and NIAID currently supports only one project dealing with rubella. This research is focused on identifying and characterizing virus gene products required for generating long-lasting immunity, as well as those associated with the expression of adverse effects.

Sources

Centers for Disease Control and Prevention. (1997). Recommended childhood immunization schedule—United States, 1997. *Journal of the American Medical Association, 277*(5), 371-372.

Centers for Disease Control and Prevention. (1997). Status report on the childhood immunization initiative: National, state, and urban area vaccination coverage levels among children aged 19-35 months—United States, 1996. *Journal of the American Medical Association, 278*(8), 622-623.

Centers for Disease Control and Prevention. (2001). Control and prevention of rubella: Evaluation and management of suspected outbreaks, rubella in pregnant women, and surveillance for congenital rubella syndrome. *Morbidity and Mortality Weekly Report, 50*(RR12), 1-23.

Centers for Disease Control and Prevention. (2002). Summary of notifiable diseases—United States, 2000. *Morbidity and Mortality Weekly Report, 49*(53), 1-102.

Cutts, F., Robertson, S., Diaz-Ortega, J., et al. (1997). Control of rubella and congenital rubella syndrome (CRS) in developing countries, Part 1: Burden of disease from CRS. *Bulletin of the World Health Organization, 75*(1), 55-68.

Pugachev, K., Abernathy, E., & Frey, T. (1997). Genomic sequence of the RA27/3 vaccine strain of rubella virus. *Archives of Virology, 142*(6), 1165-1180.

Ray, P., et al. (1997). Risk of chronic arthropathy among women after rubella vaccination. Vaccine Safety Datalink Team. *Journal of the American Medical Association, 278*(7), 551-556.

Reuman, P., Sawyer, M., Kuter, B., et al. (1997). Safety and immunogenicity of concurrent administration of measles-mumps-rubella-varicella vaccine and PedvaxHIB vaccines in healthy children twelve to eighteen months old. *Pediatric Infectious Disease Journal, 16*(7), 662-667.

Robertson, S., Cutts, F., Samuel, R., et al. (1997). Control of rubella and congenital rubella syndrome (CRS) in developing countries, Part 2: Vaccination against rubella. *Bulletin of the World Health Organization, 75*(1), 69-80.

Slater, P. E. (1997). Chronic arthropathy after rubella vaccination in women: False alarm? *Journal of the American Medical Association, 278*(7), 594-595.

Tingle, A. J., et al. (1997). Randomised double-blind placebo-controlled study on adverse effects of rubella immunization in seronegative women. *Lancet, 349*(9061), 1277-1281.

World Health Organization. (1996). *State of the world's vaccines and immunization.* Geneva, Switzerland: WHO Press.

MENINGOCOCCAL DISEASE

Introduction

Neisseria meningitidis (NM) is the leading cause of bacterial meningitis and continues to be a major public health problem, not only in the United States, but also worldwide. The organism also causes pneumonia (frequently caused by serogroup Y), conjunctivitis, sinusitis, and myocarditis. Although the disease has a more severe impact on children and young adults, all age groups are susceptible to infection. In the United States, there are an estimated 3,000 cases per year involving meningococcal serogroups B, C, and recently Y. However, in other parts of the world, the number of cases is much higher. For example, in sub-Saharan Africa during the 1996 epidemics caused by serogroup A, more than 200,000 cases were reported, with 20,000 deaths; the role of malnutrition as a contributory factor has never been addressed adequately. The case fatality for meningococcal disease in the United States remains high, approximately 12 percent, but is higher for individuals less than 1 year old or greater than 65 years old, and for individuals in sub-Saharan Africa. Significant proportions of the children who survive infections caused by NM have permanent side effects, such as deafness. A significant change in the burden of disease within the past 20 years is the increased incidence among individuals 15 to 24 years of age, particularly among college freshmen living in dormitories. As

such, the Advisory Committee on Immunization Practices has recommended that healthcare providers and college staff advise students about the availability and benefits of the licensed vaccine. The emergence of new strains of meningococci and penicillin-resistant meningococci in the United States has further complicated the picture and caused serious public health concerns.

A major gap in understanding the pathogenesis of meningococcal disease is the relationship between carriage of meningococci and invasive meningococcal disease. Most meningococci possess a polysaccharide capsule, which forms the basis of classification into serogroups. The presence of the capsule helps the organisms resist phagocytosis. Studies show that the capsule not only alters the adherence of the organisms to leukocytes, but also alters the interaction with lysosomes within the cells. An additional, recently discovered virulence mechanism is the ability of meningococci to escape protective immunity by switching capsules via genetic transformation. The organisms also carry pili that facilitate adherence to host cells and possess a large number of OMPs, including Opc and Opa, which appear to mediate invasion of epithelial cells. Further, some of these proteins (e.g., the pili and Opas) show considerable antigenic variation. This phenomenon of antigen variation poses a challenge for the immune system and for vaccine development. The organisms are also capable of secreting proteins (e.g., FrpA and FrpC) with potential toxicity and IgA protease, which can cleave human IgA; however, the role of these molecules in pathogenesis is still not clear. Another important virulence factor is endotoxin. Unlike the endotoxin of enterobacteria, this molecule contains short sugar chains and hence is termed LOS. Studies indicate that LOS is important for colonization in the nasopharynx. Additionally, the release of meningococcal LOS contributes to the hypotension and shock associated with fulminant meningococcemia. Also, LOS and other meningococcal components can induce a variety of cytokines and other mediators of the immune response that have a significant impact on the course of the infection.

Research Accomplishments

In the past two decades, several studies have been conducted to examine the immunopathogenesis of host and pathogen interactions and how such information could be used in the development of vaccines. For example, although meningococci are carried asymptomatically in the nasopharynx of 5 to 10 percent of normal individuals during nonendemic periods, it is still not clear why some individuals become susceptible to invasive meningococcal disease. It is known that individuals with complement deficiencies, who are malnourished or immunosuppressed, or who are asplenic patients, are particularly at high risk. The results of a study designed to address the issue of genetic predisposition to meningococcal disease suggest that there is a genetic inheritance pattern among families with respect to the amount of cytokines produced. These results also suggest that the type of cytokines produced may be associated with the risk of fatal disease. Other studies have demonstrated the presence of decreased plasma levels of coagulation factors and increased expression of cellular adhesion molecules in meningococcal patients, and that IL-12, TNF, and interferon gamma may contribute to natural immunity. The results of another study aimed at understanding the mechanisms of genetic susceptibility suggest that genetic variants of the mannose-binding lectin (MBL), a plasma protein involved in complement activation, may also be associated with susceptibility to the disease. Further, a recent study in children with severe meningococcal diseases indicating that protein C activation is impaired may explain the lack of regulation of intravascular thrombosis. An important recent advance was the sequencing of the genome of NM serogroups A, B, and C. It is expected that this should provide insights into the virulence capacity of the organism, a better understanding of phase variation, and an understanding of the mechanism that controls the expression of virulence determinants.

Progress in Vaccine Development

The currently licensed vaccines based on purified capsular polysaccharides from four major serogroups (A, C, W135, and Y) are moderately immunogenic, but the immune response, in general, is of short duration and cannot be boosted upon reimmunization. Also, polysaccharide vaccines do not elicit an immune response in children less than 2 years of age. Interestingly, group A capsular polysaccharide vaccine is moderately immunogenic in this age group; the underlying mechanism of this unique response is not clear. A current attractive strategy in vaccine development is to use polysaccharide-protein conjugate vaccines to enhance the immunogenicity of the polysaccharide moiety and to induce memory. In one study in the United Kingdom, it was observed that meningococcal group C conjugate vaccine is immunogenic in infants and also induces a memory response. This vaccine has now been recommended for routine immunization schedule, and its introduction in the United Kingdom in 1999 had a tremendous impact on the incidence of the disease. Conjugate vaccine trials are underway in the United States, and it is expected that such a vaccine will become available in 4 years.

There are no licensed vaccines for group B meningococcal infections in the United States, and the development of vaccines against group B strains remains problematic. Unlike the other meningococcal capsular polysaccharides, the group B polysaccharide is poorly immunogenic in infants and adults. Further, there are important concerns that a polysaccharide vaccine might induce immunopathology, such as the formation of cross-reactive autoantibodies to specific oligosaccharides also found on mammalian cells. For example, antigroup B polysaccharide antibodies cross-react with the neural cellular adhesion molecule, a membrane glycoprotein involved in cell-cell adhesion. Such concerns have prompted the pursuit of alternative strategies for group B vaccine development using mainly meningococcal OMPs, targeting lactoferrin and transferrin-binding proteins, and modifying sugar moieties on the capsular polysaccharide. Studies indicate that OMPs can induce protection. For

instance, it has been shown in an infant rat model that antibodies to PorA proteins are protective against meningococcal infections. Protein-based vaccines have been used in clinical trials in Cuba, Brazil, Chile, and Norway, with efficacies ranging from 50 to 80 percent. Unfortunately, these vaccines induced no protection in children, and the immune response was of short duration. Efforts to identify a common protective protein antigen for serogroup B has thus far been unsuccessful; however, research continues using newer approaches to identify and develop potential candidates. For example, in a recent study using computer analysis to identify regions of the NM genome that encodes novel surface exposed proteins, 600 novel proteins were predicted. The results of further studies showed that at least 25 of these proteins induce bactericidal antibodies in mice. More importantly, some of these proteins are highly conserved in several meningococcal strains tested, and can induce protection against lethal challenge in mice. Other current vaccine approaches include: 1) Multivalent OMP vesicle vaccine in which vaccine strains are constructed by recombinant DNA techniques to express three different PorA proteins, which is currently undergoing clinical trials; 2) A/B (chemically modified group B polysaccharide)/C combination vaccine; and 3) anti-idiotype group B vaccine.

Challenges

The development of a new and improved vaccine, in the context of an optimal adjuvant/delivery system that is safe and immunogenic in children, would have a tremendous impact in decreasing the incidence of the disease. Development of a vaccine against group B meningococci remains a major challenge. In addition, because of the low incidence of the disease, clinical trials of vaccine efficacy are often difficult to conduct. Another important task is to understand why certain individuals within a given population succumb to the fatal disease and others do not. Studies using a number of adjuvants, including monophosphoryl lipid A and Quil A, and neisserial porins to enhance the immune response to meningococcal vaccines represent a significant advance; however, more studies are needed to analyze the effects on Ig subclasses. Also, basic research studies should be encouraged to analyze the biological, structural, and molecular aspects of potential virulence factors and to identify novel bacterial components that may serve as potential vaccine targets.

Sources

Ada, G. (2001). Vaccines and vaccination. *New England Journal of Medicine, 345,* 1042-1053.

Centers for Disease Control and Prevention. (1996). Serogroup Y meningococcal disease—Illinois, Connecticut, and selected areas, United States, 1989-1996. *Morbidity and Mortality Weekly Report, 45* (46), 1010-1014.

Faust, S. N., et al. (2001). Dysfunction of endothelial protein C activation in severe meningococcal sepsis. *New England Journal of Medicine, 345,* 408-416.

Fusco, P. C., Michon, F., Tai, J., & Blake, M. (1997). Preclinical evaluation of a novel group B meningococcal conjugate vaccine that elicits bactericidal activity in both mice and nonhuman primates. *Journal of Infectious Diseases, 175,* 364-372.

Jack, D. L., Read, R. C., Tenner, A. J., Frosch, M., Turner, M. W., & Klein, N. J. (2001). Mannose-binding lectin regulates the inflammatory response of human professional phagocytes to *Neisseria meningitidis* serogroup B. *Journal of Infectious Diseases, 184,* 1152-1162.

Poolman, J. T. (1995). Development of a meningococcal vaccine. *Infectious Agents and Disease, 4,* 13-28.

Rappuoli, R. (2001). Conjugates and reverse vaccinology to eliminate bacterial meningitis. *Vaccine, 19,* 2319-2322.

Robbins, J. B., Schneerson, R., & Szu, S. (1995). Perspective: Hypothesis: Serum IgG is sufficient to confer protection against infectious diseases by inactivating the inoculum. *Journal of Infectious Diseases, 171,* 1387-1398.

Romero, J. D., & Outschoorn, M. (1997). The immune response to the capsular polysaccharide of *Neisseria meningitidis* group B. *Zentralbl Bakteriol, 285,* 331-340.

Semba, R., Bulterys, M., Munyeshuli, V., Gatzingi, T., Saah, A., Chao, A., & Dushimimana, A. (1996). Vitamin A deficiency and T-cell subpopulations in children with meningococcal disease. *Journal of Tropical Pediatrics, 42,* 287-290.

Virji, M. (1996). Meningococcal disease: Epidemiology and pathogenesis. *Trends in Microbiology, 4,* 466-469.

Westendrop, R. G. J., Langermans, J. A. M., Huizinga, T. W. J., Elouali, A. H., Verweij, C. I., Boomsma, D. I., & Vanderbrouke, J. P. (1997). Genetic influence on cytokine production and fatal meningococcal disease. *Lancet, 349,* 170-173.

Wise, J. (1999). UK introduces new meningitis C vaccine. *BMJ, 319,* 278.

Moraxella Catarrhalis

M. catarrhalis, once thought to be a harmless commensal organism, has become recognized over the last decade as an important human pathogen. Today, *M. catarrhalis* is the third most common cause of bacterial otitis media in children, after *S. pneumoniae* and nontypeable *H. influenzae*. Otitis media is a major cause of morbidity in the pediatric population in developed countries and is the most frequent diagnosis made by healthcare providers regarding this age group in the acute healthcare setting. It is estimated that 3.5 million episodes of otitis media per year are caused by *M. catarrhalis*. An effective otitis media vaccine most likely will need to provide immunity to all three organisms. *M. catarrhalis* is also a frequent cause of sinusitis in this age group. In adults, this organism is an important cause of LRIs, particularly in the setting of COPD, where it has become the third most common bacterial agent responsible for acute exacerbation of COPD. The organism also plays a significant role in other LRIs in adults, including pneumonia and laryngotracheobronchitis, and is infrequently the cause of septicemia, meningitis, and endocarditis in immunocompromised adults.

Work has progressed rapidly during the past several years to identify two major OMPs (OMP CD and OMP E) associated with *M. catarrhalis*. Both proteins are considered potential vaccine candidates to prevent infections caused by this bacterium. So far, the genes have been cloned and the characteristics of these proteins have been studied. These proteins are abundantly expressed on the bacterial surface and show a high degree of similarity from strain to strain. These two characteristics are important as potential vaccine antigens. A protein antigen is likely to be immunogenic in infants, and this is an important consideration in preventing otitis media. Work is in progress to define the precise structure and epitopes of these proteins and to test rigorously whether antibodies to these proteins will protect against infection caused by *M. catarrhalis*.

It was recently shown that the UspA1 protein of the *M. catarrhalis* bacterium is an adhesin that allows this organism to attach to human epithelial cells. This finding makes it likely that UspA1 is involved in the ability of *M. catarrhalis* to colonize the human upper respiratory tract (i.e., the nasopharynx), which is the first crucial step in the production of disease by this pathogen. If this is the case, then antibodies to UspA1, raised in response to vaccination with purified UspA1 protein, could prevent this organism from establishing a foothold in the body, thereby eliminating disease.

An important finding about the UspA1 protein is that it forms structures that actually stick out from the surface of the *M. catarrhalis* bacterium. These pili represent the first parts of the bacterium to encounter human cells when it enters the nasopharynx. This finding also means that antibody directed against the UspA1 protein can bind readily to this protein and exert a protective effect. A second important finding is that the portion of the UspA1 protein that is involved in the ability of this bacterium to bind to human cells is located in the front half of the protein. The UspA1 protein is a very big molecule, and this new piece of information will allow scientists to focus vaccine development efforts on the relevant portion of this protein.

Two other highly conserved OMPs also have been investigated as potential vaccine candidates. Both of these antigens, referred to as B1 and LBP, are iron-regulated proteins found on the surface of this gram-negative pathogen in response to iron-limiting conditions in its environment. Several studies have been conducted demonstrating the importance of these surface proteins and their exposed epitopes in the pathogenesis of disease and for survival in the host.

Finally, efforts are underway to develop a serotyping system based on the iron-repressible OMP B2, which has a high degree of antigenic and sequence heterogeneity. Restriction fragment length polymorphism analysis indicates that the pattern of variable and constant areas in the B2 gene is a general pattern among all strains of *M. catarrhalis*. Developing such a serotyping system for strains of *M. catarrhalis* will be important to understand the epidemiology of infection to guide future vaccine studies with this organism.

Suggested Reading

Aebi, C., et al. (1996). Expression of the CopB outer membrane protein by *Moraxella catarrhalis* is regulated by iron and affects iron acquisition from transferrin and lactoferrin. *Infection and Immunity, 64*, 2024-2030.

Campagnari, A. A., Ducey, T. F., & Rebmann, C. A. (1996). OMP B1, an iron-repressible protein conserved in the outer membrane of *Branhamella* (*Moraxella*) *catarrhalis*, binds human transferin. *Infection and Immunity, 64*, 3920-3924.

Cope, L. D., et al. (1999). Characterization of the *Moraxella catarrhalis* uspA1 and uspA2 genes and their encoded products. *Journal of Bacteriology, 181*, 4026-4034.

Lafontaine, E. R., Cope, L. D., Aebi, J. L., Latimr, G. H., McCracken, J. R., & Hansen, E. J. (2000). The UspA1 protein and a second type of UspA2 protein mediate adherence of *Moraxella catarrhalis* to human epithelial cells *in vitro*. *Journal of Bacteriology, 182*, 1364-1373.

Murphy, T. F. (1996). *Branhamella catarrhalis*: Epidemiology, surface antigenic structure, and immune response. *Microbiological Reviews, 60*, 267-279.

MYCOPLASMA PNEUMONIAE

Background

In the United States, about 15 million respiratory infections, including atypical pneumoniae and tracheobronchitis, are caused by *Mycoplasma pneumoniae* each year. *M. pneumoniae* is the leading cause of pneumonia in older children and young adults, but it also affects adults and elderly individuals. This microorganism is responsible for 25 percent of all cases of pneumonia requiring hospitalization, and 50 percent of all pneumonias in closed populations, and is the second leading cause of tracheobronchitis in children. *M. pneumoniae* is also responsible for extrapulmonary complications such as arthritis and has been associated with chronic asthma. Related organisms, such as *Mycoplasma hominis* and *Ureoplasma urealyticum*, cause pulmonary diseases in neonates.

Mycoplasmas are wall-less prokaryotes that are biosynthetically deficient in several respects. Therefore, they must rely on the microenvironment provided by the host to obtain essential metabolites (nucleotides, fatty acids, sterols, and amino acids)

needed for growth. Mycoplasmas possess a circular double-stranded DNA chromosome ranging from 600 to 1,300 kilobases, with complex genetic recombination systems and large genome families. The organism has a tremendous capacity to generate antigenic and phase variations that may be important in disease pathogenesis and tissue tropism, but this characteristic poses a special challenge for vaccine development.

Although mycoplasmas are responsible for a variety of important diseases in humans and various animal species, experimental vaccines have not affected the spread of infection, possibly the result of the organism's ability to develop antigenic changes at high frequency. This difficulty in controlling the infection may be due also to a lack of understanding about the host response to infections caused by mycoplasmas. Because previous studies indicate that patients with impaired humoral immunity suffer chronic sinopulmonary disease due to mycoplasma, it is generally held that antibody plays a role in immunity. However, the role of cell-mediated immunity has not been investigated adequately.

Research Accomplishments

Most studies within the last 2 decades have been focused on understanding the molecular biology of the organisms and on elucidating the molecular mechanisms of pathogenesis and the host responses in an effort to improve the methods of diagnosis and to develop better prevention and treatment strategies. An important resource in current understanding of mycoplasmal-host-cell interactions has been the development of *in vitro* and organ culture systems using fluoresence, confocal, conventional, and scanning electron microscopy, as well as new strides made in imaging technologies. Studies using these tools have provided considerable information in virulence strategies. In recent years, intense effort has been made to understand the mechanisms of mycoplasmal attachment to host epithelial cells, an event that has been described as cytadherence. The process of cytadherence is pivotal to the survival of *M. pneumoniae*, and its ability to persist in the host. The mycoplasmal attachment organelle has been identified. Molecular characterization studies continue on the P1 adhesin protein, which is densely clustered at the attachment organelle, and on a series of cytadherence-associated proteins (HMW1-3). The complete genome of *M. pneumoniae* has been sequenced, and it is anticipated that this will advance significantly understanding and knowledge about the physiological and genetic characteristics and may provide new leads for vaccine development.

Progress in Vaccine Development

Considerable efforts also have been made in the development of vaccines against infections caused by *M. pneumoniae*. Earlier challenge studies in the late 1960s conducted in human volunteers demonstrated that an inactivated *M. pneumoniae* vaccine was moderately protective, but these studies have not been developed further. Studies done in chimpanzees indicated that animals immunized with a formalin-inactivated vaccine or an acellular extract developed milder disease and lower colonization rates with mycoplasma compared with unimmunized controls. Because only partial protection was observed in such experiments, more studies are needed to increase the level of protection expressed. Some of the early vaccine studies were problematic because of the development of immunopathological reactions following challenge with live organisms. It is believed that this autoimmune response was mediated by cellular immunity. However, studies are still needed to clarify the roles of humoral and cell-mediated immunity in generating optimal immunity. An experimental vaccine derived from *Mycoplasma pulmonis* (the agent of murine mycoplasmosis) has been shown to induce protective antibodies; however, other approaches are still necessary.

Challenges

Studies should continue in order to understand the epidemiology of diseases caused by *M. pneumoniae*, to understand the molecular pathogenesis, and to develop powerful diagnostic technology. Indeed, the diagnosis of *M. pneumoniae* has been hampered by the lack of standardization of rapid methods. It is critical that new targets for intervention are identified, and appropriate animal models are developed. For example, it would be useful to understand the involvement of proteases in mycoplasmal growth, to evaluate the use of protease inhibitors on infections caused by mycoplasmas, or to assess newly developed candidate vaccines. There is a tremendous gap in understanding the role of humoral and cell-mediated immune responses. For example, studies should be conducted to examine the role of Th1 versus Th2 subpopulations in resistance or susceptibility to infection. In addition, it is important that the role of cytokines and inflammatory mediators as well as cellular adhesion molecules and mechanisms of T-cell activation be clarified. Further, the significance of immunopathological reactions in the development of chronic diseases associated with *M. pneumoniae* needs to be investigated. Besides the efforts to understand the host immune response, the ability of the organism to develop antigenic changes remains a major challenge in vaccine development.

Sources

Barile, M., Grabowski, M., Kapatais-Zoumbois, K., Brown, B., Hu, P., & Chandler, D. (1994). Protection of immunized and previously infected chimpanzees challenged with *Mycoplasma pneumoniae*. *Vaccine, 12,* 707-714.

Baseman, J. B., & Tully, J. G. (1997). Mycoplasmas: Sophisticated, reemerging, and burdened by their notoriety. *Emerging Infectious Diseases, 3,* 21-32.

Cassell, G. (1998). Infectious causes of chronic inflammatory diseases and cancer. *Emerging Infectious Diseases, 4,* 475-487.

Cimolai, N., Mah, D., Taylor, G., & Morrison, B. (1995). Bases for the early immune response after rechallenge or component vac-

cination in an animal model of acute *Mycoplasma pneumoniae* pneumonitis. *Vaccine, 13,* 305-309.

Clyde, W. A. (1983). *Mycoplasma pneumoniae* respiratory disease symposium: Summation and significance. *Yale Journal of Biology and Medicine, 56,* 523-527.

Dybvig, K., & Voelker, L. (1996). Molecular biology of mycoplasmas. *Annual Review of Microbiology, 50,* 25-57.

Hammerschlag, M. R. (2001). *Mycoplasma pneumoniae* infections. *Current Opinions in Infectious Diseases, 14,* 181-186.

Himmelreich, R., Plagens, H., Hilbert, H., Reiner, B., & Herrmann, R. (1997). Comparative analysis of the genomes of the bacteria *Mycoplasma pneumoniae* and *Mycoplasma genitalium*. *Nucleic Acids Research, 25,* 701-712.

Romero-Arroyo, C. E., Jordan, J., Peacock, S. J., Willby, M. J., Farmer, M. A., & Krause, D. C. (1999). *Mycoplasma pneumoniae* protein P30 is required for cytadherence and associated with proper cell development. *Journal of Bacteriology, 181,* 1079-1087.

Seggev, J., Sedmak, G., & Kurup, V. (1996). Isotype-specific antibody responses to acute *Mycoplasma pneumoniae* infection. *Annals of Allergy, Asthma & Immunology, 77,* 67-73.

Smith, C., Freidewald, W., & Chanock, R. (1967). Inactivated Mycoplasma pneumoniae vaccine. *Journal of the American Medical Association, 199,* 103-108.

PARAINFLUENZA VIRUS

The human parainfluenza viruses (HPIVs) consist of four serotypes (HPIV1 to 4). They are common seasonal respiratory pathogens that cause a range of diseases from mild URIs to life-threatening LRIs. HPIV3 is the second leading cause of bronchiolitis and pneumonia in infants and children less than 6 months of age, and also causes croup and laryngitis in infants and children. In contrast, most of the illness caused by HPIV1 and HPIV2 occurs after 6 months of age. HPIV4 has been associated with mild upper respiratory tract illness in children and adults. Recently, HPIVs have been reported to cause severe lower respiratory tract disease in bone marrow transplant recipients and in lung transplant recipients.

Although development of a vaccine to prevent parainfluenza infections has been a high priority at NIAID (see Appendix A, table of priority vaccines from first *Jordan Report*), a licensed vaccine is not available yet. The first *Jordan Report* indicated that a subunit vaccine for HPIV3 was being developed. The basis of this approach involved the protective antigens of HPIVs, i.e., the hemagglutinin-neuraminidase (HN) glycoprotein (the attachment protein) and the fusion (F) glycoprotein. Several PIV3 vaccine candidates have been produced by either purifying the HN and F proteins from native virus or by recombinant technology. Animal studies of these vaccines in hamsters and cotton rats have demonstrated protection against live virus challenge. A trivalent vaccine containing HN and F proteins of 1, 2, and 3 adjuvanted with aluminum phosphate elicited neutralizing antibodies in mice. Although these studies provide the basis for continued development of a PIV subunit vaccine, progress has been impeded by weak immunogenicity of purified proteins in immunologically naive subjects and the need for a safe adjuvant.

A number of alternative methodologies have been pursued for PIV vaccine development. A vaccine consisting of formalin-inactivated PIV was evaluated in infants in the 1960s. Although this vaccine was safe (i.e., no enhanced disease was observed), it was not sufficiently immunogenic to be protective. A more recent approach to vaccine development involves live-attenuated parainfluenza strains from either human or bovine origin. A wild-type HPIV3 strain was cultivated at low temperature for 45 passages, and mutant strains of different passage number were evaluated in nonhuman primates. Because the HPIV3cp45 virus was shown to be more attenuated than other strains in these studies, this strain was selected for human clinical trials. The safety, infectivity, and immunogenicity of HPIV3cp45 have been evaluated in a phase I, randomized, double-blind, placebo-controlled study in children 6 months to 10 years of age. The vaccine was well tolerated when administered intranasally to seropositive and seronegative children. This study indicated that the HPIV3cp45 vaccine is satisfactorily attenuated, infectious, immunogenic, and phenotypically stable. A phase II study is in progress to further evaluate this promising vaccine candidate.

Another approach to protect against infection with HPIV3 has been the use of bovine PIV3 (BPIV3) as a candidate live-virus vaccine. There are several reasons for this strategy. First, BPIV3 is antigenically related to HPIV3, as shown by sequence analyses and cross-neutralization studies of HN and F proteins of HPIV3 and BPIV3. In addition, the natural host range restriction of replication in humans results in an attenuated phenotype. This approach to immunization against viral pathogens, employing an antigenically related animal virus as a vaccine for humans, has been described as "Jennerian" and has been successful for other viral pathogens. Studies in cotton rats and nonhuman primates led to human trials. Results of these studies confirmed the attenuated phenotype and demonstrated induction of an immune response. The first study involved administration of BPIV3 to adults. This clinical trial demonstrated that the vaccine was avirulent and that replication of the virus was restricted. This clinical trial was followed by several studies in infants and children, which are briefly summarized here. A phase I, randomized, double-blind, placebo-controlled BPIV3 clinical trial was conducted initially in 6- to 60-month-old seropositive infants and children and then subsequently in seronegative infants and children. A second dose of BPIV3 vaccine was administered 2 months after the initial dose to a subset of sernonegative infants and children. A second study evaluated the BPIV3 vaccine in a larger group of seronegative infants and children, divided into groups of 2- to 6-month-old infants and 6- to 36-month-old infants and children. Most recently, a phase II clinical trial was conducted in which the BPIV3 vaccine was administered at ages 2, 4, 6, and 12 to 15 months. In these clinical trials, the BPIV3 vaccine was administered intranasally. All studies indicate that this live-virus vaccine is attenuated, infectious, immunogenic, and phenotypically stable in infants and children, and this approach should be further evaluated.

Reverse genetics is the most significant scientific advance in the development of a PIV vaccine. For the PIVs, this technology was first reported in 1997 with the recovery of infectious HPIV3 from viral genome cDNA. During the past few years, reverse genetic systems have been reported for the recovery of BPIV, PIV1, and PIV2 from cDNA. This methodology has been used successfully to identify regions of cold-passaged PIV and BPIV that contribute to the attenuation phenotype. Once identified, the attenuating mutations can be introduced into cDNA. Thus, using this technology the genetic basis of attenuation has been defined and is being used to construct improved attenuated vaccine candidates. In addition, recombinant viruses produced using reverse genetics can be modified by replacement of protective antigens from heterologous PIV strains to develop additional vaccine candidates. Recombinant chimeric PIVs that contain the attenuating mutations from well-characterized PIV vaccine candidate viruses and protective antigens of other PIV strains have been generated. For example, rBPIV3 was derived from BPIV3 cDNA and used to construct rB/HPIV3, a chimeric virus in which the F and HN genes of BPIV3 were replaced with their HPIV3 counterparts. Another recombinant live-virus vaccine candidate, designated as rHPIV3-1cp45, contains the attenuated background of the rHPIV3cp45 virus together with the HN and F protective antigens of HPIV1. Reverse genetics also was used to construct rPIV3-1.2HN, a bivalent vaccine virus against HPIV1 and HPIV2, using a recombinant HPIV3 backbone. These chimeric vaccine viruses are promising candidates for protection against PIV illness.

Another Jennerian vaccine to be considered is the use of Sendai virus to protect against HPIV1, since these viruses have a close antigenic relatedness. Studies on immunogenicity and level of attenuation are in progress.

A number of vaccines to protect against HPIV disease are in various stages of development. The most promising are the live-attenuated virus constructs generated using reverse genetics. Research conducted by NIAID investigators at the Laboratory of Infectious Diseases has resulted in major advances in PIV vaccine development that have led to the construction of live-attenuated virus vaccine candidates with great potential. The success of this approach is based on the capability of these viruses to induce a balanced immune response that includes serum and mucosal virus-neutralizing antibodies as well as cellular-mediated and innate immunity.

Sources

Clements, M. L., Belshe, R. B., King, J., et al. (1991). Evaluation of bovine, cold-adapted human, and wild type human parainfluenza type 3 viruses in adult volunteers and chimpanzees. *Journal of Clinical Microbiology, 29,* 1175-1182.

Durbin, A. P., Hall, S. L., Siew, J. W., et al. (1997). Recovery of infectious human parainfluenza virus type 3 from cDNA. *Virology, 235,* 323-332.

Ewasyshyn, M., Cates, G., Jackson, G., et al. (1997). Prospects for a parainfluenza virus vaccine. *Pediatric Pulmonology, 16* (Suppl.), 280-281.

Haller, A. A., Miller, T., Mitiku, M., & Coelingh, K. (2000). Expression of the surface glycoproteins of human parainfluenza virus type 3 by bovine parainfluenza virus type 3, a novel attenuated virus vaccine vector. *Journal of Virology, 74,* 11626-11635.

Hoffman, M. A., & Banerjee, A. K. (1997). An infectious clone of human parainfluenza virus type 3. *Journal of Virology, 71,* 4272-4277.

Hurwitz, J. L., Soike, K. F., Sangster, M. Y., et al. (1997). Intranasal Sendai virus vaccine protects African green monkeys from infection with human parainfluenza virus-type one. *Vaccine, 15,* 533-540.

Karron, R. A., Makhene, M., Gay, K., et al. (1996). Evaluation of a live attenuated bovine parainfluenza type 3 vaccine in two- to six-month-old infants. *Pediatric Infectious Disease Journal, 15,* 650-654.

Karron, R. A., Wright, P. F., Hall, S. L., et al. (1995). A live attenuated bovine parainfluenza virus type 3 vaccine is safe, infectious, immunogenic and phenotypically stable in infants and children. *Journal of Infectious Diseases, 171,* 1107-1114.

Karron, R. A., Wright, P. F., Newman, F. K., et al. (1995). A live human parainfluenza type 3 virus vaccine is attenuated and immunogenic in healthy infants and children. *Journal of Infectious Diseases, 172,* 1445-1450.

Lee, M., Greenberg, D. P., Yeh, S. H., et al. (2001). Antibody responses to bovine parainfluenza virus type 3 (PIV3) vaccination and human PIV3 infection in young infants. *Journal of Infectious Diseases, 184,* 909-913.

Newman, J. T., Surman, S. R., Riggs, J. M., et al. (2002). Sequence analysis of the Washington/1964 strains of human parainfluenza virus type 1 (PHIV1) and recovery and characterization of wild-type recombinant HPIV1 produced by reverse genetics. *Virus Genes, 24,* 77-92.

Schmidt, A. C., McAuliffe, J. M., Huang, A., et al. (2000). Bovine parainfluenza virus type 3 (3) fusion and hemagglutinin-neuraminidase glycoproteins make an important contribution to the restricted replication of 3 in primates. *Journal of Virology, 74,* 8922-8929.

Schmidt, A. C., Wenzke, D. R., McAuliffe, J. M., et al. (2002). Mucosal immunization of rhesus monkeys against respiratory syncytial virus subgroups A and B and human parainfluenza virus type 3 by using a live cDNA-derived vaccine based on a host range-attenuated bovine parainfluenza virus type 3 vector backbone. *Journal of Virology, 76,* 1089-1099.

Tao, T., Davoodi, F., Cho, C. J., et al. (2000). A live attenuated recombinant chimeric parainfluenza virus (PIV) candidate vaccine containing the hemagglutinin-neuraminidase and fusion glycoproteins of PIV1 and the remaining proteins from PIV3 induces resistance to PIV1 even in animals immune to PIV3. *Vaccine, 18,* 1359-1366.

Tao, T., Davoodi, F., Surman, S. R., et al. (2001). Construction of a live-attenuated bivalent vaccine virus against human parainfluenza virus (PIV) types 1 and 2 using a recombinant PIV3 backbone. *Vaccine, 19,* 3620-3631.

PSEUDOMONAS AERUGINOSA

Background

Pseudomonas aeruginosa is an opportunistic organism as well as a pathogen for patients with CF, a disease that usually presents itself in early childhood. CF patients have a mutant gene that does not allow the movement of chloride across the cell wall, and the clinical presentation resulting from this defect is that of excessive mucus production and impaired mucociliary clearance. As a consequence, there is the development of a variety of microbial infections, mainly *P. aeruginosa* and *Burkholderia cepacia,* the latter associated with lung deterioration. Significant advances have been made in the management of CF patients through diet and physiotherapy and by treatment with recombinant human deoxyribonuclease (rhDNase) I to relieve airway obstruction. Now, many CF patients survive to adulthood; the life expectancy is approximately 30 years. CF affects 30,000 children and young adults worldwide, with 400 deaths each year. Although there has been considerable progress in the use of gene therapy to correct the basic genetic defect of CF at the molecular level, there is no evidence that gene therapy alters the course of Pseudomonas infection in this population, so preventive approaches, such as the development of safe and effective vaccines, are needed. Efforts to control these infections with antibiotics and better pulmonary therapy have done little to reduce the high mortality associated with *P. aeruginosa* pneumonia; however, immunotherapeutic interventions with active vaccination or passive therapy may have a significant impact on the development of sepsis and on survival.

While *P. aeruginosa* is a special problem for CF patients, it also contributes to the high mortality rates in patients with emphysema, cancer, AIDS, and serious burns. Studies indicate that although *P. aeruginosa* is not the most common bacterial pathogen in AIDS patients, the presence of the organism is usually associated with fatality. The reason for the extraordinary pathogenicity of *P. aeruginosa* in these patients is not clear; however, it is possible that a variety of virulence factors produced by *P. aeruginosa* may account for the high mortality rates. Such virulence factors may play a role in colonization, tissue invasion, or the inhibition of a variety of immune responses. A major virulence factor produced by *P. aeruginosa* is an exopolysaccharide or alginate. Alginate not only encapsulates the infecting bacteria, thereby protecting them from antibiotic treatment or from attack by host immune responses, but also enables the bacteria to adhere to epithelial cells of the lung and enhances the opportunity for further colonization and invasion. Other virulence factors associated with Pseudomonas infections include cell-associated structures, such as pili, as well as secreted products, such as exotoxin A, exoenzyme S, hemolytic phospholipase, and proteases. Expression of these virulence factors is highly regulated, which probably accounts for the ability of *P. aeruginosa* to cause such a wide variety of infections in vastly different host environments. In addition to the expression of virulence determinants, *P. aeruginosa* in the lungs of CF patients grows in biofilms, and this may explain the difficulty encountered in treatment with antibiotics. In this regard, new approaches are in development aimed at killing the organisms within the biofilms.

Research Accomplishments

During the past 2 decades, significant advances have been made in understanding the pathogenesis of *P. aeruginosa* infections in patients with CF, as well as understanding the molecular and cellular basis of the CF defect. Several ideas have been suggested to explain the relationship between the CF gene defect and susceptibility to *P. aeruginosa*, including impaired killing of *P. aeruginosa* by host defensins, presumably due to the high salt content in the secretions in CF patients; low production of nitric oxide, an important defense mechanism; reduced uptake of *P. aeruginosa* in CF respiratory epithelial cells; and reduced sialylation of epithelial glycoconjugates, resulting in reduced adherence of organisms. Indeed, a number of studies have been conducted to examine these ideas. For example, studies by NIAID-supported investigators show that leukocytes from delta 508 homozygous CF patients are deficient in the uptake of *P. aeruginosa*. Also, the results of a recent NIAID-supported study showed that the intracellular organelle, trans-Golgi network, is hyperacidified in CF lung epithelial cells, resulting in increased adherence of *P. aeruginosa*. The studies further show that correction of the hyperacidification by normalizing the pH leads to decreased bacterial adherence.

Studies carried out by NIAID-supported investigators, designed to examine the significance of chronic malnutrition in CF patients, indicate that diet-induced protein calorie malnutrition alters the clearance of *P. aeruginosa* from the lung. Also, mal-nourished animals show excessive inflammation in response to *P. aeruginosa*, relative to normal animals, presumably due to the failure to produce anti-inflammatory cytokine IL-10. These results are consistent with the view that nutritional deficiency contributes to compromised immune defenses and bacterial colonization and excessive inflammation in the respiratory tract of CF patients. Thus, future treatment efforts for CF patients should also consider nutritional supplementation.

Studies conducted to examine the inflammatory changes associated with *P. aeruginosa* infections show that CF patients have high levels of proinflammatory cytokines (e.g., IL-1, 8, and TNF-a) in the lung environment relative to the levels in healthy individuals. By contrast, the levels of anti-inflammatory cytokines, such as IL-10, are low in CF patients as compared to those in healthy individuals. Indeed, experimental animal model studies show increased pathology associated with *P. aeruginosa* infection in IL-10 knockout mice. Molecular analysis of signal transduction events suggests that *P. aeruginosa* induces epithelial cell production of IL-8 by activation of NFkB. Cells with CF mutations have significant endogenous levels of activated NFkB. These inflammatory changes must be taken into account in the design of preventive procedures, such as vaccines against *P. aeruginosa*.

Considerable attention has been focused on the mechanisms by which the organisms sense, integrate, and process information from their surroundings. This process, described as quorum sensing, is used by bacteria for cell-cell communication and has been shown to be important in the pathogenesis of diseases caused by *P. aeruginosa*. Studies now indicate that certain of the extracellular virulence factors are controlled by a system of quorum-sensing molecules. Quorum sensing is also involved in the formation of bacterial biofilms. There are essentially two components to the system: A small diffusible signal molecule, typically N-acyl homoserine lactone in gram-negative bacteria; and a second molecule, a transcriptional activator protein. Recent studies by NIAID-supported investigators indicate that quorum-sensing mutants are less virulent in animal models than their wild-type/normal *P. aeruginosa* strains. Such studies should enhance understanding of the interactions between bacterial biofilms and host responses. Another recent study designed to understand the differences between free-living *P. aeruginosa* and those in biofilms, and to understand why biofilms are resistant to antibiotics, has yielded useful information. Using DNA microarray analysis, the investigators showed that only a few key genes are differentially expressed in biofilms; however, at least one of these genes is involved in morphology and antibiotic sensitivity of biofilms. Because of the increasing difficulty to treat the organism, particularly once the biofilms are fully formed, these findings, and the anticipation that the studies may lead to the development of targets for therapeutic intervention, represent important advances.

Recent advances have been made in understanding the actions of type III secretory proteins of *P. aeruginosa*. These proteins are also found in several pathogenic strains of gram-negative bacteria, including Salmonella, Shigella, and Yersinia, and are integral to the virulence of gram-negative bacteria. Recently, it was demonstrated that the expression of type III secretory proteins, in particular PcrV, in clinical isolates of *P. aeruginosa* is associated with mortality and morbidity in CF patients.

Progress in Vaccine Development

Significant advances have been made in the development of vaccines against *P. aeruginosa*. Several surface proteins and polysaccharides have been demonstrated to be safe and immunogenic in small phase I and II studies and have been shown to generate protective immunity in various animal model systems. First, HMW polysaccharides and mucoid exopolysaccharide (MEP) vaccine preparations have been tested in humans. In addition, experiments are in progress to enhance the immunogenicity of MEP by conjugation to protein carriers. Investigators also have pursued the use of recombinant OMPs as vaccines against *P. aeruginosa* infections. The results of experiments using a hybrid vaccine, containing protective epitopes of OMPs F and I, indicated that the vaccine was highly immunogenic and protective against *P. aeruginosa* infections in mice, especially when expressed as a plant virus. In clinical studies, recombinant OMP I was found to be safe and immunogenic in human volunteers. However, the use of OMPs as vaccines against *P. aeruginosa* infections requires further study. Recent studies in mice using a DNA vaccine based on an OMP indicate that antibodies produced were specific for the protein and that injection of the vaccine was protective in a mouse model of *P. aeruginosa* infection. Third, oral immunization with killed *P. aeruginosa* vaccine preparation protected naive animals against challenge with live bacteria. Despite these encouraging results, most studies done to date have demonstrated immunogenicity without protective efficacy. Besides active immunization, the use of passively administered antibodies is an attractive alternative in that many patients susceptible to infections with *P. aeruginosa* are immunocompromised and do not respond adequately to active immunization. In this regard, a recent study reported that human anti-Pseudomonas LPS antibodies generated in transgenic mice are opsonic for the uptake and killing of bacteria by human polymorphonuclear leukocytes.

Challenges

For CF patients, a vaccine should induce an immune response that would prevent mucosal colonization of *P. aeruginosa* and/or elicit a response against virulence factors associated with adherence. A better understanding of the molecular regulation of *P. aeruginosa* virulence factors, and in particular, the interaction of *P. aeruginosa* with host cells as well as the overall host immune response to infections should provide valuable information for vaccine design. Indeed, the availability of the *P. aeruginosa* genome, and new technological approaches should make these goals feasible. Researchers are now using genetic tools, such as *P. aeruginosa* microchips, to examine bacterial virulence factors and to develop better vaccine candidates. In addition, DNA arrays are being used to identify bacterial genes in clinical specimens. Clearly, study comparability will require standardization of these newer approaches.

Sources

Amura, C. R., Fontan, P. A., Sanjuan, N., & Sordelli, D. (1994). The effect of treatment with interleukin-1 and tumor necrosis factor on *Pseudomonas aeruginosa* lung infection in a granulocytopenic mouse model. *Clinical Immunology and Immunopathology, 73,* 261-266.

Cripps, A. W., Dunkley, M. L., & Clancy, R. L. (1994). Mucosal and systemic immunization with killed *Pseudomonas aeruginosa* protects against acute respiratory infection in rats. *Infection and Immunity, 62,* 1427-1436.

Hemachandra, S., Kamboj, K., Copfer, J., Pier, G., Green, L. L., & Schreiber, J. R. (2001). Human monoclonal antibodies against *Pseudomonas aeruginosa* lipopolysaccharide derived form transgenic mice containing megabase human immunoglobulin loci are opsonic and protective against fatal Pseudomonas sepsis. *Infection and Immunity, 69,* 2223-2229.

Holder, I. A., Neely, A. N., & Frank D. W. (2001). PcrV immunization enhances survival of burned *Pseudomonas aeruginosa*-infected mice. *Infection and Immunity, 69,* 5908-5910.

Johansen, H. K. (1996). Potential of preventing *Pseudomonas aeruginosa* lung infections in cystic fibrosis patients: Experimental studies in animals. *APMIS, 63*(Suppl.), 5-42.

Mansouri, E., Gabelsberger, J., Knapp, B., Hundt, E., Lenz, U., Hungerer, K. D., Gilleland, H. E., Staczek, J., Domdey, H., & von Specht, B. U. (1999). Safety and immunogenicity of a *Pseudomonas aeruginosa* hybrid outer membrane protein F-1 vaccine in human volunteers. *Infection and Immunity, 67,* 1461-1470.

Meynard, J. L., Barbut, F., Guiguet, M., Batise, D., Lalande, V., Lesage, D., Guiard-Schmid, J. B, Petit, J. C., Frottier, J., & Meyohas, M. C. (1999). *Pseudomonas aeruginosa* infection in human immunodeficiency virus infected patients. *Journal of Infection, 38,* 176-181.

Pier, G. B., DesJardin, D., Grout, M., Garner, C., Bennet, S., Pekoe, G., Fuller, S., Thornton, M. O., Harkonen, W., & Miller, H. C. (1994). Human immune response to *Pseudomonas aeruginosa* mucoid exopolysaccharide (alginate) vaccine. *Infection and Immunity, 62,* 3972-3979.

Poschet, J. F., Boucher, J. C., Tatterson, L., Skidmore, J., Van Dyke, R. W., and Deretic, V. (2001). Molecular basis for defective glycosylation and Pseudomonas pathogenesis in cystic fibrosis lung. *Proceedings of the National Academy of Sciences, 98,* 13972-13977.

von Specht, B., Knapp, B., Hungerer, K., Lucking, C., Schmit, A., & Domdey, H. (1996). Outer membrane proteins of *Pseudomonas aeruginosa* as vaccine candidates. *Journal of Biotechnology, 44,* 145-153.

Whiteley, M., Bangera, M. G., Bumgarner, R. E., Parsek, M. R., Teitzel, G. M., Lory, S., & Greenberg, E. P. (2001). Gene expression in *Pseudomonas aeruginosa* biofilms. *Nature, 413,* 860-864.

RESPIRATORY SYNCYTIAL VIRUS

Respiratory syncytial virus (RSV) is the single most important cause of severe lower respiratory tract infection in infants and young children, the elderly, and the immunocompromised. It is a common cause of winter outbreaks of acute respiratory disease. RSV infects repeatedly and causes disease throughout life, including a wide array of respiratory symptoms from rhinitis and otitis media to pneumonia and bronchiolitis, with the latter two diseases having significant morbidity and mortality. In the United States, 3.5 to 4 million children younger than 4 years of age acquire RSV infection annually. It is estimated that RSV accounts for 100,000 hospitalizations annually in infants of less than 1 year of age. Although the number of RSV-associated hospitalizations did not change significantly over the past 2 decades, the number of RSV-associated deaths in the United States has decreased over the same period from 4,500 to no more than 510 per year. RSV infects nearly all children by 2 years of age, with re-infections during later childhood and adulthood that are generally associated with milder disease. Recently, RSV has been recognized as a significant cause of severe respiratory infections in the elderly, with outbreaks that are complicated with pneumonia reported among institutionalized elderly patients. It is estimated that there are 60,000 RSV-associated hospitalizations per year in the United States among the elderly. Severe RSV infections are also a problem in immunocompromised patients of any age, especially transplant recipients. There is recent evidence of a link between RSV infection and the development of asthma.

Although development of a vaccine to prevent RSV infections has been a high priority at NIAID (see Appendix A, table of priority vaccines from first *Jordan Report*), a licensed vaccine is not yet available. The development of an RSV vaccine is a difficult but important priority. The most significant obstacle to developing a vaccine against RSV infections is the unexpected enhanced disease that resulted from vaccination of children with a formalin-inactivated whole RSV vaccine in the 1960s. Recipients who were seronegative at the time of vaccination experienced lower respiratory tract disease of increased incidence and severity upon subsequent natural infection. To develop an effective vaccine, it is imperative to understand the protective as well as the disease-enhancing immune responses to RSV. Research efforts have been focused on the individual components of these responses, including cell-mediated events as well as production of serum and secretory antibodies. Although much has been learned about these components, a safe and effective vaccine that induces protective immunity and does not cause enhanced disease is not yet available. An effective vaccine could be useful in reducing morbidity, reducing the frequency of hospitalization, and decreasing the death rate. Vaccine candidates under development are evaluated in animal models first, followed by adults, immune children, older nonimmune children, younger nonimmune children, and susceptible infants.

There are two RSV strain subgroups, A and B. A successful vaccine would induce resistance to subgroup A and B strains of RSV. The major protective antigens of RSV are the F and attachment (G) glycoproteins found on the surface of RSV. The proteins induce neutralizing antibodies that protect against wild-type RSV infection. The F surface protein is highly conserved among the RSV subgroups, and functions to promote fusion of the virus and host cell membranes. The major difference between RSV subgroups A and B is the G protein, which is responsible for attachment of RSV to a susceptible cell. Although there is 47 percent amino acid sequence diversity between RSV A and RSV B G proteins, the G protein contains a central conserved domain that is flanked by two hypervariable regions.

Purified F protein (PFP) has been developed as a potential vaccine candidate by Wyeth-Lederle Vaccines. PFP-1 and PFP-2 are subunit vaccines that were tested in various populations in phase I and II human clinical trials. In studies with 12- to 48-month-old RSV seropositive children, PFP-1 and PFP-2 have been shown to be safe and immunogenic. These studies were not designed to evaluate vaccine efficacy.

Subunit vaccines may be particularly useful in specific groups of high-risk children and adults. A pilot study in children with CF demonstrated that PFP-2 vaccine induced a significant antibody response and a significant reduction in the number of lower respiratory tract illnesses. In addition, studies demonstrated that PFP-2 vaccine is safe and immunogenic in ambulatory adults over age 60, and in seropositive children with bronchopulmonary dysplasia.

A phase II double-blind, controlled, multicenter study of the safety, immunogenicity, and effectiveness of the PFP-3 subunit vaccine was conducted in RSV seropositive children with CF. The vaccine was safe and immunogenic; however, the study did not demonstrate a reduction in the incidence of lower respiratory tract illness in vaccinees.

Maternal immunization using a purified F protein subunit vaccine is a strategy being evaluated to protect infants younger than 6 months of age from RSV disease. The rationale is based on reports of efficient transfer of specific maternal neutralizing antibodies to infants, and demonstration of the prophylactic value of high-titer anti-RSV polyclonal antiserum or humanized monoclonal antibody administered to high-risk children (protection against lower respiratory tract RSV disease and hospitalization). The advantages of maternal immunization are that babies less than 6 months old are most at risk for RSV infection, but are least responsive to vaccines; pregnant women respond well immunologically to vaccines; and placental transfer of maternal antibody occurs naturally during the third trimester. A phase I double-blind, placebo-controlled study was conducted with 35 healthy third trimester pregnant women who were randomized in a 2:1 ratio to receive either PFP-2 vaccine or saline placebo. The vaccine was safe and immunogenic. Transplacental transfer of maternal neutralization antibodies to RSV was efficient. Infants born to vaccine recipients were healthy and did not experience adverse events related to maternal immunization.

The G protein fragment of RSV is the basis of a subunit vaccine being developed by scientists at the Centre d'Immunologie Pierre Fabre. A novel recombinant vaccine candidate, BBG2Na, has been constructed by fusing the conserved central domain of the G protein (G2Na) of RSV Long strain to BB (the albumin-binding region of streptococcal G protein). A clinical trial was conducted in 108 healthy adults. The BBG2Na vaccine was found to be safe, well tolerated, and immunogenic.

A subunit RSV vaccine consisting of the F, G, and M proteins is being developed by Aventis Pasteur. The primary target of this vaccine is prevention of significant respiratory disease in RSV non-naive study populations. Two phase I clinical trials have been conducted in healthy 18- to 45-year-old adults that have supported the safety and immunogenicity of this product. The first trial compared an aluminum phosphate formulation of the vaccine (n=30) with aluminum phosphate control (n=10). The second trial compared the aluminum phosphate formulation (n=10) with a formulation containing a new adjuvant poly[di(carboxylatophenoxy)phosphazene] (PCPP) (n=30) in a different sample of young, healthy adults. Both vaccines were well tolerated and immunogenic. Larger phase II studies in adult populations are either planned or underway.

Other subunit vaccines in preclinical development include:

- Recombinant chimeric RSV FG glycoprotein vaccines adsorbed onto aluminum hydroxide gel with or without the addition of 3-deacylated monophosphoryl lipid A

- F protein formulated with alum with or without G protein (from subtypes A and B)

- Synthetic peptide of the conserved region of the G protein with or without cholera toxin as a mucosal adjuvant

- Recombinant fragment (BBG2Na) of the G protein formulated with dimethyldioctadecylammonium bromide, a nasal adjuvant

- Recombinant fragment of the G protein in a lipsome-encapsulated formulation, prepared by including a variety of different lipids

- Mimotope (peptide that mimics the antigenicity) of a conserved and conformationally determined epitope of the F protein recognized by an anti-RSV monoclonal antibody (MAb19) that neutralizes RSV

A live-attenuated RSV vaccine that could be delivered to the respiratory mucosa has been the basis of another approach to vaccine development. Intranasal immunization with a live RSV vaccine has the potential to induce systemic and local immunity and to protect against upper and lower respiratory disease. Early attempts included cold passage, cold adaptation, chemical mutagenesis, temperature-sensitive selection, and combinations of these methods. NIAID scientists at the Laboratory of Infectious Diseases in collaboration with Wyeth-Lederle Vaccines have developed live-attenuated vaccine candidates. Several promising mutants derived from wild-type strain RSV A-2 (strain A2, subgroup A) were evaluated in seropositive children and older seronegative children. From these studies, RSV vaccine candidate *cpts* 248/404 (a cold-passaged, temperature-sensitive mutant of a human RSV A strain) was shown to be safe and immunogenic and attenuated when administered intranasally in a placebo-controlled, randomized, double-blind trial in RSV seropositive and seronegative infants and children. However, when this vaccine was administered to 1- to 2-month-old RSV naive infants, mild-to-moderate upper respiratory congestion resulted, indicating that more attenuation was needed. In order to construct more-attenuated vaccine candidates, the technology of reverse genetics was employed. This powerful tool is the most significant scientific advance in recent years to facilitate vaccine development. By using reverse genetics, the genetic basis for RSV attenuation was determined, which provided the basis for the construction of defined attenuated vaccine viruses with improved genetic stability. Examples include strains rA2cp248/404?SH and rA2cp248/4041030?SH that are being evaluated in infants 4 to 12 weeks of age. To date, the pattern of nasal congestions observed with *cpts* 248/404 has not been seen. This study demonstrates the progress that has been made in developing appropriately attenuated recombinant RSV vaccines for infants.

Reverse genetics also has been used to expedite the development of RSV vaccines to protect against RSV subgroup B. One approach has been to replace the G and F genes of recombinant RSV A-2 with the G and F genes of strain B1 of subgroup B. Another approach has been to construct a strain that expresses the RSV subgroup B gene in a recombinant subgroup A virus backbone. The rB/HPIV3-RSV-A and -B chimeric viruses are promising vaccines with the potential of protecting infants and children against RSV and PIV3 infections; these vaccines have been constructed with reverse genetics by employing the BPIV as a backbone in which the HPIV3 protective antigens have been inserted as well as the protective antigens of RSV (see Parainfluenza Virus section for more information about rB/HIV3).

A vaccine strategy to be considered for protecting adults against RSV illness is a combination of a live-attenuated vaccine with a subunit vaccine. This alternative approach was used because previous studies of PRP-2 in ambulatory and institutionalized adults over 60 years of age demonstrated that the vaccine was safe and moderately immunogenic in healthy older adults, but relatively less immunogenic in the institutionalized elderly. Thus, a clinical trial was conducted in which *cpts* 248/404 and PFP-2 were administered to healthy young adults and healthy elderly adults using simultaneous and sequential vaccination schedules. Both vaccines were well tolerated; however, the *cpts* 248/404 vaccine appeared to be overattenuated. Future studies that combine PFP-2 with a less attenuated RSV vaccine would be desirable.

The prospects for the future for RSV vaccines are encouraging. Ongoing studies are focused on furthering the understanding of protection and immunopotentiation of RSV disease to provide the scientific basis required for the rational design of candidate RSV vaccines. Subunit vaccines have been shown to be safe and immunogenic in seropositive children, pregnant women, and adults (including those over 60). They have great potential use in adults and specific groups of high-risk children (CF) and for protecting infants via maternal immunization. Different adjuvants are currently being studied to augment immunogenicity of subunit vaccines. Live-attenuated vaccine candidates also have been shown to be safe and immunogenic. New methods in biotechnology (reverse genetics) are now available to provide tools for designing vaccines with defined mutations to achieve desired levels of attenuation that are genetically stable.

Sources

Bastien, N., Trudel, M., & Simard, C. (1999). Complete protection of mice from respiratory syncytial virus infection following mucosal delivery of synthetic peptide vaccines. *Vaccine, 17,* 832-836.

Brandt, C., Power, U., Plotnicky-Gilquin, H., et al. (1997). Protective immunity against respiratory syncytial virus in early life after murine maternal or neonatal vaccination with the recombinant G fusion protein BBG2Na. *Journal of Infectious Diseases, 176,* 884-891.

Crowe, J. E., Jr. (1995). Current approaches to the development of vaccines against disease caused by respiratory syncytial virus (RSV) and parainfluenza virus (PIV). *Vaccine, 13,* 415-421.

Crowe, J. E., Jr., Bui, P. T., London, W. T., et al. (1994). Satisfactorily attenuated and protective mutants derived from a partially attenuated cold-passaged respiratory syncytial virus mutant by introduction of additional attenuating mutations during chemical mutagenesis. *Vaccine, 12,* 691-699.

Falsey, A. R., & Walsh, E. E. (1996). Safety and immunogenicity of a respiratory syncytial virus subunit vaccine (PFP-2) in ambulatory adults over age 60. *Vaccine, 14,* 1214-1218.

Gonzalez, I. M., Karron, R. A., Eichelberger, M., et al. (2000). Evaluation of a live attenuated *cpts* 248/404 RSV vaccine in combination with a subunit RSV vaccine (PFP-2) in healthy young and older adults. *Vaccine, 18,* 1763-1772.

Groothuis, J. R., King, S. J., Hogerman, D. A., et al. (1998). Safety and immunogenicity of a purified F protein respiratory syncytial virus (PFP-2) vaccine in seropositive children with bronchopulmonary dysplasia. *Journal of Infectious Diseases, 177,* 467-469.

Groothuis, J. R., Simoes, E. A. F., Levine, M. J., et al. (1993). Prophylactic administration of respiratory syncytial virus immune globulin to high-risk infants and young children. The Respiratory Syncytial Virus Immune Globulin Study Group. *New England Journal of Medicine, 329,* 1524-1530.

Hancock, G. E., Smith, J. D., & Heers, K. M. (2000). Serum neutralizing antibody titers of seropositive chimpanzees immunized with vaccines coformulated with natural fusion and attachment proteins of respiratory syncytial virus. *Journal of Infectious Diseases, 181,* 1768-1771.

Herlocher, M. L., Ewasyshyn, M., Sambhara, S., et al. (1999). Immunological properties of plaque purified strains of live attenuated respiratory syncytial virus (RSV) for human vaccine. *Vaccine, 17,* 172-181.

Huang, Y., & Anderson, R. (2002). Enhanced immune protection by a liposome-encapsulated recombinant respiratory syncytial virus (RSV) vaccine using immunogenic lipids from *Deinococcus radiodurans. Vaccine, 20,* 1586-1592.

Jin, H., Clarke, D., Zhou, H., et al. (1998). Recombinant human respiratory syncytial virus (RSV) from cDNA and construction of subgroup A and B chimeric RSV. *Virology, 251,* 206-214.

Karron, R. A., Wright, P., Belshe, R. B., et al. (2002). *Evaluation of live rRSV A2 vaccines in infants and children.* Abstract 1638 presented at the Society of Pediatric Research, Baltimore, MD.

Klinguer, C., Beck, A., De-Lys, P., et al. (2001). Lipophilic quaternary ammonium salt acts as a mucosal adjuvant when co-administered by the nasal route with vaccine antigens. *Vaccine, 19,* 4236-4244.

Munoz, F. M., Piedra, P. A., Maccato, M., et al. (2001). *Respiratory syncytial virus purified fusion protein-2 (PFP-2) in pregnancy* (p. 158). Abstract presented at RSV After 45 Years, Segovia, Spain.

Murphy, B. R., & Collins, P. L. (2002). Live-attenuated virus vaccines for respiratory syncytial and parainfluenza viruses: Applications of reverse genetics. *Journal of Clinical Investigation, 110,* 1-7.

Murthy, K., Salas, M., Welliver, R., et al. (2001). *Maternal immunization with respiratory syncytial virus vaccine protects neonates from viral infection* (p. 69). Abstract presented at RSV After 45 Years, Segovia, Spain.

Piedra, P. A., Grace, S., Jewell, A., et al. (1996). Purified fusion protein vaccine protects against lower respiratory tract illness during the respiratory syncytial virus season in children with cystic fibrosis. *Pediatric Infectious Disease Journal, 15,* 23-31.

Piedra, P. A., Maccato, M., Jewell, A. M., et al. (1994). *Maternal/cord neutralizing antibody titers to respiratory syncytial virus subtypes A and B and their relationship to the circulating RSV subtypes* [Abstract H39]. 34th ICACC Meeting.

Piedra, T. (2000). *Viral infections in cystic fibrosis.* Presented at the 14th Annual North American Cystic Fibrosis Conference, Baltimore, MD.

Power, U. F., Nguyen, T. N., Rietveld, E., et al. (2001). Safety and immunogenicity of a novel recombinant subunit respiratory syncytial virus vaccine (BBG2Na) in healthy young adults. *Journal of Infectious Diseases, 184,* 1456-1460.

Prince, G. A., Capiau, C., Deschamps, M., et al. (2000). Efficacy and safety studies of a recombinant chimeric respiratory syncytial virus FG glycoprotein vaccine in cotton rats. *Journal of Virology, 74,* 10287-10292.

Sales, V. (2001). *Safety and immunogenicity of a respiratory syncytial virus subtype A (RSV A) vaccine in adults—Two phase I studies.* Presented at the IV International Symposium on Respiratory Viral Infections, Curacoa.

Schmidt, A. C., Wenzke, D. R., McAuliffe, J. M., et al. (2002). Mucosal immunization of rhesus monkeys against respiratory syncytial virus subgroups A and B and human parainfluenza virus type 3 by using a live cDNA-derived vaccine based on a host range-attenuated bovine parainfluenza virus type 3 vector backbone. *Journal of Virology, 76,* 1089-1099.

Shay, D. K., Holman, R. C., Roosevelt, G. E., et al. (2001). Bronchiolitis-associated mortality and estimates of respiratory syncytial virus-associated deaths among U.S. children, 1979-1997. *Journal of Infectious Diseases, 183,* 16-22.

Sigurs, N., Bjarnason, R., Sigurbergsson, F., et al. (1995). Asthma and immunoglobulin E antibodies after respiratory syncytial virus bronchiolitis: A prospective cohort study with matched controls. *Pediatrics, 95,* 500-505.

Steward, M. W. (2001). The development of a mimotope-based synthetic peptide vaccine against respiratory syncytial virus. *Biologicals, 29,* 215-219.

Suara, R. O., Piedra, P. A., Glezen, W. P., et al. (1966). Prevalence of neutralizing antibody to respiratory syncytial virus in sera from mothers and newborns residing in The Gambia and in the United States. *Clinical and Diagnostic Laboratory Immunology, 3,* 477-479.

Whitehead, S. S., Hill, M. G., Firestone, C. Y., et al. (1999). Replacement of the F and G proteins of respiratory syncytial virus (RSV) subgroup A with those of subgroup B generates chimeric live attenuated RSV subgroup B vaccine candidates. *Journal of Virology, 73,* 9773-9780.

Wright, P. F., Karron, R. A., Belshe, R. B., et al. (2000). Evaluation of a live, cold-passaged, temperature-sensitive, respiratory syncytial virus vaccine candidate in infancy. *Journal of Infectious Diseases, 182,* 1331-1342.

SMALLPOX

As concerns increase about the use of biological agents in acts of terrorism or war, Federal health agencies are evaluating existing measures and stepping up new ones to protect the public from the health consequences of such an attack. Smallpox virus (*Variola major*) is considered one of the most dangerous potential biological weapons because it is easily transmitted from person to person, and few people carry full immunity to the virus. Although a worldwide immunization program eradicated smallpox disease decades ago, small quantities of smallpox virus still exist in a few research laboratories around the world.

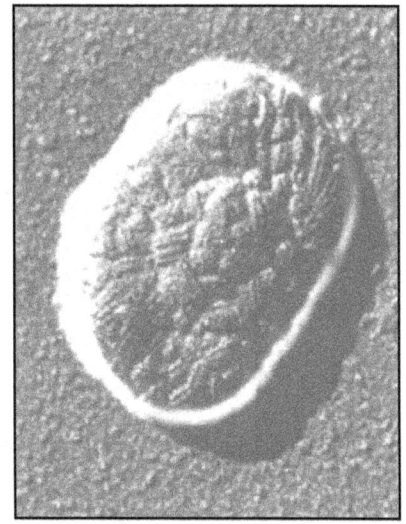

Variola major

With smallpox eradicated, vaccinations against the disease have not been required in the United States for nearly 30 years. Those who did receive a vaccination 3 decades ago are believed to have little immunity to the virus left, and people born in the United States since that time have not been vaccinated at all. No new smallpox vaccine had been manufactured in almost 20 years; with no market for the vaccine, the private sector lost interest in the product and showed little interest in producing a next generation vaccine.

The classic smallpox vaccine licensed in the United States was prepared from calf lymph. The vaccine was made with 1950s methods and is not a sterile product. It produces significant side effects and is currently contraindicated in such populations as the immune suppressed, pregnant, and the very young. Currently available supplies of smallpox vaccine in the United States are limited to about 15 million doses. The anticipated need to control a U.S. outbreak is 40 million doses, and the international need is undetermined but substantial.

Federally sponsored research to counter the threat of smallpox is progressing rapidly and will be accelerating in the year ahead. Major research efforts [cofunded by NIAID with the Centers for Disease Control and Prevention (CDC) and the Departments of Defense and Energy] include the following:

- Extending the usefulness of the currently available, older vaccine (by doing human studies to determine whether available stocks can be "stretched")

- Developing a safe, sterile smallpox vaccine grown in cell cultures using modern technology

- Exploring development of a vaccine that can be used in all segments of the civilian population (e.g., immune-suppressed individuals, pregnant mothers)

- Increasing knowledge about the genome of smallpox and related viruses

During the past year, significant progress has been made in the nation's ability to have vaccine available to vaccinate every American, if necessary. Results from a NIAID-supported clinical trial indicate that the existing U.S. supply of smallpox vaccine—15.4 million doses—could successfully be diluted up to five times and retain its potency, effectively expanding the number of individuals it could protect from the contagious disease. The trial, conducted through the NIAID VTEUs, compared full-strength Dryvax smallpox vaccine to five- and tenfold diluted vaccine in 680 young adults with no history of smallpox vaccination. More than 97 percent of all participants in the trial responded with a vaccine "take," a blister-like sore at the injection site that serves as an indirect measure of the vaccine's effectiveness. The investigators found no significant difference in the take rate of the three doses. This study is an important component of the Department of Health and Human Services' goal of having enough smallpox vaccine to vaccinate every American. In addition, to ensure that sufficient vaccine becomes available to protect the entire U.S. population, a contract established in 2000 by CDC with Acambis (Cambridge, MA) to produce and maintain a stockpile of 40 million doses of a new, MRC-5 (a diploid human lung cell line suitable for the production of viral vaccines) cell culture-grown vaccinia vaccine was modified to reflect the need for expanded and accelerated production and human testing. The revised goal is to produce more than 50 million doses by the end of 2002, with increased surge capacity

for production of more than 180 million doses annually from 2003 on. Pilot lot production of the new vaccine is now underway, as are phase I clinical trials. Phase II and III clinical trials are scheduled to begin later in 2002. Acambis expects to license the new vaccine by the end of 2003; however, it will be available for emergency use as an investigational new drug (IND) product as soon as it is manufactured. A second contract has been awarded to Acambis, in partnership with Baxter (Vienna, Austria), for production of 155 million doses of Vero cell culture-produced vaccinia vaccine for delivery by the end of 2002. The expanded use of the Dryvax vaccine, coupled with production of new vaccine from these two contracts, should result in sufficient vaccine for the entire U.S. population by the end of 2002.

Studies are now underway to examine if Dryvax can be diluted and used in non-naive adults and in children. Other vaccines based on second- and third-generation smallpox vaccines, such as a more-attenuated strain of vaccinia called MVA, also should move into clinical trials in the coming year.

STREPTOCOCCUS PNEUMONIAE

In the United States, pneumococcal infections are responsible for an estimated 500,000 cases of pneumonia and 40,000 deaths annually, and are associated with as many as 7 million cases of otitis media. Serious invasive diseases caused by *S. pneumoniae* include pneumonia, sepsis, and meningitis. The overall incidence of invasive pneumococcal disease in the United States is estimated to be 15 to 30 cases per 100,000 population. The rate varies significantly, however, as a function of age and ethnicity. Overall, the rates in children less than or at 2 years of age (160 per 100,000) and in the elderly (50 to 83 per 100,000) are much higher than the rate in immunocompetent adults. The case fatality rate among the elderly is 30 to 40 percent, despite the use of antibiotics. Disease rates in blacks are three- to fivefold higher than rates in whites, and as much as tenfold higher in Native Americans than in whites.

The conventional vaccine for pneumococcus consists of a mixture of 23 different capsular polysaccharides. While this vaccine is very effective in young adults who are normally at low risk of serious disease, it is only about 60 percent effective in the elderly. In children less than 2 years of age, the vaccine is ineffective and is not recommended due to the inability of this age group to mount an antibody response to the pneumococcal polysaccharides. Antimicrobial drugs such as penicillin have diminished the risk from pneumococcal disease. However, the increasing presence of antimicrobial-resistant forms of *S. pneumoniae* has promoted an even greater need for immunoprophylactic approaches to protect against serious invasive disease and colonization. Furthermore, many individuals, especially those at high risk for infection, do not receive the required immunizations against *S. pneumoniae*. Therefore, additional strategies are needed to improve the access of these patients to vaccination, with special emphasis being placed on immunizing adults while maintaining a commitment to vaccinate children.

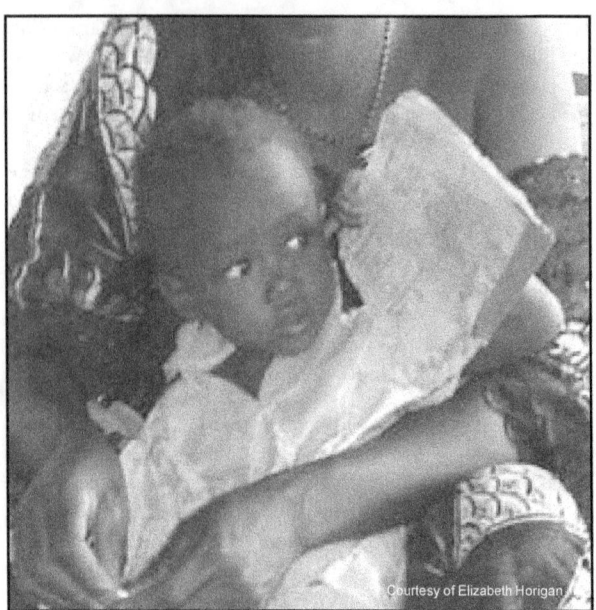

Courtesy of Elizabeth Horigan

A child holding his medical records while he waits to be vaccinated as part of the Gambia Pneumococcal Study. This study in 16,000 Gambian children is designed to determine whether 3 doses of 9-valent pneumococcal conjugate vaccine can significantly reduce the occurence of x-ray confirmed pneumonia

Recently, a pneumococcal 7-valent conjugate vaccine (Prevnar®), manufactured by Wyeth-Lederle Pediatrics, was licensed for use in toddlers and children under the age of 2, as well as older children with weakened immune systems or otherwise at high risk. This represents the first pneumococcal vaccine licensed directly for use in infants, and is now recommended as part of the routine vaccination schedule along with 10 other vaccines. Previously licensed vaccines were only effective in adults. In clinical trials, this conjugate vaccine was shown to be safe and prevent invasive pneumococcal disease when administered along with routine infant immunizations. The results from a large-scale, controlled, double-blind efficacy trial in southern California involving 38,000 children demonstrated the vaccine to be 97 percent effective in preventing serotype-specific invasive pneumococcal disease in children less than 5 years of age. The study also showed that the vaccine reduced common ear infections overall by 7 percent and multiple ear infections by 23 percent. An additional study in Finland further substantiated these findings by showing that the same vaccine caused an overall reduction in the occurrence of otitis media by 6 percent, a 34 percent reduction in otitis caused by *S. pneumoniae,* a 57 percent reduction in otitis caused by the seven serotypes contained in the vaccine, and a 20 percent reduction in the need for ear tubes. While the reduction in the number of cases of otitis may appear small and disappointing, in the U.S. pediatric population, this reduction translates into very large numbers (i.e., 1.2 million of 20 million cases of otitis per year) on a scale that could reduce healthcare costs by $300 to 500 million annually. One

disconcerting finding associated with the Finnish trial was an approximately 30-percent increase in nonvaccine-type pneumococcal disease. This represents the first time anyone has shown replacement disease (as opposed to carriage) following the use of a pneumococcal conjugate vaccine in a clinical trial.

Unpublished efficacy data have been provided recently for a third large-scale clinical trial in which 40,000 infants from South Africa were randomized to receive either a placebo or a 9-valent pneumococcal conjugate vaccine manufactured by Wyeth-Lederle. The results demonstrate an efficacy for vaccine-type pneumococcal invasive disease of approximately 85 percent and 58 percent for infants who are HIV negative and HIV positive, respectively. Radiographic pneumonia with consolidation revealed efficacies of 22 percent and 6 percent for infants who are HIV negative and HIV positive, respectively.

Several potential pneumococcal vaccine candidates are currently under investigation, including conjugate vaccines that incorporate different carrier proteins from the standard diphtheria and tetanus toxoids, such as surface protein D isolated from a strain of nontypeable *H. influenzae.*

Other pneumococcal antigens, such as pneumococcal surface protein (Psp)A and PspC, autolysin, pneumolysin, hyaluronate lyase, pneumococcal surface antigen A, choline binding protein A, and several neuraminidase enzymes, also are being considered as potential vaccines or drug targets. Highly conserved versions of these protein-based vaccines may offer a greater degree of protection against invasive and noninvasive forms of pneumococcal disease either alone or in conjunction with other protein/enzyme vaccines, the licensed pneumococcal conjugate vaccine, or the capsular polysaccharide vaccines. For example, PspA has been shown to elicit antibodies in mice that protect against a challenge 100 times the minimal lethal dose (LD_{50}). Passive protection experiments with these antibodies also protect, suggesting a significant role of this protein in the pathogenesis of disease. The protein-based vaccines also may provide a more comprehensive approach to dealing with *S. pneumoniae* by stimulating broader antibody responses, including mucosal immunity, to the various 92 serotypes associated with the organism. With this in mind, it is possible that these protein vaccines may improve the ability of immunocompromised populations (e.g., HIV patients, diabetics, organ transplantation patients, sickle cell disease patients) and the elderly, particularly the chronically ill and nursing home populations, to respond more vigorously to pneumococcal antigens. Because pneumococcal disease has a three- to tenfold increased incidence in Native Americans, Alaska Natives, and African Americans of all age groups compared to Caucasian populations, efforts to improve the vaccination status of these ethnic/minority groups are ongoing.

One area of particular concern following the use of conjugate pneumococcal vaccines in children is the reported increase in nasopharyngeal carriage of and disease from nonvaccine serotypes of pneumococci. There are preliminary data to indicate that candidate protein vaccines most likely will contribute significantly to eliminating and/or controlling replacement serotypes, observed following the use of conjugate vaccines such as Prevnar®, especially in cases of otitis media.

Additional exciting data have demonstrated that intranasal immunization with pneumococcal antigens can lead to protection against pneumococcal disease, and more importantly, against pneumococcal carriage in the nasal passages of mice. This discovery may be critical to the eventual control of pneumococcal disease. Pneumococci are spread by person-to-person contact. They are found in the nasal passages of between 10 and 50 percent of humans, depending on age and health status, with children generally being the primary reservoir. In most cases, carriage does not result in disease, but in some cases the pneumococci invade from the nasal tissue to cause pneumonia, ear infections, eye infections, or meningitis. Vaccines that could prevent carriage would be able to prevent the spread of pneumococci and ultimately its ability to causes disease.

For reasons not well understood, the overwhelming majority of penicillin-resistant, multidrug-resistant *S. pneumoniae* isolates express a select few of the 90 different capsular types associated with the pneumococcus. These capsular types are predominantly 6B, 9V, 14, 19F, and 23F. The restriction of these dangerous drug-resistant bacteria to such a few serotypes raised the hopes that appropriate conjugate vaccines, which include these few serotypes, could corner the most dangerous strains of *S. pneumoniae*. Recent work led to the discovery of how resistant bacteria could break out of this corner. The process involves the transfer of DNA molecules containing genetic determinants of new capsular types from multidrug-resistant strains to strains containing different capsular polysaccharides. In a recent outbreak of multidrug-resistant pneumococcal disease among AIDS patients in New York, a most unusual phenomenon occurred—the appearance of a widely spread multidrug-resistant pneumococcal strain that usually expresses the 23F capsule, but this time, in these isolates, acquired the capsular type 3. The bacterium was resistant to all the useful antibiotics currently used against pneumococci except vancomycin. A simple test, using a mouse model, showed that these capsular type 3 "transformants" of the multidrug-resistant pneumococcus have increased their virulence capacity more than a millionfold over that of the same bacterium when it carries the usual 23F capsule. Wide-scale deployment of pneumococcal vaccines may produce a selective pressure for this type of capsular switch among clinical isolates. The above finding emphasizes the importance of increased international surveillance for resistant pneumococci.

Suggested Reading

Advisory Committee on Immunization Practices. (1997). Prevention of pneumococcal disease: Recommendations of the ACIP. *Morbidity and Mortality Weekly Report, 46,* 1-24.

Black, S., Shinefield, H., Fireman, B., et al. (2000). Efficacy, safety, and immunogenicity of a heptavalent pneumococcal conjugate vaccine in children. *Pediatric Infectious Disease Journal, 19,* 187-195.

Briles, D. E., et al. (2000). Immunization of humans with rPspA elicits antibodies that passively protect mice from fatal infection with *Streptococcus pneumoniae* bearing heterologous PspA. *Journal of Infectious Diseases, 182,* 1694-1701.

Coral, M. C. V., et al. (in press). Families of pneumococcal surface protein A (PspA) of *Streptococcus pneumoniae* invasive isolates recovered from Colombian children. *Emerging Infectious Diseases.*

Eskola, J., Kilpi, T., Palmu, A., et al. (2001). Efficacy of a pneumococcal conjugate vaccine against acute otitis media. *New England Journal of Medicine, 344,* 403-409.

Jedrzejas, M. J. (2001). Pneumococcal virulence factors: Structure and function. *Microbiology and Molecular Biology Reviews, 65,* 187-207.

Kirk, M., & Chan-Tack, M. D. (2001). Influenza and pneumococcal immunization rates among a high-risk population. *Southern Medical Journal, 94,* 323-324.

Lipsitch, M., et al. (2000). Competition among *Streptococcus pneumoniae* for intranasal colonization in a mouse model. *Vaccine, 18,* 2895-2901.

Lucas, A. H., Moulton, K. D., Tang, V. R., & Reason, D. C. (2001). Combinatorial library cloning of human antibodies to *Streptococcus pneumoniae* capsular polysaccharides: Variable region primary structures and evidence for somatic mutation of Fab fragments specific for capsular serotypes 6B, 14, and 23F. *Infection and Immunity, 69,* 853-864.

Malley, R., et al. (1999). Intranasal immunization with killed unencapsulated whole cells prevents colonization and invasive disease by capsulated pneumococci. *Infection and Immunity, 67,* 4320-4325.

Overturf, G. D., & American Academy of Pediatrics, Committee on Infectious Diseases. (2000). Technical report: Prevention of pneumococcal infection, including the use of pneumococcal conjugate and polysaccharide vaccines and antibiotic prophylaxis. *Pediatrics, 106,* 367-376.

Santosham, M., et al. (2001, April 28-30). *Pneumococcal 7-valent conjugate vaccine prevents carriage among high-risk Native Americans.* Abstract presented at the meeting of the Society for Pediatric Research, Baltimore, MD.

TETANUS

Despite long-established and effective vaccines for tetanus, childhood and neonatal tetanus remain significant worldwide problems. A more simplified approach for immunizing children could greatly facilitate the delivery of these vaccines, decrease the barriers to immunization, and improve immunization rates.

One interesting area that has shown great promise is the use of the skin as a mechanism for the delivery of vaccines. Transcutaneous immunization (TCI) involves the introduction of antigens along with an adjuvant using a topical application to intact skin. This new technology offers many advantages over parenteral injections, such as eliminating the risk of needle-borne diseases and reducing the complications related to physical skin penetration.

Investigators are developing several novel approaches for the delivery of vaccines via the skin. One approach involves incubating expression vectors with the outer layer of skin in a noninvasive mode. Noninvasive vaccination onto the skin (NIVS) requires no needle injections and no specially trained personnel. These investigations have demonstrated that topical application of an adenovirus vector encoding either the tetanus toxin C-fragment (tet-C) or the influenza A virus hemagglutinin (HA) by using a patch could elicit specific humoral immune responses against either tet-C or HA in rodents and nonhuman primates. Subfragments of the antigen DNA can be found in other areas of the skin or in deep tissues after localized gene delivery by a patch. Results suggest that a transient but productive wave of antigen expression within the outer layer of skin may be able to broadcast specific signals to activate the immune system. In addition, data have been presented indicating that animals with preexposure to adenovirus can still be vaccinated by adenovirus-mediated NIVS. It is conceivable that anti-adenovirus immunologic components may not be able to reach the surface of the skin in sufficient quantities for counteracting applied vectors. These studies suggest that vaccines may be inoculated by simply applying a "vaccine patch" containing concentrated adenovirus recombinants that encode specific antigens. The patch would be applied to the outer layer of skin, which is a convenient target site and an immunocompetent area for the delivery of vaccines. The possibility of eliciting specific immune responses after the delivery of noninvasive vaccines provides the impetus for translating patch-based, noninvasive vaccination into routine vaccination programs in a wide variety of clinical settings.

Another approach in the development of this technology involves the use of cholera toxin (CT), which, when applied to the skin surface, acts as an adjuvant for the coadministered antigens diphtheria toxoid and TT. The observation that CT placed on the skin in a saline solution could induce a potent anti-CT response suggests that CT might act as an adjuvant for coadministered proteins on the skin. Studies are now in progress to determine the optimal dose and concentration of diphtheria and tetanus antigens required for TCI, the optimal ratio of antigen to adju-

vant, and whether coadministering various antigens with CT interferes with the immune response to each individual component. One interesting and recent study in sheep found that the concurrent administration of CT (adjuvant) with TT delivered transcutaneously could induce specific systemic antibody responses to both antigens, whereas mucosal IgA antibody responses were absent. This is in contrast to the results observed following an intramuscular immunization with TT with alum where systemic antibody levels were higher and mucosal IgA responses were observed.

Other novel antigen delivery systems have been developed in recent years, including a new technique of antigen encapsulation that renders antigens, formerly ineffective when administered orally, into potent immunogens. This new encapsulation process avoids the use of organic solvents, protects the antigens during their passage through the stomach, and releases the antigens in a "burst" into the small intestine. With the aid of certain excipients, antigen presentation to Peyer's patches in sufficient quantity results in a vigorous immune response that is comparable to that produced by a parenterally administered antigen with an adjuvant such as alum. Numerous successful oral immunization studies have been carried out in mice with a number of antigens encapsulated by this new technique. In atopic humans, an encapsulated allergen (i.e., short ragweed extract) has been administered orally and induces significant immune responses.

Mice given three doses orally of encapsulated TT on Days 0, 1, and 2 demonstrated an increase in the anti-TT antibody response after the primary immunization, and a significant anamnestic response following a boost with the encapsulated vaccine on Days 42, 43, and 44. Ragweed-sensitive patients, who received escalating or maintenance daily doses for up to 8 weeks, responded with a remarkable increase in allergen-specific IgG that was similar to the immune response observed with high-dose, long-term, subcutaneously administered allergen. No toxicity was observed among the volunteers.

A phase I/II clinical trial with the encapsulated TT has been completed in healthy adults with prevaccine anti-tetanus antibody titers <2 IU/ml. The objectives of this study were to show that the encapsulated antigens can elicit a booster response in humans and to compare the immune response following oral immunization to that obtained with standard intramuscular immunization with TT. There were no serious adverse events that appeared to be associated with the microencapsulated, TT material in normal healthy adults. Anti-TT antibody responses, as measured by a neutralizing antibody assay, were minimal and not significant at all dose levels tested. As expected, most individuals immunized with dT vaccine intramuscularly responded rapidly with significant increased titers to both antigens. It is likely that a single oral administration of the microencapsulated vaccine may not be sufficient to stimulate the mucosal immune response. In addition, it may be necessary to alum adsorb the tetanus antigen to make it more immunogenic.

Other projects designed to produce a needle-free tetanus immunization have involved the use of an adenovirus recombinant carrier encoding the immunogenic but nontoxic tetanus toxin C-fragment. The use of a single dose administered either intranasally or by an epicutaneous patch can provide 100-percent and 80-percent protection, respectively, against a lethal challenge of live *Clostridium tetani*. The use of needle-free approaches for vaccinating against tetanus can provide a very safe, cost-effective, and compliant-friendly way to protect the public, especially in developing countries, against this deadly disease.

Sources

Chen, D., Colditz, I. G., Glenn, G. M., & Tsonis, C. G. (2002). Effect of transcutaneous immunization with co-administered antigen and cholera toxin on systemic and mucosal antibody responses in sheep. *Veterinary Immunology and Immunopathology, 86,* 177-182.

Flanagan, M., Wang, C., & Michael, J. G. (1993). Characterization of the immune response following the oral administration of modified antigen in an adjuvant-free system (abstract). *Journal of Immunology, 150,* 35.

Glenn, G. M., Rao, M. R., Matyas, G. R., & Alving, C. R. (1998). Immunization through the skin using cholera toxin. *Nature, 391,* 851.

Glenn, G. M., Scharton-Kersten, T., Vassell-Vassell, R., Mallet, C. P., Hale, T. L., & Alving, C. R. (1998). Transcutaneous immunization with cholera toxin protects mice against lethal mucosal toxin challenge. *Journal of Immunology, 161,* 3211-3214.

Hammond, S. A., Guebre-Xabier, M., Yu, J., & Glenn, G. M. (2001). Transcutaneous immunization: An emerging route of immunization and potent immunostimulation strategy. *Critical Reviews in Therapeutic Drug Carrier Systems, 18,* 501-526.

Litwin, A., Flanagan, M., Entis, G., Gottschlich, G., Easch, R., Garside, P., & Michael, J. G. (1996). Immunologic effects of encapsulated short ragweed extract: A potent new agent for oral immunotherapy. *Annals of Allergy, Asthma & Immunology, 77,* 132-138.

Shi, Z., Zeng, M., Yang, G., Siegel, F., et al. (in press). Adenovirus as a carrier for needles-free vaccination against tetanus. *Vaccine.*

TUBERCULOSIS

Despite significant advances in tuberculosis research and treatment strategies worldwide, tuberculosis remains one of the leading killers in infectious diseases. Failure to eradicate tuberculosis worldwide is attributable to a number of factors, including insufficient public health infrastructure; poverty; homelessness; crowding; drug abuse; and the HIV coepidemic, which not only speeds up the pathogenesis of tuberculosis in HIV-infected patients, but significantly increases the chance for conversion of asymptomatic *Mycobacterium tuberculosis* infection to active tuberculosis. Infection with *M. tuberculosis*, in most cases, results in an asymptomatic colonization with the bacterium, which is controlled by the immune system (latent or persistent infection). Weakening of the immune system can result in reactivation of bacterial growth and progression to active tuberculosis. Development of effective vaccines to prevent either primary infection with *M. tuberculosis* or progression to active disease remains a priority for NIAID. In 1998, the U.S. Department of Health and Human Services Advisory Council for Elimination of Tuberculosis (ACET), U.S. National Vaccine Program Office, and NIAID of NIH convened a workshop to develop a national strategy and research plan for the development of effective vaccines against tuberculosis, the Blueprint for Tuberculosis Vaccine Development.

Despite available chemotherapy to treat tuberculosis effectively and prevent death by this disease, the duration of treatment (6 to 9 months), and drug-related adverse events frequently lead to noncompliance and treatment failures, which in turn often result in the development and spread of drug-resistant tuberculosis. A combination of active case finding, drug treatment via directly observed treatment short course (DOTS), and vaccination is considered the most effective means by which tuberculosis could be eliminated as a global public health burden.

The only currently available tuberculosis vaccine, *Mycobacterium bovis* BCG, was developed almost 100 years ago. Despite its lack of consistent efficacy to prevent adult pulmonary tuberculosis, this vaccine is used worldwide and protects to a reasonable degree against disseminated tuberculosis in infants.

Changes in this Research Area in 20 Years

Until the early 1980s, tuberculosis in the United States had been steadily declining. A sudden increase in new cases was reported between 1986 and 1992, followed once again by a decline. It was realized that this resurgence of tuberculosis was attributable largely to a deteriorating public health infrastructure and was also coincident with the HIV epidemic. In 1993, tuberculosis was declared a global health emergency by WHO. Subsequent to these events, research funding and interest in this disease increased steadily, and significant advances have been made in the understanding of tuberculosis immunology and vaccinology. During the past 10 years, a number of global organizations, including NIH, have increased significantly their financial support for tuberculosis research and vaccine development. NIH alone has increased funds for tuberculosis research from $3.6 million per year in 1991 to $56 million per year in 2001. The European Commission's Tuberculosis Vaccine Cluster, a collaboration between academic and industrial entities, has dedicated EU 5 million for research to better understand tuberculosis vaccine efficacy, as well as to develop and evaluate preclinical vaccine candidates. Action TB, an international open research collaboration established in 1993 and coordinated by GlaxoSmithKline, has allocated £20 million from 1993 to 2003 to fund translational tuberculosis research programs, including the identification and development of vaccine candidates and surrogate markers of protection. The Bill and Melinda Gates Foundation has contributed $20 million to research leading to the development of an effective new tuberculosis vaccine (2000 to 2005).

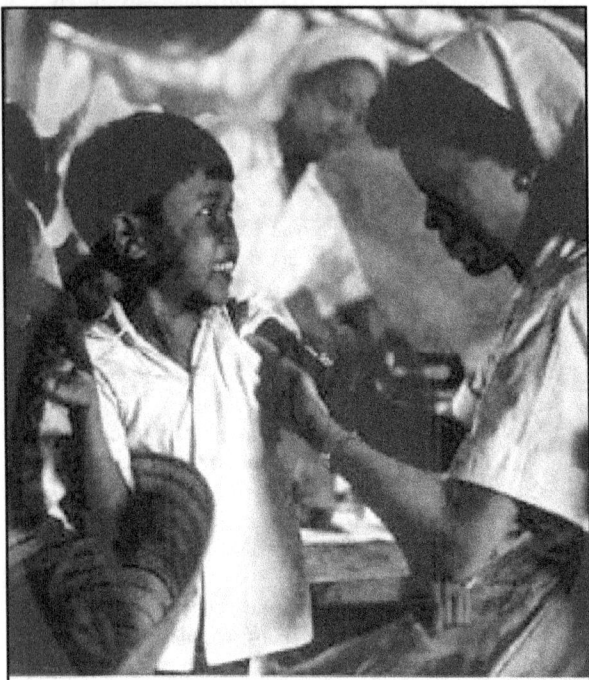

BCG VACCINATION HAS BEEN GIVEN TO MILLIONS

At the end of the war a campaign was started to give BCG vaccination to people threatened by tuberculosis. This work is still going on in many countries with assistance from WHO and UNICEF. Ninety million have been vaccinated.

3

Courtesy of NLM

Research in vaccine development was especially boosted in recent years by the publication of the complete sequence of the *M. tuberculosis* genome, as well as by the availability of genetic tools that allowed production of recombinant mycobacterial strains to aid in vaccine development and evaluation.

Overall, significant efforts have been made to understand and reevaluate BCG field trials worldwide and to understand the cause(s) of varying efficacy for this vaccine in different populations and geographic areas. This interest led to the development of advanced animal models of *M. tuberculosis* infection in an attempt to mimic more closely human disease in animals and to possibly predict vaccine efficacy from animal studies. From these experiments, it became clear that the pathogenesis of tuberculosis varies among different animal models of infection

and disease and that a number of immunological factors modulate disease outcome after infection with *M. tuberculosis*.

Through the development and refinement of these models, which now extend from rodents (mice and guinea pigs) to rabbits and nonhuman primates, researchers continue to gain insight into immunological factors that are

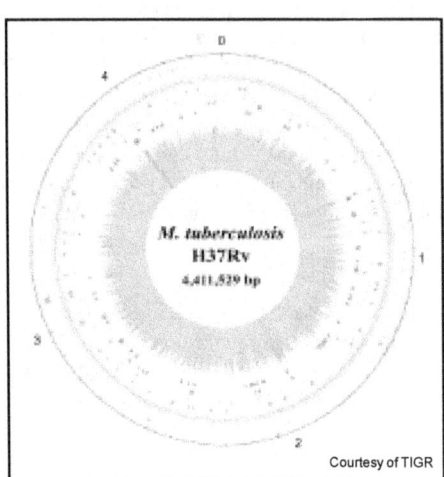

Courtesy of TIGR

Genome for M. Tuberculosis

involved in the development of active disease versus asymptomatic, controlled infection. This enhanced understanding of small animal models of tuberculosis has enabled the testing of more than 170 potential vaccine candidates over the past 5 to 10 years. These potential candidates comprise a number of vaccine classes: Recombinant BCG and live-attenuated *M. tuberculosis* strains, various other live vectors (bacterial and viral), subunit vaccines, DNA vaccines, and approaches to improve upon the use of BCG through adjunctive immunotherapy and prime-boost strategies. BCG is usually administered once early in life. However, since the protective efficacy of BCG appears to diminish with time, investigations are underway to determine whether alternative routes of administration and/or revaccination or boosting with protein antigens would reactivate immunological memory and prevent reactivation disease. Since about one-third of the world's population is infected with *M. tuberculosis*, and many of these individuals also received childhood BCG vaccinations, this strategy may prove critical in the prevention of disease progression from asymptomatic infection, especially in areas where there is a high prevalence of HIV co-infection.

Several candidates that appear to protect against virulent *M. tuberculosis* in small animal models equally well or better than BCG are being prepared to enter early human clinical trials. These include a recombinant BCG vaccine expressing the 30 kD major secretory protein of *M. tuberculosis*, Ag85B; a fusion protein composed of immunodominant *M. tuberculosis* peptides; a multi-epitope subunit vaccine/adjuvant combination; and a boost strategy using Ag85A expressed from a viral vector after primary BCG vaccination.

Most Significant Scientific Advances in Tuberculosis Vaccine Research

The most significant scientific advances in tuberculosis vaccine research include the development of genetic tools in mycobacteria and the sequencing of the *M. tuberculosis* genome. These advances, combined with the development of advanced animal models, allow targeted selection of candidate genes, creation of mutant mycobacterial strains, and evaluation *in vivo*. Recently, this research was further augmented through the establishment of the Structural Genomics Consortium, funded by NIH and led by Los Alamos National Laboratory, whose goal is to determine the three-dimensional structure of more than 400 *M. tuberculosis* proteins. Advances toward a more thorough understanding of tuberculosis immunology are also enabling a more detailed re-evaluation of the varying efficacy of BCG. From this, hypotheses have emerged as to the parameters that may be important in protection against tuberculosis. These hypotheses have guided strategies to arrive at a vaccine superior to BCG. The current efforts have culminated in the first set of candidate vaccines to enter human trials since BCG was introduced in 1921.

BCG Tice (Organon, Inc.) is licensed, but not recommended for inclusion in tuberculosis vaccination and control programs in the United States. Worldwide, a variety of BCG strains are available and widely delivered under the Expanded Programme on Immunization (EPI) as antituberculosis vaccines.

Several tuberculosis vaccine candidates are scheduled to be evaluated in humans within the next few years. One, a BCG-prime/modified virus Ankara (MVA)-Ag85 boost strategy is about to enter phase I testing in the United Kingdom. Others, as noted above, should enter early human testing within the next 1 to 2 years. Strategies to develop immunotherapeutic adjuvants have also resulted in clinical trials. For example, *Mycobacterium vaccae* has been administered as an adjunct to regular chemo-therapy in several recent trials and is currently under study in HIV-infected individuals in Tanzania.

Challenges for the Development of a Vaccine for Tuberculosis

The majority of research toward new and improved vaccines has only occurred during the last decade. Hence, little historical experience in tuberculosis vaccinology is available that can be used as guidance for the development or improvement of new tuberculosis vaccines. Although, and largely because, tuberculosis vaccine research has made tremendous advances over the last 10 to 15 years, a number of critical questions are arising whose answers should remarkably speed tuberculosis vaccine development:

- What is the basis of asymptomatic colonization (or latency, persistence) and what does it mean from the standpoint of bacterial physiology and host response? To answer this question, improved animal models that specifically mimic latency as seen in humans, or alternatively, strategies to derive relevant answers from human tissue need to be developed.

Types of Vaccine Candidates

Type	Pros	Cons	Promise
rBCGs (expressing cytokines, protective Ags, listeriolysin)	Safe Inexpensive	Safe in immuno-compromised?	MODERATE/HIGH
Live, attenuated M.tb (auxotrophs)	Mimics natural infection	Safety must be shown	MODERATE
Other myco-bacteria (vaccae, microti, habana)	Safe	Not strongly immunogenic	LOW

Types of Vaccine Candidates (2)

Type	Pros	Cons	Promise
Non-mycobacterial living vectors (Salmonella, Vaccinia expressing M.tb Ags)	Novel delivery methods possible	No evidence yet of immunity better than BCG	MODERATE
Subunit vaccines; fusions (proteins, peptides, lipids, CHOs)	Safe Well-characterized Easily manufactured Can generate strong immunity	Likely to require multiple doses and adjuvant	MODERATE/HIGH
DNA vaccines	•Easy to manufacture; inexpensive; stable	Unproven efficacy Needs adjuvant Safety concerns	MODERATE/HIGH

Courtesy of Ann Ginsberg and Christine Sreemore

- What factors can serve as markers of immunoprotection in humans to allow assessment of immunogenicity in clinical trials? Only with the aid of data from human vaccine trials will researchers be able to refine animal models and identify what immune parameters need to be established for further vaccine development. For these reasons, it is critical that vaccine candidates are quickly evaluated for safety and efficacy in human trials, and any subsequent findings used to devise more targeted vaccine strategies.

- What is the importance of co-infections and comorbidity in patients at high risk for *M. tuberculosis* infection and progression to active disease? Will a vaccine that was developed in laboratory animals be effective in these real-life settings?

- What role will diagnostics play in the development of tuberculosis vaccines? Since delayed-type hypersensitiv-ity (DTH) testing is not a reliable measure of infection or cure, identification of the appropriate patient population remains a challenge. For this reason, diagnostics development needs to remain closely coupled with immunology and vaccinology research to produce, in parallel, essential tools for the successful conduct of clinical evaluation of candidate vaccines.

- How does BCG work in children? This is a currently understudied but important aspect of vaccine development. Little is known about general or tuberculosis-specific differences in immune response and vaccine efficacy among infants, children, and adults. It is recognized that tuberculosis presents clinically quite differently in young children than in adults and that BCG efficacy differs significantly in these populations.

- Since it will not be ethical to conduct a placebo controlled clinical trial with an experimental vaccine, what treatment regimens will the patient populations receive during this trial? How will this influence the ability to assess efficacy of the vaccine or even the outcome measures of the trial? How can effectual studies be designed to minimize the sample size and study duration? Who will fund such challenging and time-consuming studies and commercialize a vaccine? At the stage of clinical evaluation, there is a large number of challenges that will influence the design of efficacy trials in humans.

- Can a tuberculosis vaccine be developed for and safely tested in HIV-positive patients?

NIAID-Supported Tuberculosis Vaccine Research

To answer the above questions, NIAID is funding not only investigator-initiated research, but solicited research on tuberculosis immunology, pathology, pathogenesis, vaccine development, target antigen identification, diagnostics, development of improved tools for epidemiological studies, and development of markers of immunoprotection. Additionally, the aforementioned Structural Genomics Consortium will determine the structure of more than 400 *M. tuberculosis* proteins through national and international collaborations and make the resulting data available to the research community.

NIAID's Tuberculosis Research Materials and Vaccine Screening Contract provides high-quality research reagents and vaccine testing services in small animal models to researchers worldwide. NIAID's Tuberculosis Research Unit and vaccine testing and evaluation units provide clinical trials infrastructure for vaccine evaluation and establishment of surrogate markers of protection nationally and internationally. A recent request for proposals seeks to establish contract resources for vaccine platform development.

Despite the many challenges remaining in tuberculosis vaccine development, a new sense of optimism is permeating the tuberculosis research and public health communities as recent research advances result in novel vaccine candidates entering human trials.

Sources

Advisory Committee for the Elimination of Tuberculosis. (1996). The role of BCG vaccine in the prevention and control of tuberculosis in the United States. A joint statement by the Advisory Council for the Elimination of Tuberculosis and the Advisory Committee on Immunization Practices. *Morbidity and Mortality Weekly Report, 45*(RR-4), 1-18.

Antonucci, G., Girardi, E., Raviglione, M. C., & Ippolito, G. (1995). Risk factors for tuberculosis in HIV infected persons: A prospective cohort study. The Gruppo Italiano di Studio Tubercolosi e AIDS (GISTA). *Journal of the American Medical Association, 274*, 143-148.

Baldwin, S. L., D'Souza, C., Roberts, A. D., Kelly, B. P., Frank, A. A., Lui, M. A., Ulmer, J. B., Huygen, K., McMurray, D. M., & Orme, I. M. (1998). Evaluation of new vaccines in the mouse and guinea pig model of tuberculosis. *Infection and Immunity, 66*, 2951-2959.

Bardarov, S., Kriakov, J., Carriere, C., Vaamonde, C., McAdam, R. A., Bloom, B. R., Hatfull, G. F., & Jacobs, W. R. (1997). Conditionally replicating mycobacteriophages: A system for transposon delivery to *Mycobacterium tuberculosis. Proceedings of the National Academy of Sciences, 94*, 10961-10966.

Behr, M. A. (2001). Comparative genomics of BCG vaccines. *Tuberculosis (Edinb), 81*, 165-168.

Behr, M. A., Wilson, M. A., Gill, W. P., Salamon, H., Schoolnik, G. K., Rane, S., & Small, P. M. (1999). Comparative genomics of BCG vaccines by whole-genome DNA microarray. *Science, 284*, 1520-1523.

Blower, S. M., Small, P. M., & Hopewell, P. C. (1996). Control strategies for tuberculosis epidemics: New models for old problems. *Science, 273*, 497-500.

Brandt, L., Feino Cunha, J., Weinreich Olsen, A., Chilima, B., Hirsch, P., Appelberg, R., & Andersen, P. (2002). Failure of the Mycobacterium bovis BCG vaccine: Some species of environmental mycobacteria block multiplication of BCG and induction of protective immunity to tuberculosis. *Infection and Immunity, 70*, 672-678.

Centers for Disease Control and Prevention. (2001). *Reported tuberculosis data in the United States, 2000.* Atlanta, GA: United States Department of Health and Human Services.

Colditz, G. A., Berkey, C. S., Mosteller, F., Brewer, T. F., Wilson, M. E., Burdick, E., & Fineberg, H. V. (1995). The efficacy of bacillus Calmette-Guerin vaccination of newborns and infants in the prevention of tuberculosis: Meta-analyses of the published literature. *Pediatrics, 96*(1Pt 1), 29-35.

Colditz, G. A., Brewer, T. F., Berkey, C. C., Wilson, M. E., Burdick, E., Fineberg, H. V., & Mosteller, F. (1994). Efficacy of BCG vaccine in the prevention of tuberculosis. Meta analysis of the published literature. *Journal of the American Medical Association, 271,* 698-702.

Cole, S. T., Brosch, R., Parkhill, J., Garnier, T., Churcher, C., Harris, D., Gordon, S. V., Eiglmeier, K., Gas, S., Barry, C. E., Tekaia, F., Badcock, K., Basham, D., Brown, D., Chillingworth, T., Connor, R., Davies, R., Devlin, K., Feltwell, T., Gentles, S., Hamlin, N., Holroyd, S., Hornsby, T., Jagels, K., & Barrell, B. G. (1998). Deciphering the biology of *Mycobacterium tuberculosis* from the complete genome sequence [published erratum: *Nature* (1998), 396, 190]. *Nature, 393,* 537-544.

Elias, D., Wolday, D., Akuffo, H., Petros, B., Bronner, U., & Britton, S. (2001). Effect of deworming on human T cell responses to mycobacterial antigens in helminth-exposed individuals before and after bacille Calmette-Guerin (BCG) vaccination. *Clinical and Experimental Immunology, 123,* 219-225.

Flynn, J. L., & Chan, J. (2001). Immunology of tuberculosis. *Annual Review of Immunology, 19,* 93-129.

Geiter, L. (2000). *Ending neglect: The elimination of tuberculosis in the United States.* Washington, DC: Committee on the Elimination of Tuberculosis in the United States, Division of Health Promotion and Disease Prevention, Institute of Medicine.

Ginsberg, A. M. (2000). A proposed national strategy for tuberculosis vaccine development. *Clinical Infectious Diseases, 30*(Suppl. 3), S233-S242.

Hoft, D. F., Brown, R. M., & Belshe, R. B. (2000). Mucosal vaccination of humans inhibits delayed type hypersensitivity to purified protein derivative but induces mycobacteria-specific interferon-gamma responses. *Clinical Infectious Diseases, 30*(Suppl. 3), S217-S222.

Horwitz, M. A., Harth, G., Dillon, B. J., & Maslesa-Galic, S. (2000). Recombinant bacillus Calmette-Guerin (BCG) vaccines expressing the *Mycobacterium tuberculosis* 30-kDa major secretory protein induce greater protective immunity against tuberculosis than conventional BCG vaccines in a highly susceptible animal model. *Proceedings of the National Academy of Sciences, 97*(25), 13853-13858.

Institute for Genomic Research. *Sequence for Mycobacterium tuberculosis strain CDC1551.* http://www.tigr.org/tigr-cripts/CMR2/GenomePage3.spl?database=gmt.

Johnson, J. L., Kamya, R. M., Okwera, A., Loughlin, A. M., Nyole, S., Hom, D. L., Wallis, R. S., Hirsch, C. S., Wolski, K.,

Foulds, J., Mugerwa, R. D., & Ellner, J. J. (2000). Randomized controlled trial of *Mycobacterium vaccae* immunotherapy in non-human immunodeficiency virus-infected Ugandan adults with newly diagnosed pulmonary tuberculosis. The Uganda-Case Western Reserve University Research Collaboration. *Journal of Infectious Diseases, 181*(4), 1304-1312.

McShane, H., Brookes, R., Gilbert, S. C., & Hill, A. V. (2001). Enhanced immunogenicity of CD4(+) T-cell responses and protective efficacy of a DNA-modified vaccinia virus Ankara prime-boost vaccination regimen for murine tuberculosis. *Infection and Immunity, 69*(2), 681-686.

National Institute of Allergy and Infectious Diseases. *Global Health Research Plan for HIV/AIDS, Malaria and Tuberculosis.* http://www.niaid.nih.gov/publications/globalhealth/global.pdf.

Orme, I. M., McMurray, D. N., & Belisle, J. T. (2001). Tuberculosis vaccine development: Recent progress. *Trends in Microbiology, 9,* 115-118.

Pelicic, V., Jackson, M., Reyrat, J. M., Jacobs, W. R., Gicquel, B., & Guilhot, C. (1997). Efficient allelic exchange and transposon mutagenesis in *Mycobacterium tuberculosis. Proceedings of the National Academy of Sciences, 94,* 10955-10960.

Perlman, D. C., El-Helou, P., & Sal, N. (1999). Tuberculosis in patients with human immunodeficiency virus infection. *Seminars in Respiratory Infections 14*(4), 344-352.

Skeiky, Y. A., Ovendale, P. J., Alderson, M. R., Dillon, D. C., Smith, S., Wilson, C. B., Orme, I. M., Reed, S. G., & Campos-Neto, A. (2000). T cell expression cloning of a *Mycobacterium tuberculosis* gene encoding a protective antigen associated with the early control of infection. *Journal of Immunology, 165,* 7140-7149.

Waddell, R. D., Chintu, C., Lein, A. D., Zumla, A., Karagas, M. R., et al. (2000). Safety and immunogenicity of a five-dose series of inactivated *Mycobacterium tuberculosis* vaccination for the prevention of HIV-associated tuberculosis. *Clinical Infectious Diseases 30*(Suppl. 3), S309-S315.

Worku, D., & Hoft, D. F. (2000). *In vitro* measurement of protective mycobacterial immunity: Antigen specific expansion of T cells capable of inhibiting extracellular growth of bacilli Calmette-Guerin. *Clinical Infectious Diseases, 30*(Suppl. 3) S257-S261.

World Health Organization. (2000). *WHO fact sheet number 104: Tuberculosis.* http://www.who.int/inf-fs/en/fact104.html.

Jordan Perspective: Acellular Pertussis Vaccines

The effort to develop an improved pertussis vaccine was associated with very turbulent times that should be remembered best for the fact that four such vaccines were licensed in the United States. They also will be remembered for leading to the creation of the National Childhood Vaccine Injury Act and for the splendid cooperation of Japanese and Swedish scientists. The effort also required perhaps the greatest amount of intercontinental air travel of any foreign vaccine trial to date. Dr. David Klein, the responsible program officer, made 36 trips to Sweden in 7 years. I am indebted to him for providing notes and comments regarding the following sequence of events (1).

Bordetella pertussis was isolated and so named in 1906 by French bacteriologists Jules Bordet and Octave Gengou who developed the first vaccine in 1912. Twelve years later, Thorvald Madsen reported some evidence of protection by crude whole-cell vaccines, and in 1942, Pearl Kendrick and colleagues at the Michigan Department of Public Health developed a combination diphtheria-tetanus-pertussis vaccine (two toxoids plus whole cells). Whole cell vaccine was licensed in the United States in 1948, with licensure of diphtheria and tetanus toxoids and whole-cell pertussis (DTP) vaccine following a year later. I still remember the name of my childhood friend who had whooping cough, but most people forgot how severe the disease is because immunization with DTP decreased the reported number of cases in the United States from more than 265,269 in 1934 to 1,010 in 1976, the year I came to the National Institutes of Health (NIH). The public became increasingly aware of the adverse reactions to DPT attributed to the whole-cell vaccines, and began to reject the vaccine despite the continuing circulation of the bacterium. Neither infection nor immunization provides lifelong immunity (2). Electing to risk disease rather than accept immunization, antivaccine movements increased in Japan, Sweden, Britain, Italy, and other countries (3).

Whole-cell vaccine usage was discontinued in Japan and Great Britain in 1974-1975; pertussis morbidity and mortality returned. To address some of the issues, an international symposium on pertussis to examine the risk-to-benefit ratio of whole-cell vaccination was held at NIH on November 1-3, 1978. Sweden discontinued immunization for pertussis the next year. In Japan, before the National Institute of Allergy and Infectious Diseases (NIAID) had listed "subcellular antigen" of pertussis as being in early development (see Table 3 in "History and Commentary"), scientists had developed an acellular vaccine and instituted routine administration of it to children 2 years of age and older in 1981 (4). Somehow, I missed the fact of this early use even after I met two scientists Drs. Hiroko and Yugi Sato who participated in the development of the acellular vaccine at the Japanese

National Institutes of Health (5) and were working in the laboratory of Dr. Charles Manclark of the Food and Drug Administration (FDA) when the need for an acellular vaccine for use in the United States became dramatically apparent.

This happened in 1982 when a Washington, DC, affiliate of NBC aired "DTP: Vaccine Roulette." There followed the formation of Determined Parents Together (DPT) by Barbara Loe Fisher, a concerned Virginia parent. NIAID responded the next year by issuing a call for proposals for development of an acellular vaccine and contracted with the Michigan Department of Public Health to do so. By 1984, vaccine manufacturers were overwhelmed with litigation; only two were still marketing whole-cell vaccine. In 1985, the publication of the book *DTP: A Shot in the Dark* by medical historian Harris L. Coulter and Ms. Fisher provided some personal insight into the problems associated with the use of DTP vaccine. Congressional hearings began on the National Childhood Vaccine Injury Act coauthored by DPT and the American Academy of Pediatrics. A public health service interagency pertussis subcommittee was formed, and a small working group from this subcommittee visited Japan to learn of its experience with acellular pertussis vaccines. NIAID broadened a contract with the National Bacteriology Laboratory of Sweden to undertake an efficacy trial of two Japanese-produced acellular vaccines in infants.

Unfortunately, the Michigan Department of Public Health, with advice from FDA staff and the Sato's, was unable to produce a satisfactory acellular vaccine. Fortunately, the public health service subcommittee successfully negotiated with two Japanese manufacturers, BIKEN and Takeda Chemical Industries, Ltd., to provide vaccines for the Swedish trials. These companies would eventually collaborate with U.S. vaccine manufacturers to produce diphtheria and tetanus toxoids and acellular pertussis (DTaP) vaccine—Japanese acellular pertussis combined with U.S. diphtheria and tetanus toxoids. The first trial to get underway in Sweden in 1986 compared pertussis toxin (PT) with PT plus filamentous hemagglutinin (FHA). They were 54 percent and 69 percent efficacious, respectively. This same year, Congress passed the National Childhood Vaccine Injury Act and mandated NIAID to accelerate development and testing of new candidate acellular vaccines with the goal of licensure.

In 1989, NIAID sought candidate vaccines from manufacturers for phase I/II trials. Nine manufacturers in 5 countries submitted 13 acellular vaccines. Sample lots were sent to the FDA's Center for Biologics Evaluation and Research to be tested for purity, and a multicenter trial was conducted at six

Laboratories in Stockholm and the Institute Superior of Sanita in Rome to perform phase III efficacy trials with vaccines selected after the phase I/II trials. All of the vaccines were trivalent-DTaP. But not all acellular (aP) components were the same in the trials that followed in Italy (7), Sweden (8), and elsewhere. *B. pertussis*, a complex organism, consists of many parts, most of which seem to be antigenic: PT, FHA, three types of agglutinogens (AGGs), and pertactin (PRN). Since extensive trials established no firm correlate of protection, vaccine manufacturers have successfully licensed products with only a single acellular component, PT (9), to as many as five. They are tabulated below:

Product Company	ACEL-IMUNE® Wyeth-Lederle*	Tripedia® Connaught/Aventis***	INFANRIX® SKB/GSK	Certiva™ NAV/Baxter**
Licensed	December 1991	August 1992	January 1997	July 1998
Antigens				
PT	+	+	+	+
FHA	+		+	+
PRN	+			
AGG2	+			
AGG3	+			

* Combined with Haemophilus influenzae type b (Hib) conjugate to make Tetramune®; licensed March 1993
** License withdrawn 2001
*** Efforts are underway by this company to license a vaccine with all five pertussis components with or without Hib and inactivated poliovirus (IPV)
GSK = GlaxoSmithKline
SKB = SmithKline Beecham
NAV = North American Vaccine

There are two other items of interest. First, continued use of whole-cell vaccine in the United States caused the pertussis disease burden to be too low to assess vaccine efficacy in the United States. In Italy and Sweden, disease rates were high, and officials were interested in participating in trials of less reactogenic vaccines. But controversy arose over why studies of vaccines that would eventually be used in the United States needed to be conducted abroad. Responsible agencies in all countries allowed the studies to continue. Today, the experimental human immunodeficiency virus (HIV) vaccines developed in the United States are being tested abroad in many countries. Second, Dr. John Robbins of the National Institute of Child Health and Human Development (NICHD), convinced that PT was the essential and only antigen needed, negotiated with other Swedish investigators in Göteburg (9) to test a DTaP vaccine produced by NAV containing only diphtheria and tetanus toxoids. Its efficacy was 71 percent and it was licensed as CertivaÔ in July 1998. Within a year, NAV was absorbed by Baxter, and the license was soon withdrawn. The other vaccines had shown efficacies ranging from 84 to 90 percent, and it had been suggested that physicians would favor vaccine with multiple pertussis antigens.

Vaccines with acellular pertussis antigens have not been associated with serious adverse events, although booster doses induce more intense, but not troublesome, local reactions.

Time from use of acellular vaccine in Japan: 10 years. Time from expressed need for improved vaccine in the United States: 9 years.

The final chapter in this saga is now being written. Because endemic disease occurs in adults in populations in which pertussis is controlled by immunization, a study was begun in 1996 to characterize the epidemiology and clinical spectrum in adults and adolescents and to determine the duration of efficacy and immunity regarding acellular pertussis vaccines.

References

1 Klein, D. L., & Heilman, C. (1996). The new pertussis vaccines. In S. H. E. Kaufman (Ed.), *Concepts in vaccine development*. New York: Walter de Gruytee.

2 Cherry, J. D. (1996). Historical review of pertussis and the classical vaccine. *Journal of Infectious Diseases, 174*(Suppl. 3), S259-S263.

3 Gangarosa, E. J., Galazka, A. M., Wolfe, C. R., et al. (1988). Impact of anti-vaccine movements on pertussis control: The untold story. *Lancet, 351,* 356-361.

4 Kimura, M., & Kuno-Sakai, H. (1988). Epidemiology of pertussis in Japan. (5th International Symposium on Pertussis). *Tokai Journal of Experimental and Clinical Medicine,* (Suppl. 13), 1-7.

5 Sato, Y., Sato, H., Izumiya, K., et al. (1982). Role of antibody to filamentous hemagglutinin and to leukocytosis promoting factors — hemagglutinin in immunity to pertussis. In L. Weinstein & B. N. Fields (Series Eds.) & J. L. Robbins, S. L. Hill, & I. C. Sadoff (Vol. Eds.), *Seminars in infectious diseases: Vol. 4. Bacterial vaccines.* New York: Thieme-Stratton.

6 Edwards, K. M., Meade, B. D., Decker, M. D., et al. (1995). Comparison of 13 acellular pertussis vaccines: Overview and serologic response. *Pediatrics, 96*(3), Part 2, 548-557.

7 Greco, D., Salmaso, A., Mastrantonio, P., et al. (1996). A controlled trial of two acellular vaccines and one whole cell vaccine against pertussis. *New England Journal of Medicine, 334,* 341-348.

8 Gustafsson, L., Hallander, H. O., Olin, P., et al. (1996). A controlled trial of two component acellular, a five component acellular, and a whole-cell pertussis vaccine. *New England Journal of Medicine, 334,* 349-355.

9 Trollfor, B., & Taranger, J. (1997). The Göteborg Pertussis Vaccine Study. In F. Brown, D. Greco, P. Mastrantonio, S. Salmaso, & S. Wassilak (Vol. Eds.), *Developments in biological standardization: Vol. 89. Pertussis vaccine trials* (pp. 49-51). Karger.

Jordan Perspective: Influenza Vaccine

Although the 1918 to 1919 pandemic of influenza near the end of World War I had increased attempts to culture the presumed causative virus, success awaited the use of the living chicken embryo. In 1933, Smith, Andrewes, and Laidlaw (1) reported the growth of the first virus, which became influenza A. In 1934, Francis (2) reported the transmission of a virus shown to be a second type, influenza B (3). Influenza C has since been shown to infect man, but is not a significant pathogen. Many animals—notably fowl, horses, and pigs—harbor, transmit, and are made ill by these viruses. All of these viruses are classified by their two surface proteins—a hemagglutinin (HA) that agglutinates erythrocytes, and a neurominidase (NA) that elutes the virus from cells. The ability to manipulate these two surface antigens has made possible the development and updating of live, attenuated influenza vaccine.

Influenza viruses are negative strand RNA viruses with a segmented genome. Segment four encodes the HA, and segment six encodes the NA. Mutation of these segments, particularly the HA, is occurring constantly, producing new antigenic variants. On occasion, co-infection of cells with a human and an animal virus may lead to the swapping of HA segments and result in a new, more virulent strain. Use has been made of the propensity of influenza virus to swap gene segments to design a live vaccine as a possible substitute for the currently used inactivated vaccine.

Such a vaccine—whole virus harvested from allantoic fluid, concentrated, and inactivated with formaldehyde—was first used with success by Francis to immunize U.S. forces during the early 1940s (4). Disruption of the viral particles and other purification procedures in subsequent years reduced the reactogenicity of the injectable vaccine, improving its uptake. As new HAs are detected by worldwide surveillance, new strains are substituted for old ones. Currently, the vaccine includes two A strains—H_1N_1 and H_3N_2—and one B strain. It is most effective in young and middle-aged adults, and less effective in young children and the elderly.

Studies in the Francis laboratory of the School of Public Health at the University of Michigan were funded in the 1940s and for a number of years thereafter by the U.S. Army through the Board for the Investigation and Control of Influenza and Other Epidemic Diseases in the Army, the forerunner of the Armed Forces Epidemiological Board (AFEB). Dr. Jonas Salk was a member of the laboratory staff who participated in the development of the inactivated vaccine. He later moved to the University of Pittsburgh where he used the same methodology to develop inactivated polio vaccine, the efficacy of which was demonstrated in the 1954 field trial coordinated by Dr. Francis.

Another member of the Francis laboratory is Dr. H. F. Maassab, whose work has been supported since 1976 by the National Institute of Allergy and Infectious Diseases (NIAID), work that made live influenza vaccines possible (5). First with influenza A (A/Ann Arbor/6/60) and then with influenza B (B/AnnArbor/1/66), he attenuated wild-type viruses by serial passage at successively lower temperatures (cold adapted) until they were no longer virulent in ferrets. These became master donor strains whose six internal genes maintained the attenuation characteristic, and whose HA and NA gene segments could be replaced by reassortment with those segments from newly emergent wild-type strains. Dr. Maassab has been able to do this repeatedly, creating live vaccines that matched the composition of the inactivated vaccine for a given season.

Since 1976, cold-adapted influenza virus vaccines (CAIVs) based on Maassab's donor strains have been tested in clinical trials conducted by NIAID scientists and others. Dr. Brian Murphy, of the NIAID Laboratory of Infectious Diseases, and associates studied intranasal installation of CAIV (6) and found that the vaccine was highly protective in adult and pediatric volunteers who were given the vaccine and then challenged with influenza (7). In clinical trials since 1993 cosponsored by Wyeth-Ayerst Research and NIAID, CAIVs, including monovalent and bivalent type A vaccine, monovalent type B vaccine, and trivalent vaccine, have been administered to more than 8,000 subjects whose ages ranged from 2 months to more than 100 years. In 1995, Aviron, as part of a Collaborative Research and Development Agreement (CRADA) with NIAID and a licensing agreement with the University of Michigan, initiated a clinical trial of a cold-adapted trivalent influenza vaccine, FluMist™. The results of this multicenter, placebo-controlled trial in children 15 to 71 months old were most impressive (8). The live vaccine was stored frozen at -20°C before being thawed. A spray applicator was used that consisted of a syringe-like device that was calibrated and divided for delivery of two 0.25 ml-aliquots (one per nostril) as a large particle spray for a total delivered volume of 0.5 ml of vaccine or placebo. One dose was administrated to 288 children; two doses to 1,314 children, 60 days apart. The vaccine efficacy was 93 percent against culture-confirmed influenza. The one-dose regimen (89 percent) and the two-dose regimen (94 percent) were protective, and the vaccine was efficacious against both strains of influenza circulating in 1996-1997, A (H_3N_2) and B. The immunized children had significantly fewer febrile illnesses, including 30 percent fewer episodes of febrile otitis media. FluMist™ also has been tested in adults, including some infected with human immunodeficiency virus (HIV). A license application is under review by the Food and Drug Administration (FDA).

Time from cold-adapted master donor strains: ± 20 years.

References

1 Smith, W., Andrewes, C. H., & Laidlaw, P. P. (1933). A virus obtained from influenza patients. *Lancet, 2,* 66-68.

2 Francis, T., Jr. (1934). Transmission of influenza by a filterable virus. *Science, 80,* 457-459.

3 Francis, T., Jr. (1940). A new type of virus from epidemic influenza. *Science, 921,* 405-406.

4 Francis, T., Jr. (1953). Vaccination against influenza. *Bulletin of the World Health Organization, 8,* 725-741.

5 Maassab, H. F., Heilman, C. A., & Herlocher, M. L. (1990).

Cold-adapted influenza viruses for use as live vaccine for man. *Advances in Biotechnological Processes, 14,* 203-242.

6 Murphy, B. R., Chalhub, E. G., Nusinoff, S. R., & Chanock, R. M. (1972). Temperature-sensitive mutants of influenza virus. II. Attenuation of its recombinants for man. *Journal of Infectious Diseases, 126,* 170-178.

7 Murphy, B. R. (1993). Use of live attenuated cold-adapted influenza. A reassortant virus vaccine in infants, children, young adults and elderly adults. *Infectious Disease in Clinical Practice, 2,* 174-181.

8 Belshe, R. B., Mandelman, P. M., Treanor, J., et al. (1998). The efficacy of live attenuated, cold-adapted, trivalent, intranasal influenza virus vaccine in children. *New England Journal of Medicine, 338,* 1405-1412.

Jordan Perspective: Pneumococcal Vaccine

This story begins with the identification in 1917 by Dochez and Avery (1) of the specific soluble substance elaborated by the pneumococcus, and subsequent studies of the substance by Avery and Heidelberger (2). In 1927, Schiemann and Casper (3) demonstrated that the substance was immunogenic in the mouse. Three years later, Francis and Tillett (4) reported the induction of antibodies in humans. The protective polysaccharide antigen had been identified.

A number of vaccine trials followed, the largest being one of a bivalent (types 1 and 2) vaccine given to more than 40,000 males in the Civilian Conservation Corps in the late 1930s. The results were inconclusive. During World War II, pneumococcal pneumonia became a problem at an Army air base in Sioux Falls, South Dakota. Fortunately, Dr. Heidelberger had continued his studies and was able to provide purified type-specific vaccines for the predominant types identified by a carrier survey. This classic study demonstrated that immunization of humans with type-specific capsular polysaccharides of selected pneumococcal types (1, 2, 5, and 7) was effective in preventing pneumonia caused by those types. Of equal interest was the observation that immunizing 50 percent of the population greatly reduced in nonimmunized subjects the incidence of pneumonia caused by the vaccine types (5).

E. R. Squibb and Sons then developed and marketed two six-valent pneumococcal capsular polysaccharide vaccines, one vaccine for use in adults, the other for use in children. These vaccines never gained widespread acceptance. Physicians in the early 1950s chose to rely on new antimicrobial agents to treat bacterial pneumonia, rather than on prevention through

immunization. In 1954, therefore, Squibb terminated its production of pneumococcal vaccine. The Biologics Control Laboratory of the National Microbiological Institute, National Institutes of Health, withdrew without prejudice Squibb's license to produce these vaccines, and Squibb subsequently abandoned all of its pneumococcal vaccine research and development programs. Perception of the need for the development of a pneumococcal polysaccharide vaccine generally diminished until Dr. Robert Austrian produced data showing that despite antibiotic treatment, the mortality rate for bacteremic pneumococcal pneumonia was still high (6). In 1967, the Infectious Diseases Advisory Committees of the National Institute of Allergy and Infectious Diseases (NIAID), of which I had just become a member, recommended to Dr. Dorland Davis, the institute's director, that funds be provided for the research and development of pneumococcal vaccine. NIAID contracted with Eli Lilly and Company to develop an experimental polyvalent polysaccharide vaccine to be tested by Dr. Robert Austrian and other investigators. In 1976, 13 years after his first report to the Association of American Physicians, Austrian informed that group of the convincing results obtained in a population of novice gold miners in South Africa (7).

Just as Eli Lilly's vaccine was being shown to be effective in South Africa, the company made a corporate decision in 1975 to stop producing it. Fortunately, Merck Sharp & Dohme intensified its efforts to develop a pneumococcal vaccine. Merck, with Dr. Maurice Hilleman leading its vaccine program, had committed itself earlier to the task of developing and producing a meningococcal polysaccharide vaccine for the Army. Merck conducted independent clinical trials among gold miners in South Africa and obtained levels of safety and efficacy comparable to those found by Austrian with the product produced by Eli Lilly. Merck applied to the Food and Drug Administration (FDA) in 1976 for a license to manufacture and market a 14-valent vaccine. The company was issued a product license on November 21, 1977, and began marketing PNEUMOVAX® in February 1978. Lederle Laboratories obtained a product license for its 14-valent vaccine in August 1979 and began marketing PNU-IMMUNE® shortly thereafter. Subsequently, 23-valent vaccines were developed and licensed in 1983. They contain 87 percent of the serotypes responsible for bacteremia pneumococcal diseases in adults worldwide and are reported to be 65 to 70 percent effective in healthy adults. Time from first successful vaccine trial: 37 years.

Such effectiveness is lacking in children (8), for T-cell-independent polysaccharide vaccines are poorly immunogenic in the young, particularly those less than 2 years of age. After the success in the late 1980s of the *Haemophilus influenzae* (Hib) polysaccharide-protein conjugate championed by Robbins and Schneerson (9), steps were taken to apply this approach to the development of a pneumococcal vaccine for children. In 1987, NIAID sought the interest of industry in manufacturing a heptavalent conjugate vaccine. Only one company, Praxis Biologics, a new venture started by Dr. Richard Smith, Professor of Pediatrics at the University of Rochester and a close associate of NIAID grantee Dr. Porter Anderson, an expert on polysaccharides, submitted a contract proposal. Merck wrote that it would proceed independently.

Combining pneumococcal conjugates was not easy. It took time going from three to five to seven serotypes, trying different proteins, and conducting phase I trials during years when Praxis was absorbed by Wyeth-Lederle Vaccines. Finally, in 2000, 21 years after the first 14-valent polysaccharide vaccine was licensed, a heptavalent conjugate vaccine was licensed. This contains the most common serotypes that cause acute otitis media (4, 6B, 9V, 14, 18C, 19F, and 23Y) conjugated to the nontoxic diphtheria toxin analogue CRM197. Two efficacy trials, one in California (10) and the other in Finland (11), have shown the vaccine to be safe and moderately effective in the prevention of otitis media caused by serotypes included in the vaccine, but the Finnish trial demonstrated an increase in the incidence of otitis media from serotypes not in the vaccine. Merck will soon submit a license application for its multivalent conjugate.

It took 5 years longer than predicted by the Institute of Medicine (IOM) (see Table 5 in "History and Commentary") to bring conjugated pneumococcal polysaccharides to licensure. It is well that vaccines are now available for children

and adults because an increasing proportion of pneumococci isolated around the world are resistant to penicillin and other antibiotics. But both vaccines can be improved (12).

References

1 Dochez, A. R., & Avery, O. T. (1917). The elaboration of specific soluble substance by pneumococcus during growth. *Journal of Experimental Medicine, 26*, 477-493.

2 Avery, G. T., & Heidelberger, M. (1923). Specific soluble substance of pneumococcus. *Journal of Experimental Medicine, 38*, 73-79.

3 Schiemann, O., & Casper, W. (1927). Sind die speztfisch präcipitablen substanzen der 3 pneumokokkentyper haptene? *Zeitschrift Für Hygiene und Infecktionskrankheiten, 108*, 220-257.

4 Francis, T., Jr., & Tillett, W. S. (1930). Cutaneous reactions in pneumonia. The development of antibodies following the interdermal injection of type-specific polysaccharide. *Journal of Experimental Medicine, 52*, 573-585.

5 Hodges, R. G., & MacLeod, C. M. (1946). Epidemic pneumococcal pneumonia. I thru V. *American Journal of Hygiene, 44*, 183-243.

6 Austrian, R. (1963). The current status of bacteremic pneumococcal pneumonia. Reevaluation of an underemphasized clinical problem. *Transactions of the Association of American Physicians, 76*, 117-125.

7 Austrian, R., Douglas, R. M., Schiffman, G., Coetzee, A. M., Koornhof, H. J., Hyden-Smith, S., & Reid, R. D. W. (1976). Prevention of pneumococcal pneumonia by vaccination. *Transactions of the Association of American Physicians, 89*, 184-192.

8 Douglas, R. M., & Miles, H. B. (1984). Vaccination against streptococcus pneumonia in childhood, lack of demonstrable benefit in young Australian children. *Journal of Infectious Diseases, 149*, 861-869.

9 Robbins, J. B., & Schneerson, R. (1940). Polysaccharide protein conjugates: A new generation of vaccines. *Reviews of Infectious Diseases, 161*, 821-832.

10 Black, S., Shinefield, H., Fireman, B., et al. (2000). Efficacy, safety and immunogenicity of pneumococcal vaccines in children. *Pediatric Infectious Disease Journal, 19*, 187-195.

11 Eskola, J., Kilpi, T., Palmu, A., et al. (2001). Efficacy of a pneumococcal conjugate vaccine against otitis media. *New England Journal of Medicine, 344*, 403-409.

12 Butler, J. C., Shapiro, E. D., & Carlone, G. M. (1999). Pneumococcal vaccines: History, current status, and future directions. *American Journal of Medicine, 107*, 695-765.

Sexually Transmitted Diseases

Sexually Transmitted Diseases

OVERVIEW

Sexually transmitted diseases (STDs) comprise a spectrum of infections that are a major, yet often ignored, area of women's health. Women, particularly adolescents, and infants are disproportionately affected by these infections. STDs also represent a major area of health disparity in the United States, with the current epidemic disproportionately affecting minority populations and lower socioeconomic groups. The rates of gonorrhea and syphilis are greater for African Americans than for non-Hispanic whites. African-American and Hispanic women suffer a proportionally greater share of the severe magnifications of these diseases, such as pelvic inflammatory disease (PID) caused by bacterial infections, and cervical cancer caused by human papillomavirus (HPV) infection. STDs have an impact on the human immunodeficiency virus (HIV) epidemic as well. Studies indicate that infection with a variety of STDs can increase the risk of HIV transmission by at least threefold to fivefold.

Apart from the HIV epidemic, STDs cause significant morbidity and mortality, as well as contribute greatly to increasing healthcare costs. Gonococcal and chlamydial infections cause PID, infertility, and ectopic pregnancy. Several common STDs adversely affect pregnancy and result in spontaneous abortion, stillbirth, chorioamnionitis, premature rupture of membranes, preterm delivery, and postpartum endometritis. Neonatal infections include gonococcal conjunctivitis, which may lead to

blindness; chlamydial pneumonia, which may lead to chronic respiratory disease; and herpes encephalitis. Moreover, genital infections attributable to HPV are causally associated with cervical cancer, the most common cause of cancer-related death in women throughout the world.

Despite recent global efforts in health education aimed at preventing the sexual transmission of HIV, STDs remain hyperendemic in many developing countries and in the inner-city populations of industrialized countries. Throughout the world, the majority of STDs are clustered in the resource-limited settings of urban and peri-urban areas, where increasing numbers of adolescents and young adults, poverty, unemployment, lack of education, perceived lower status of women, and social disintegration fuel the epidemic spread of STDs.

A consensus has emerged that the prevention of sexually transmitted HIV infection and the prevention of the major sequelae of STDs in women and infants mandate a global initiative for the prevention and control of STDs. Among other things, this initiative will depend on the development of safe, effective vaccines that prevent infection, disease, and/or sequelae. Currently, except for hepatitis B infection, no such vaccines exist.

GONORRHEA

In the last 20 years, great strides have been made in research on *Neisseria gonorrhoeae*, the pathobiology of gonorrhea, and the prevention of this disease. These advances were made possible by developments in molecular biology technology, the genome sequencing initiative, and an infusion of talented young investigators into the field.

Pilus as a Vaccine Target and Antigenic Variation in *N. gonorrhoeae*

In the 1970s, scientists had a simplistic view that immunizing the populace with the major surface antigens of *N. gonorrhoeae* would stimulate protective and, hopefully, lasting immunity to infection. This attitude was not unreasonable given what was then known about immunization in general. The pilus was chosen as the most likely vaccine candidate because it was immunogenic, it was a major structure on the surface of the bacterium, and because it promoted bacterial attachment to human cells. A number of trials were initiated in military recruits to study the efficacy of a pilus-based vaccine. These studies showed that the pilus could induce immunity in volunteers. Unfortunately, this immunity only protected the volunteers against infection by a limited number of bacterial strains.

STD	Incidence (Estimated number of new cases every year)	Prevalence* (Estimated number of people currently infected)
Chlamydia	3 million	2 million
Gonorrhea	650,000	Not Available
Syphilis	70,000	Not Available
Herpes	1 million	45 million
Human Papillomavirus (hpv)	5.5 million	20 million
Hepatitis B	120,000	417,000
Trichomoniasis	5 million	Not Available
Bacterial Vaginosis**	Not Available	Not Available

* No recent surveys on national prevalence for gonorrhea, syphilis, trichomoniasis or bacterial Vaginosis have been conducted.

** Bacterial Vaginosis is a genital infection that is not sexually transmitted but is associated with sexual intercourse.

Source: CATES, 1999

STD Table

Genetic studies were initiated around the time of the pilus-based vaccine trials. These studies revealed that the pilin gene undergoes tremendously high rates of antigenic variation, leading to antigenic changes of pilin, the subunit that makes up the pilus structure. This explains why volunteers immunized with the pilus were immune only to limited strains of the species: The bacterium changes the antigenic character of the pilus at high frequency, and in so doing, escapes from the host immune response. Further work indicated that antigenic variation occurs at many levels, affecting many of the bacterial coat proteins. This phenomenon of antigenic variation is analogous to what happens to the flu virus, only the bacterial process is much more complicated and affects many more proteins.

Porin: A Major Virulence Factor and Vaccine Target

The porin, a protein on the surface of *N. gonorrhoeae*, serves as a portal of entry for small compounds, i.e., porin pores allow nutrients to enter the bacterial cell. Porin also has the interesting property of inserting into the membrane of human cells, and in so doing, sending signals to the host cell. (How these signals affect the cell is unclear at present.) The porin protein does not undergo large-scale antigenic variation, i.e., porins from a wide number of strains are antigenically similar to each other. Thus, porin promises to be a good vaccine target. Toxicity studies indicate that porins are safe immunogens. However, preliminary trials indicate that while porins can induce an antibody response in humans, the antibodies thus derived do not kill the bacteria.

No vaccines are presently in human trials, nor are any licensed for use. The discoveries that there is antigenic variation in *N. gonorrhoeae* and that porins are not a protective immunogen have turned the attention of investigators to other approaches to identify vaccine and pharmacological candidates. Much work now centers on the activities of the bacterium when it is in close association with host cells in the body.

Identifying the Bacterium's Achilles' Heel: The Development of Cell Culture Systems

For years, *N. gonorrhoeae* was thought to exist only on the mucosal surfaces of humans, i.e., the dogma was that this bacterium does not invade cells. This view was derived in part from the lack of suitable animal models to study gonococcal disease. In the 1980s and 1990s, a variety of cell culture systems were developed for studying *N. gonorrhoeae*. These cell systems, representing different anatomical sites that are susceptible to *N. gonorrhoeae* infection, make it possible to study numerous aspects of the infection process. Using these systems, scientists have discovered that the life cycle of the bacterium does have an intracellular stage and that the bacterium not only adheres to the epithelial cell, but also enters it, transits across its length, and exits into the subepithelial space. It is at this latter site that the symptoms of the disease are actually elicited.

Identifying the Bacterium's Achilles' Heel: Human Challenge Studies

Complementing these cell culture systems is the human challenge system. This system, developed in the late 1980s, is designed to study early events in a *N. gonorrhoeae* infection of the urethra. The system is limited to studies of infections in the adult male urethra and to early times of infection. Nevertheless, experiments using this system have already revealed important aspects of a gonorrhea infection. They show that iron from human transferrin is important for the establishment of infection. They also show that antigenic variation occurs during early stages of the infection.

Identifying the Bacterium's Achilles' Heel: Cell Biology and Receptor Studies

The last decade saw the application of cell biology approaches to understanding the life cycle of *N. gonorrhoeae*. These studies have revealed how certain secreted bacterial enzymes remodel the normal cell and deactivate its infection-fighting capabilities. Studies also have identified numerous bacterial receptors on the surfaces of human cells. The cell normally uses these receptors in its normal day-to-day function. Yet *N. gonorrhoeae* has succeeded in using these receptors for its own gain. Upon contact with these receptors, the bacterium sends signals into the cell. These signals, in the form of protein phosphorylation and $Ca2^+$ fluxes, trigger cascades of biochemical reactions within the cell, all designed to fool the cell into internalizing the bacterium and keeping it safe from harm by innate cellular defense systems.

Studies have also revealed how the bacterium manages to outcompete the human host for certain nutrients. For instance, *N. gonorrhoeae* requires iron for growth and infectivity. At the mucosal surfaces, iron is derived mainly from the host protein transferrin. During infection, the bacterium reduces cellular levels of transferrin receptor, a protein that binds and internalizes transferrin, and allows iron uptake. In so doing, the bacterium makes transferrin more readily available for its own use.

Identifying the Bacterium's Achilles' Heel: How Bacteria Send Signals to Host Cells

Many bacteria, including *N. gonorrhoeae*, are known to move along solid or semisolid surfaces. This process is known as twitching motility, named for the manner of the movement. Twitching motility requires the bacterial type IV pilus and helps the microbes to spread across and colonize the mucous layer on the surface of cells in the body. Recent studies on the fundamental nature of twitching motility have shed light on how bacteria move. The knowledge gained from these studies is applicable to a wide variety of other pathogenic bacteria that express type IV pili. It is also likely to shed valuable light on how motility on the mucosal surfaces may send signals into the host cell to perturb normal cell functions.

N. gonorrhoeae moves by extending the pilus, a filamentous structure, onto a substrate, such as the membrane of a cell, then pulling the pilus back into its body. This process is analogous to a climber using a grappling hook to ascend a mountain. The pilus retraction process occurs at a tremendous force. Similar forces placed artificially on the membrane of human cells in culture induce changes to cell morphology, perturb normal biochemical pathways, and change gene expression patterns. Pilus retraction during bacterial attachment is likely to generate forces on the cell membrane and stimulate biochemical pathways that fool the cell into internalizing the bacteria. Future work along these lines will undoubtedly uncover more targets for pharmacological intervention in this disease. Other pathogens express retractable type IV pili, among them are enteropathogenic *Escherichia coli*, the causative agent of diarrheal disease, and *Pseudomonas aeruginosa*, a pathogen that affects cystic fibrosis and burn patients. Studies on *N. gonorrhoeae* pilus retraction will undoubtedly benefit research programs on other microbial pathogens.

Identifying the Bacterium's Achilles' Heel: Genome Sequence of *N. gonorrhoeae*

A great help to investigators in the field has been the completion of the genome sequence of this bacterium. Today, investigators interested in certain genes and proteins can simply search the genome database for their items of interest. Cumulatively, this database has saved scientists from having to put in thousands of hours of laborious laboratory work to identify their targets.

Identifying the Bacterium's Achilles' Heel: Future Challenges

Information gathered on *N. gonorrhoeae* illustrates an important point about this bacterium: It has evolved numerous means to propagate itself and survive in humans. Previous efforts to develop vaccines against gonococcal infection failed because actions were taken in the absence of an adequate knowledge base. Future challenges in vaccine development will require the expansion of this database, and the careful selection of possible vaccine targets.

The lack of an animal model for gonorrheal disease hampers the search for suitable vaccine and pharmacological targets. *N. gonorrhoeae* has an exquisite tropism for the human body. This preference for infecting humans is due to the specificity of the bacterium for numerous human receptors as well as its requirement for human forms of such nutrients as transferrin and lactoferrin iron. The bacterium also causes a wide range of diseases at multiple anatomical sites of the human body. Thus, developing suitable animal models that replicate gonococcal diseases will be a difficult and challenging task. Since this effort is not a high-yield proposition, many talented researchers have avoided taking on such challenges.

Cell culture systems have been of tremendous help in understanding the life cycle of *N. gonorrhoeae*. Current knowledge is mostly on the initial phase of an infection process, i.e., adherence and cell entry. Little is known about the intracellular activities of the bacterium or about the mechanisms that contribute to the carrier state. The latter is an important part of the disease process. Carriers are more likely to transmit the disease than people with overt infections, and women carriers are more likely to develop PID and infertility. At the moment, most cell culture studies use cells grown on a solid substrate, the plastic bottom of a culture dish. Future progress in *N. gonorrhoeae* vaccine research will require the refinement of these culture systems to mirror the conditions of the different mucosal epithelia found on the human body. (For instance, polarized epithelial cell cultures replicate the architecture of the epithelial mucosa.) As is the case for animal models, developing such culture systems is difficult, time consuming, and a low-yield proposition.

The fields of cell biology, signal transduction, and microbial pathogenesis are converging and finding common languages. Many of the proteins and biochemical cascades used by the cell for normal function are redirected by *N. gonorrhoeae* for its own purposes. The challenge is to identify the molecular pathways usurped by the bacterium and define the end result of this interference since elements in these pathways may serve as vaccine and/or pharmacological targets. In addition, the design of any vaccine and/or pharmacological agent will have to take into account whether the treatment itself will interfere with host cell function.

Finally, the advent of microarray technology will be of tremendous help in vaccine development. For instance, microarray analysis of *N. gonorrhoeae* gene expression during the different stages of adhesion and invasion will identify new bacterial proteins that are upregulated during the infection process. Some of these proteins are likely to be good vaccine targets. Microarray analysis of epithelial cell genes that are up- or downregulated during *N. gonorrhoeae* infection will also be extremely valuable. Such studies will reveal host proteins and signal cascades that are perturbed or usurped by the bacteria during infection. Some of these cellular proteins are also likely to be good vaccine or pharmacological targets.

Microarray analysis is a double-edged sword. If performed with stringency and precision, this technology will yield invaluable information. If it is performed by inexperienced individuals and with incomplete gene arrays, the information will be misleading at best. Microarray analysis, therefore, should not be imported into every laboratory. It is a difficult technology requiring expert technical knowledge ranging from nucleic acid chemistry to statistics. This technology is best provided by core facilities.

CHLAMYDIA

More cases of STD are caused by *Chlamydia trachomatis* than by any other bacterial agent, making *C. trachomatis* infection an enormous public health problem in the United States and throughout the world. *C. trachomatis* infects men and women, in the majority of cases causing silent, asymptomatic infection that can persist for many years. Men with asymptomatic infection serve as carriers of the disease, spreading the infection, but only rarely suffering long-term health consequences as a result. Women are at tremendous risk of serious complications of infection. Acute infection with Chlamydia can result in PID, a serious and painful syndrome that often leads to permanent damage of the reproductive tract and a dramatic increase in the likelihood of infertility and/or ectopic (tubal) pregnancy. *C. trachomatis* infection in the United States has always accounted for a significant percentage of STD, but the number of infected individuals has exploded over the past 20 years. Various studies have estimated that there are 4 to 5 million new cases each year and that between 3 and 5 percent of women are infected at any time with *C. trachomatis*. Among inner city adolescent females, the incidence rate can be as high as 30 percent. As this population enters childbearing age, there will be not only devastating reproductive health problems in these women, but also tremendous economic costs associated with treatment. Previously, the costs of treating and caring for patients with PID ranged from $2 to $6 billion annually, and the estimates for 2000 are as high as $10 billion.

One significant difficulty in curtailing Chlamydia infections is the ability to diagnose infections rapidly. Most sexually active patients are not screened routinely by primary care providers. Even in cases where Chlamydia is suspected, the test must be sent to a specialized laboratory for evaluation. This lack of diagnosis is particularly discouraging in that the organisms respond well to antibiotic therapy and can even be treated with a single dose of certain drugs. Increased awareness and routine screening of at-risk populations would have a significant impact on these infections and their cost. Infection that remains undetected in girls and women causes damage to the reproductive system that is often not treatable using antibiotics. Once this damage arises, costly invasive measures are the only treatment for infertility, and these are not successful in many patients.

A safe vaccine administered prior to adolescence that is effective through childbearing age would have a significant impact on the acquisition and spread of this disease and the cost of the resulting pathology. There are no vaccine candidates presently in human trials; however, the development of such vaccines is an active area of research. One of the major successes of this work has been the identification of several components of *C. trachomatis* that stimulate protective immune responses. Although exciting, the protection that results from immunizing experimental animals with any one of these components is not complete. These components also appear to stimulate different arms of the immune system. Most researchers now believe that an effective vaccine must incorporate multiple Chlamydia-derived components that stimulate multiple arms of the immune system. Identification of these components has been greatly assisted in the past 3 years by the availability of the complete genome sequence of *C. trachomatis*. The ability to examine every gene in the organism has allowed for identifying and

testing candidate proteins based on their similarity to proteins important in immunity to other bacterial pathogens.

Despite these efforts to develop candidate vaccines, three major impediments have remained unresolved. First, the amount and quality of information obtainable by infecting experimental animals with *C. trachomatis* is limited. The Chlamydia organism that does infect mice is not the same as those that infect people, it causes different pathology and responds differently to immune pressure in the host. Conversely, strains that commonly infect people do not cause severe disease in mice. Second, there is significant concern that the use of a Chlamydia vaccine in people will result in side effects. Many of the serious complications of infection are thought to result not from the infection itself, but from the effects of the immune system attempting to control the infection. A vaccine that stimulates immunity might also cause the same destruction of the reproductive tract seen during actual infection. Third, *C. trachomatis* cannot be manipulated genetically. Many approaches to creating new vaccines depend on weakening live organisms by disrupting specific functions, thereby rendering the organism harmless. These weakened bacteria can then be used as vaccines to stimulate immunity to the virulent organisms. These genetic approaches have not been possible with *C. trachomatis*. Hopefully, research over the next few years will allow investigators to overcome each of these barriers in order to generate effective and safe vaccines.

GENITAL HERPES

The concept of what may constitute protective immunity has improved through studies of animal and human immune responses to genital herpes simplex virus (HSV) infection. More sophisticated vaccine products have resulted from advances in molecular virology and immunology. The sequences of HSV

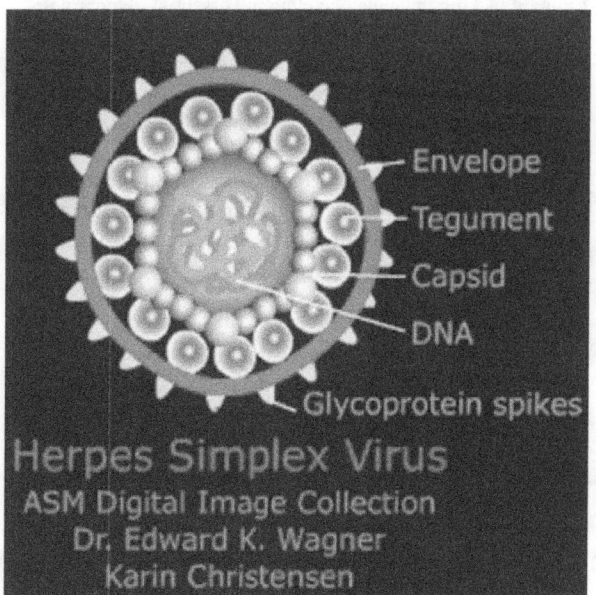

Envelope
Tegument
Capsid
DNA
Glycoprotein spikes

Herpes Simplex Virus
ASM Digital Image Collection
Dr. Edward K. Wagner
Karin Christensen

types 1 and 2 (HSV-1 and HSV-2) have been elucidated and used to prepare a variety of vaccine candidates, including subunit, genetically attenuated, replication-impaired, nucleic acid (DNA)-based, and vectored vaccines. Adjuvant research has yielded new strategies for boosting immune responses to candidate vaccines. New adjuvants used in herpes vaccine research include 3-deactylated monophosphoryl lipid A (3-dMPL), MF59, and immunostimulatory nucleic acid sequences (CpGs). Improved understanding of the epidemiology of genital herpes has facilitated clinical trial designs. Animal model studies first showed that vaccines could be used to reduce the frequency of clinically apparent and inapparent (virus shedding in the absence of obvious lesions) recurrent genital HSV infections. Trials in humans subsequently confirmed the animal studies and provided the first controlled clinical data supporting the concept of vaccine immunotherapy for the treatment of patients with persistent viral infections.

There have been two important related advances. The first was the demonstration that a subunit vaccine (a glycoprotein D product developed by GlaxoSmithKline) could afford significant protection against genital herpes disease. The second was the observation that the protection was seen only in women. Gender-specific (female) protection was also seen with another subunit vaccine (a product containing HSV-2 glycoproteins B and D developed by Chiron Corporation), although the protection was transient.

There are no licensed vaccines for the treatment or prevention of genital herpes. There are two vaccines in human trials. A subunit vaccine developed by GlaxoSmithKline Biologicals contains recombinant truncated HSV-2 glycoprotein D and alum plus 3-dMPL. The vaccine has been tested for the prevention of genital herpes disease in two large phase III trials in adults. There are plans for an additional phase III trial. A replication-impaired HSV-2 mutant lacking the gene encoding the essential glycoprotein gH was developed by Xenova Research, Ltd., (formerly Cantab Pharmaceuticals, PLC) as a disabled infectious single-cycle (DISC) virus vaccine. The DISC vaccine was shown to be immunogenic and well tolerated in phase I trials in the United Kingdom and the United States. It has been tested in a phase II trial in the United States as a therapeutic vaccine for the treatment of patients with frequently recurring genital herpes. There are plans for further development of the Xenova Research, Ltd., product as a prophylactic vaccine.

The pathogenesis of genital herpes involves initial infection of epithelial cells and rapid spread of the virus to sensory ganglion neurons where a persistent (latent) infection is established. Reactivation of the latent infection causes symptomatic and asymptomatic recurrent infections that can result in spread to susceptible sexual partners, and in the case of the pregnant woman, perinatal transmission. One challenge with regard to developing a herpes vaccine is defining the expected benefit of vaccination: Is prevention of disease without necessarily preventing acute and latent infection sufficient or must the vaccine protect against infection? Ideally, a vaccine would protect the genital epithelium against infection; however, at this time, it is uncertain whether current technology can produce a product that will induce durable protection of epithelial surfaces. An alternative strategy would be to protect the ganglion neurons

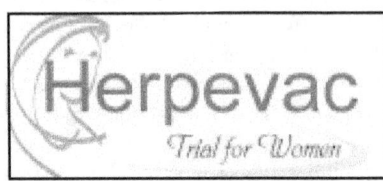

In Winter 2002 NIAID will launch an HSV vaccine efficacy study in women.

from acute and latent infection and thereby prevent subsequent spread, but further research is needed in order to understand how to engender protection of the ganglia. Other areas of research that would facilitate development of a vaccine to control genital herpes include: Defining immune correlates to protection, defining the role of local (genital) immune responses in protection and exploring how vaccines can induce these local responses, understanding the effect of prior HSV-1 nongenital infection on the risk of acquiring HSV-2 genital infection, determining whether a vaccine that affords partial protection against disease and reduces the magnitude of latent infection can result in fewer recurrent infections and less spread of the virus in the population, and understanding why subunit vaccines afforded only gender-specific protection.

HUMAN PAPILLOMAVIRUS

The past 20 years has been an explosive time in understanding the natural history of HPV infection and the role that HPV plays in cervical and other anogenital cancers. In the early 1980s, the first genital HPV types were molecularly cloned from benign genital warts and from cancers. Today, more than 50 genital types have been identified and they are classified as either high risk or low risk based on the likelihood that they will be found in cancers. Genital HPV infection has been shown to be extremely common, with approximately 50 percent of women (and likely men) becoming infected. Infection with either high or low-risk HPVs is often subclinical, but a portion of individuals with low-risk types, particularly HPV 6 or 11, will develop genital warts, whereas a subset of women with high-risk HPVs will develop preneoplastic lesions [dysplasia/cervical intraepithelial neoplasia (CIN)/squamous intraepithelial lesions]. Pap smear screening and treatment can prevent most of these lesions from progressing to cancer, and the majority of infections will be self-limiting. However, rapidly growing lesions, inadequate screening, or treatment failure can result in malignancy. It is now clear that almost 100 percent of squamous cell cancers (SCCs) of the cervix; the majority of adenocarcinomas of the cervix; and SCC of the vulva, vagina, penis, and anus harbor high-risk HPVs, with HPV 16 accounting for 50 percent of the cancers. Vaccination to prevent HPV infection, or as a therapy to modulate disease, would not only have tremendous importance in reducing the burden of anogenital cancer, but would have a huge impact on public health by reducing the need for screening and intervention.

There have been tremendous advances in vaccine research that have followed three avenues: 1) Prophylactic vaccines to prevent infection, 2) therapeutic vaccines to treat cancer patients, and 3) therapeutic vaccines to prevent progression. Animal studies have shown that protection against infection can be achieved with neutralizing antibodies. These antibodies are directed against conformational epitopes on the surface of the virus. Importantly, research has shown that virus-like particles (VLPs), lacking viral DNA, can be made in the laboratory, and these particles elicit neutralizing antibodies. Thus, VLPs are good candidates for prophylactic vaccines. The rationale behind developing therapeutic vaccines is based on the fact that all HPV-associated cancers or premalignant lesions express the viral oncoproteins E6 and E7. Thus, vaccine strategies that can generate T cells that kill E6/E7 expressing cells could have a therapeutic benefit.

Currently, there are no licensed vaccines for the prevention or treatment of genital HPV; however, there are a number of candidate vaccines that are in various stages of clinical trials. HPV VLPs, either as a single type (usually HPV 16) or in combination (types 6, 11, 16, and 18), are being tested in several trials to prevent infection. Merck reported preliminary results from a phase II trial that provided encouraging evidence of protection. Similar trials using VLPs, or chimeric VLPs to which a piece of E7 has been added, are being undertaken by Medimmune/SmithKline, Medigene/Schering, and the intramural arm of the National Cancer Institute (NCI). Preclinical research or early trials are investigating other recombinants to deliver the coat protein. There are also a large number of trials of potential therapeutic vaccines. Vaccination of women who have advanced cervical cancer using a recombinant virus that contained E6/E7 was reported, and more studies are underway in patients with cancer and CIN. Peptides or portions of E6/E7 with adjuvant or linked to other immunostimulatory proteins are being tried by Xenova Research, Ltd.; Stressgen; University of Leiden; NCI; and others.

There are many challenges to the development of HPV vaccines. As for all STD vaccines, a major challenge is how to develop a vaccine that will provide protection at the mucosal surface of the genital tract. The current strategies are based on creating a massive systemic response that will seep into the genital tract when trauma occurs. It may be necessary to find new ways to specifically target the immune response to the genital tract. Duration of the vaccination response is also important; initial vaccination will occur before the onset of sexual activity and must be protective for many decades of potential exposure. Another issue to consider is the multiplicity of HPV types; while four types are responsible for approximately 80 percent of cancers, the remaining 20 percent involve a large number of other types. The challenges facing therapeutic HPV vaccines are even greater, as the underlying mechanisms that mediate regression are less well understood than for prevention. One problem is that HPV is a virus that only infects epithelial cells, and those cells are good at avoiding the immune system by having only limited contact with the immune system and by interacting poorly with the immune cells. Once the HPV lesion has become cancerous, further changes block the ability to present the E6/E7 antigens for recognition, even if immune cells are present. Finally, the highest incidence of cervical cancer is in the developing world; thus, HPV vaccines should be simple and affordable.

SYPHILIS

The inability to cultivate *Treponema pallidum* on artificial medium historically has been the principal deterrent to advances in syphilis research. The advent of recombinant DNA technology in the early 1980s, more specifically the expression of *T. pallidum* antigens in *E. coli*, was key to circumventing this impediment. Throughout the 1980s, work in a number of laboratories led to the identification and subsequent molecular characterization of the major B and T-cell treponemal immunogens recognized during syphilitic infection. In addition to comprising potential vaccine candidates, a number of these molecules have shown considerable promise as serodiagnostic antigens. For some of these cloned proteins, sequence similarity with proteins of other prokaryotes made it possible to deduce cellular location and physiological function. On the whole, however, the lack of sequence homologies at this early stage in the molecular era emphasized the "genetic gulf" that exists between *T. pallidum* and nonspirochetal bacteria.

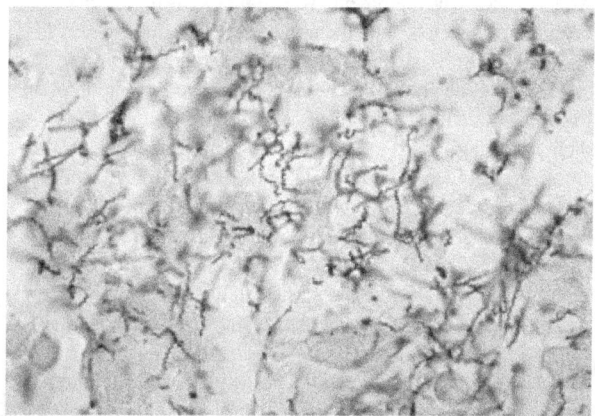

Syphilis

DNA sequence analysis of cloned *T. pallidum* proteins in the late 1980s led to a discovery that has had far reaching consequences for the field. It was found that many of these protein immunogens have lipids covalently bound to their N-termini. In addition to markedly altering the physical properties of these proteins by providing hydrophobic membrane tethers, the lipid components also were found to confer proinflammatory properties of considerable relevance to the disease process. We now know that these lipoproteins are potent activators of innate immune cells (i.e., macrophages, dendritic cells, and endothelial cells), that these activities are lost if the proteins are not lipid modified, and that these molecules activate immune cells by interacting with the pattern recognition receptors CD14 and toll-like receptor 2. From the standpoint of the host, activation of the innate immune response is a double-edged sword. It is beneficial because it sounds the danger signal that alerts host defenses to the presence of an invader, stimulating potentially protective local and systemic immune responses. At the same time, the resulting inflammatory processes are likely to be the principal cause of the tissue damage that gives rise to disabling clinical manifestations. The presence of large numbers of activated lymphocytes and macrophages within primary syphilitic lesions (chancres) is a major factor in their ability to serve as cofactors for sexual transmission of the acquired immunodeficiency syndrome (AIDS) virus.

Investigators entered the molecular era assuming that the outer membrane of *T. pallidum* was similar to those of gram-negative bacteria. It also was widely assumed that the immunogenic proteins identified using recombinant DNA techniques were surface exposed. On the other hand, an extensive body of evidence predating the molecular era demonstrated that the syphilis spirochete's surface reacts poorly with the specific antitreponemal antibodies present in human syphilitic sera. The existence of these two mutually exclusive notions about the treponemal surface emphasized the need for a detailed examination of *T. pallidum* ultrastructure. The resulting studies have yielded a model of *T. pallidum* molecular architecture with important consequences for understanding syphilis pathogenesis as well as vaccine development. According to this model, the syphilis spirochete's outer membrane contains an extremely low density of membrane proteins (now often referred to as rare outer membrane proteins). The highly immunogenic lipoproteins, in contrast, are located in the periplasmic space, anchored via their N-terminal lipids to the cytoplasmic membrane, where they are inaccessible to antibodies. The paucity of surface-exposed antigenic targets, coupled with the sequestration of the proinflammatory lipoproteins, is believed to explain, at least in part, why the spirochete so successfully disseminates throughout the body and establishes persistent, even lifelong, infection in some individuals (hence the nickname stealth pathogen).

The past several years of syphilis research have been dominated by the quest for rare outer membrane proteins. This extensive effort is motivated by the belief that identification of these surface antigens is the key to vaccine development. Given the low cellular abundance of these molecules, and the limited numbers of organisms obtainable, it is not surprising that this work has posed an enormous challenge. Throughout the 1990s, a number of creative strategies evolved for identifying these molecules, and promising vaccine candidates have been identified. Indeed, several of these proteins have been shown to confer partial protection in the experimental rabbit model. This work recently received a tremendous boost with the availability of the *T. pallidum* genomic sequence. With the bacterium's entire genetic blueprint available, syphilis researchers now can catalog all of its outer membrane protein candidates as a prelude to assessing their cellular locations and protective capacities. The syphilis vaccine that has eluded investigators for decades could be at hand in the not too distant future, although the research is still far from human trials. It also must not be overlooked that the syphilis genome has provided investigators with many novel insights into the bacterium's strategy for physiological survival within the host and, hopefully, will yield the information needed for its successful *in vitro* cultivation, another longstanding objective of syphilis research.

In the 1930s, syphilis was designated the principal public health problem facing the United States. Following World War II, with the introduction of penicillin as the mainstay of syphilotherapy, syphilis rates plummeted. However, from the 1970s and into the early 1990s, the disease staged an impressive comeback, with African Americans bearing a hugely disproportionate share of the disease burden. The recognition that syphilitic genital ulcers dramatically increase the sexual transmission of HIV further amplified the disease's importance as a public health threat. Fortunately, as a result of the 7-to-10-year cyclic nature of syphilis epidemics within the United States, along with the reinvigorated efforts of public health workers, syphilis rates are now at a historic low. Buoyed by these trends, the Centers for Disease Control and Prevention (CDC) has implemented an aggressive campaign to eliminate syphilis from the United States. Developments emanating from basic and clinical research, including improved diagnostics, effective new oral therapeutic regimens, tools for the molecular typing of *T. pallidum* strains, and hopefully a safe and effective syphilis vaccine, are expected to complement epidemiologically based strategies for disease eradication.

Vector-Borne & Zoonotic Infections

Vector-Borne and Zoonotic Infections

OVERVIEW

Arthropod-borne infectious diseases are responsible for a large and growing proportion of the mortality and morbidity throughout the world. Diseases such as malaria, dengue fever, Japanese encephalitis, yellow fever, West Nile fever, and leishmaniasis affect untold millions of people in the world's poorest nations, where the opportunity for intervention is most limited. In the United States, these diseases are emerging as increasingly significant sources of morbidity, but death is extremely rare. The combination of adequate early diagnosis and treatment maintains a very low transmission rate. In developing countries, these resources are not always available, and alternative means must be found to interrupt transmission and prevent disease. Immune-based methods to accomplish these goals include development of vaccines against the pathogens to protect the humans who are exposed, vaccines to block transmission of the pathogens by killing them inside their arthropod vectors, and vaccines against the vectors themselves. Among the most promising vaccine development efforts underway at present are a transmission-blocking vaccine against Lyme disease, a protective vaccine against malaria, and immunological approaches to preventing the establishment of leishmanial parasites inside the human lymphocytes.

ANTHRAX

Background

Anthrax is a life-threatening bacterial disease caused by *Bacillus anthracis*, a gram-positive bacillus that produces heat-resistant spores. Anthrax is rare in humans and occurs in two natural forms (cutaneous and systemic), mainly among those who come in close contact with animals or their products. Cutaneous anthrax is characterized by an inflamed carbuncle covered by a black eschar. If not treated, the bacilli may spread to regional lymph nodes and then to the bloodstream, resulting in systemic anthrax. Systemic anthrax, which is nearly always fatal, also may develop from initial sites of infection in either the lung (from the inhalation of spores) or the gut (from eating contaminated meat). Death results from edema, massive hypotension, shock, and pulmonary edema in the case of inhalation anthrax.

Natural epidemics of pulmonary anthrax are rare. Since the threat of using anthrax as a bioterrorism agent has been demonstrated, outbreaks of pulmonary anthrax must be suspected as originating from the deliberate release of spores into the atmosphere. This can result in an enormous number of fatalities within a short period of time, well before diagnosis is possible.

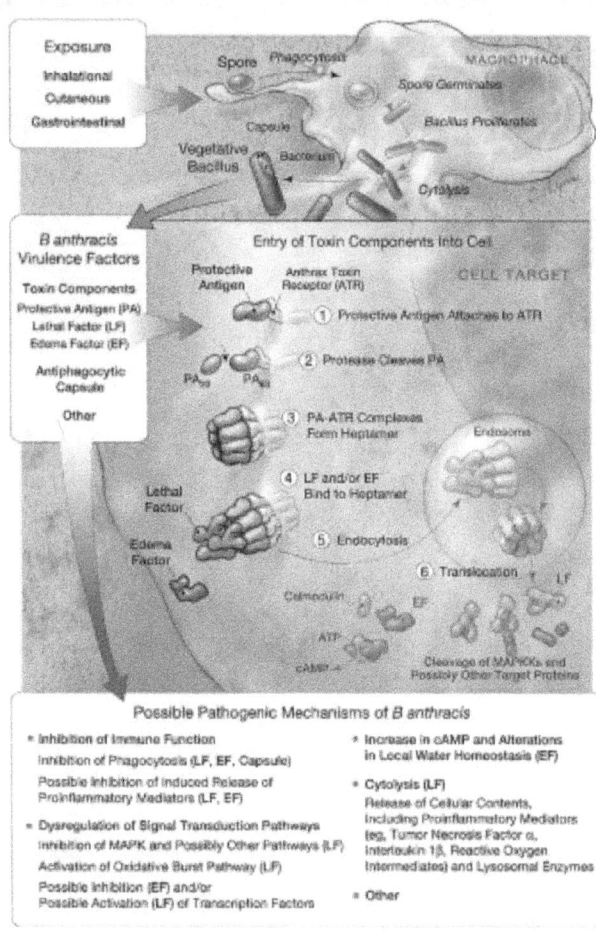

Possible Pathogenic Mechanisms of *B anthracis*

Current Status of Research and Development

In response to the threat of using various bacterial pathogens as agents of bioterrorism, the National Institute of Allergy and Infectious Diseases (NIAID) formed the Working Group on Anthrax Vaccines (WGAV) to review the current status of anthrax vaccines in 1999. Anthrax Vaccine Adsorbed (AVA), which was licensed for human use in 1970, is the only vaccine available for anthrax. It is an alum-adsorbed, killed-cell vaccine with a shelf life of less than 1 year. It was designed mainly for use in textile workers to protect against cutaneous anthrax (wool sorter's disease), scientists working with anthrax, and veterinarians, and is administered as six injections over an 18-month period. The efficacy of AVA for preexposure vaccination against pulmonary anthrax has only been demonstrated in animal models, and the results of recent preclinical studies show that after as few as two immunizing doses it is able to confer protection against inhalation spore challenge in nonhuman primates.

Roughly 2 million doses of the vaccine have been administered, mostly to U.S. military personnel. But some service members have raised concerns about the vaccine's safety and efficacy, and more than 400 military personnel have refused the shots, worried that vaccination could be connected to complaints of chronic fatigue, memory loss, and other health problems. These concerns prompted Congress to request a National Academies study of the vaccine's adverse reactions, long-term health implications, gender differences in reactions, and effectiveness against inhalation exposure. The committee concluded that while the current anthrax vaccine is safe and effective, it does have certain drawbacks. It relies on older vaccine technology and requires a cumbersome dosing schedule.

The results of preclinical studies conducted by investigators at the U.S. Army Medical Research Institute of Infectious Diseases (USAMRIID) have established that it is the protective antigen (PA) of *B. anthracis* that induces significant protective immunity against inhalation spore challenge, and that PA is the component of AVA responsible for generating such immunity. The gene for PA has been cloned and inserted into a nonspore-forming, avirulent strain of *B. anthracis,* as well as into an *Escherichia coli* vector expression system. This enables the production of large amounts of purified recombinant PA (rPA) for use as a vaccine. The administration of two intramuscular injections of rPA (50ug or 5ug with alhydrogel as adjuvant) induces 90- to 100-percent protective immunity against inhalation spore challenge in rabbits and monkeys within 3 months after immunization. Levels of serum immunoglobulin G (IgG) antibodies against PA, as well as toxin-neutralizing antibodies, parallel the degree of protective immunity generated in response to rPA upon inhalation spore challenge. The safety of the anthrax vaccines has been publicly debated for the past few years. Reports from scientific reviews conducted by the Department of Defense, the Institute of Medicine, and the U.S. Army concluded that no patterns of unexpected local or systemic adverse events were identified in individuals who had received AVA.

During the 2001 anthrax mail attacks, AVA was not initiated immediately as standard of care for potential exposures because of the limited availability of vaccine. Later in the fall it was offered under investigational new drug procedures for postexposure contacts.

Recent scientific findings with the discovery of the crystalline structure of the lethal and edema factor and the sequencing of the *B. anthracis* genome are certain to provide further tools for researchers in the development of new and improved anthrax vaccines.

On the basis of these and other findings, WGAV recommended that NIAID support joint, collaborative studies with USAMRIID to conduct phase I clinical trials on the safety and efficacy of an rPA vaccine for humans. Such studies are now underway.

Sources

Hanna, P. (1998). Anthrax pathogenesis and the host response. *Current Topics in Microbiology and Immunology, 225,* 13-35.

Inglesby, T. (2002). Anthrax as a biological weapon. *Journal of the American Medical Association, 287*(17), 2236.

Ivins, B. E., Pitt, M. L., Fellows, P. F., Farchaus, J. W., Benner, G. E., Waag, D. M., Little, S. F., Anderson, G. W., Jr., Gibbs, P. H., & Friedlander, A. M. (1998). Comparative efficacy of experimental anthrax vaccine candidates against inhalation anthrax in rhesus monkeys. *Vaccine, 16,* 1141-1148.

McBride, B. W., Mogg, A., Telfer, J. L., Lever, M. S., Miller, J., Turnbull, P. C., & Baille, L. (1998). Protective efficacy of a recombinant protective antigen against *Bacillus anthracis* challenge and assessment of immunological markers. *Vaccine, 16,* 810-817.

Singh, Y., Ivins, B. E., & Leppla, S. H. (1998). Study of immunization against anthrax with the purified recombinant protective antigen of *Bacillus anthracis. Infection and Immunity, 66,* 3447-3448.

DENGUE

Dengue viruses are the most widespread arthropod-borne viruses (arboviruses). They are members of the Flaviviridae family, which includes more than 70 related but distinct viruses, most of which are mosquito borne. Other major pathogens in this family include yellow fever and Japanese encephalitis viruses. In 2002, dengue was present on most continents, and more than one-half of all United Nations member states (discussed below) were threatened by dengue. Epidemics continue to emerge, and this

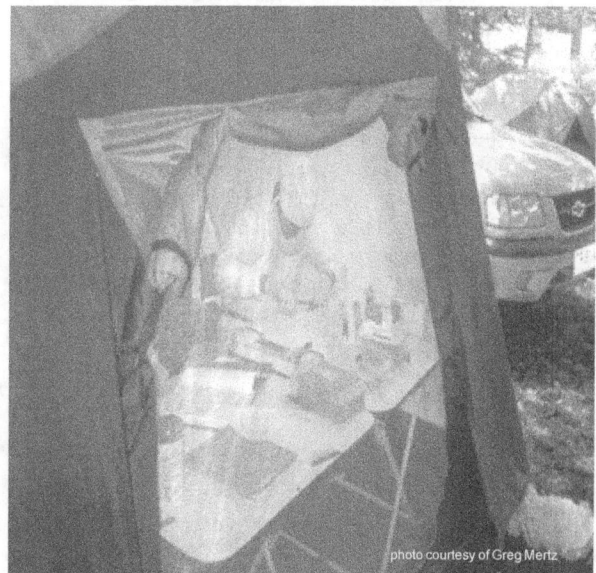

NIAID researchers working on dengue in Brazil.

virus causes severe infections in areas where periodic epidemics did not previously occur. The disease will continue to spread as newly urbanized areas become infested with mosquito vectors. In those areas where dengue is endemic, more than 1.5 billion people (including about 600 million children) are at risk. It is estimated that between 35 and 60 million people are infected with dengue, and that 2,000 to 5,000 children die from dengue annually. These figures most likely underestimate the scope of this problem.

There are four closely related, but serologically distinct, dengue viruses (types 1 through 4). Because there is no cross-protection between the four types, a population could experience a dengue-1 epidemic in one year, followed by a dengue-2 epidemic the next. Primary infection with any serotype often causes a debilitating, but usually nonfatal, form of illness. To date, limited antiviral drug chemotherapy studies have not proved successful; consequently, most currently used forms of therapy for uncomplicated dengue are supportive in nature.

Some infected patients experience a much more severe and often fatal form of the disease, called dengue hemorrhagic fever (DHF), the most severe form of which is referred to as dengue shock syndrome (DSS). Unlike other infectious diseases, the presence of antibodies after recovery from one type of dengue infection is believed to predispose some individuals, under certain incompletely understood circumstances, to the more severe form of disease (DHF/DSS) through immune-enhancement when infected by a different dengue virus serotype. Although all age groups are susceptible to dengue fever, DHF is most common in children.

Dengue viruses are prevalent throughout the tropics, where the urban-dwelling mosquito *Aedes aegypti* is a major vector. Other related mosquitoes, such as *Aedes albopictus*, are also efficient vectors. Although the virus may circulate in endemic cycles, it periodically causes acute, widespread epidemics in which large percentages of the population may be infected. An example is the 1987 epidemic in Thailand, which officially involved 174,285 cases; most were children younger than 15 years of age. Dengue caused 1,007 reported deaths among these children. That year in Thailand, dengue was the third-leading cause of illness in children, and the leading cause of childhood death. DHF has emerged as an important public health problem in Southeast Asia as new waves of epidemics occur; this appears to be happening in the Western Hemisphere and the Pacific Islands as well.

In the Americas, the first epidemic of cases of severe DHF occurred in 1981. The illness was associated with a dengue-2 epidemic in Cuba that followed the dengue-1 epidemic of 1977. During the 1981 outbreak in Cuba, 116,151 hospitalized cases of dengue fever were reported, and 10,312 cases were classified as severe DHF; 158 deaths (many in adults) were reported. More recently, the Caribbean and South and Central America have experienced frequent outbreaks of dengue, with cases of fatal

DHF now commonly reported from many countries. Most U.S. residents become infected with dengue during travel to tropical areas. However, as larger epidemics have occurred in northern Mexico, portions of the southern United States have experienced increased importation of dengue cases. Local transmission of dengue has been documented in Texas in 1999. Furthermore, a U.S.-based epidemic of dengue started in Hawaii in 2001, and continues into early 2002 with more than 100 cases reported. The 1999 Texas outbreak was limited by focusing on avoidance of *A. aegypti* mosquitoes. In Hawaii, the vector appears to be *A. albopictus*, which is a less efficient vector for dengue.

Dengue continues to spread or emerge in areas previously considered not to be endemic, but usually is not associated with major outbreaks of the disease. The westward expansion of dengue in Asia was first documented in the late 1980s by the increased epidemics in India and Sri Lanka. Africa and the Middle East also were considered to be areas with a low incidence; however, dengue emerged in these areas in the early 1990s, as demonstrated by the widespread occurrence of dengue infections in U.S. military personnel stationed in Somalia, as well as by reports of dengue in Saudi Arabia.

Because attempts to eradicate mosquito vectors have not been successful in developing countries, the control of dengue will be possible only after an efficient vaccine has been developed. Clearly, the phenomenon of immune-enhancement may be a major problem in developing an effective dengue vaccine. It suggests that instead of a monotypic vaccine, a multivalent vaccine against all four serotypes of the dengue virus may have to be prepared to avoid inducing monotypic-enhancing antibodies that might lead to DHF associated with subsequent natural infections caused by other dengue types. The potential risks of administering a live-attenuated vaccine to a population with preexisting enhancing antibodies are another potential problem that remains to be examined in a systematic manner.

NIAID is now funding several projects that address basic virological and immunological aspects of flavivirus infections in general, and dengue infections in particular. The Centers for Disease Control and Prevention (CDC) has had a large, successful program focusing on applied dengue research. The World Health Organization (WHO) is also funding vaccine development programs, and dengue vaccine development programs are in place at a limited number of vaccine manufacturers and small biotechnology companies. The U.S. Army has had a productive, long-term research program aimed at developing a dengue vaccine.

Progress in dengue research has been slowed mainly because these viruses grow poorly in cell culture, and there is no acceptable animal model for DHF. NIAID funds several extramural and intramural projects studying basic virological and immunological aspects of flaviviruses, such as yellow fever, dengue, West Nile fever, and Japanese encephalitis viruses. Discoveries from these projects cross-fertilize vaccine studies on these viruses. Some of the most promising basic molecular studies that might be applied to the development of an improved dengue vaccine revolve around the development of full-length, infectious dengue cDNAs. Information from studies using the infectious clone has been combined with sequence immunological data to yield new insights into important antigenic regions on the dengue virion. The recent determination of the three-dimensional structure of the E protein of another flavivirus (tick-borne encephalitis virus) and dengue has allowed formulation of an even more sophisticated model for understanding antigenicity and pathogenicity of flaviviruses. It is hoped that this research can yield efficient and less costly ways to manufacture safe flavivirus vaccines.

Flavivirus vaccine research has focused on five areas: Live-attenuated or inactivated vaccines, infectious clone-derived vaccines, immunogens vectored by various recombinant systems, subunit immunogens, and nucleic acid vaccines.

A promising set of live-attenuated dengue vaccines has been developed in Thailand, with support of WHO. Preliminary trials in adults and children in Thailand were encouraging, with the tetravalent vaccine inducing broadly cross-reacting antibody in 80 to 90 percent of the subjects. This vaccine has been transitioned to commercial development by agreements with Pasteur Merieux Connaught. Commercial lots have been manufactured and testing is underway in collaboration with Walter Reed Army Institute of Research (WRAIR).

Because of the success of flavivirus inactivated vaccines against Japanese encephalitis in Japan, and tick-borne encephalitis in Australia, attempts have been made to develop a killed dengue vaccine. However, because of difficulties in growing high titers of dengue in cell culture, early attempts to make inactivated products were not successful. Recently, WRAIR scientists have used certified Vero cells and serum-free media to grow dengue to high titers. A prototype dengue-2 inactivated vaccine purified and concentrated from these cells induces protective levels of antibodies in mice and monkeys. Further testing is planned.

Infectious clones of dengue, Japanese encephalitis, West Nile fever, and yellow fever are being combined to produce chimeric vaccines, and preliminary studies are very encouraging. In one of these programs, scientists at the National Institutes of Health (NIH) and in Australia also have attempted to alter the genetic structure of the dengue clone to produce live-attenuated vaccine candidates. Mouse and monkey trials have been encouraging, and a number of potential vaccine candidates are entering clinical trials.

The most advanced studies of flavivirus immunogens delivered by poxvirus vectors have been with Japanese encephalitis virus to deliver antigenic Japanese encephalitis proteins to humans in phase I trials. Further studies are needed, but these vectors induce cellular and antibody immunity against Japanese encephalitis. Preexisting immunity to the vector attenuated the response. To avoid this problem, vaccinia virus recombinants

also have been used to generate subviral particles containing dengue and Japanese encephalitis antigens. These particles elicit antibody in mice, but their potential as vaccines is still being explored.

Subunit vaccines for a variety of flaviviruses have been prepared in *E. coli*, baculovirus, yeast, and insect cell systems. Generally, the experience with dengue-containing *E. coli* products, and some other expressed products, was not promising. With *E. coli*-dengue products, mice produced good antibody titers, but monkey studies were not as successful. One lesson learned was that flavivirus proteins require extensive processing and folding during maturation. Studies to fine tune various expression systems to yield more stable flavivirus immunogens are in progress, and baculovirus-expressed products and products from Drosophila cells appear promising in early mouse testing.

Preliminary studies have been reported on a new nucleic acid vaccine for St. Louis encephalitis, a related flavivirus, and dengue and West Nile fever. PreM and E proteins have been expressed under control of various promoters. Mice immunized with this product developed low levels of antibody, but were protected against a live virus challenge. Research by the CDC (Ft. Collins) and the U.S. Navy is attempting to further develop this approach for dengue. In the near future, this exciting area undoubtedly will be a focus of expanded vaccine research efforts.

Sources

Barrett, A. D. (1997). Japanese encephalitis and dengue vaccines. *Biologicals, 25*(1), 27-34.

Barrett, A. D. (1997). Yellow fever vaccines. *Biologicals, 25*(1), 17-25.

Centers for Disease Control and Prevention. (2002). Imported dengue—United States, 1999 and 2000. *Morbidity and Mortality Weekly Report, 51*(13), 281-282.

Chambers, T., Tsai, T., Pervikov, Y., & Monath, T. (1997). Vaccine development against dengue and Japanese encephalitis: Report of a World Health Organization meeting. *Vaccine, 15*(14), 1494-1502.

Shope, R., & Meegan, J. (1997). Arboviruses. In A. Evans & R. Kaslow (Eds.), *Viral infections of humans* (pp. 151-183). New York: Plenum Publishing Corporation.

World Health Organization. (1996). *State of the world's vaccines and immunization*. Geneva, Switzerland: WHO Press.

JAPANESE ENCEPHALITIS

Japanese encephalitis is endemic in parts of China, India, Korea, Nepal, Thailand, Vietnam, Kampuchea, Myanmar, the Philippines, Taiwan, Indonesia, Malaysia, Bangladesh, and Sri Lanka and poses a risk to U.S. travelers and the U.S. military. Infection with this mosquito-borne virus in endemic areas is common; however, clinical disease occurs in only 1 of every 300 to 1,000 infections. These clinical cases have a case fatality rate of up to 40 percent, with severe neurological sequelae occurring in 10 to 30 percent of survivors. Like the closely related yellow fever and dengue viruses, Japanese encephalitis virus circulates in endemic cycles, which periodically erupt into major epidemics. Consequently, the incidence of infections caused by Japanese encephalitis virus varies substantially and ranges from 10,000 to more than 50,000 cases worldwide per year. Estimates of about 1,000 cases per year have been reported in India, Nepal, and Sri Lanka. An annual morbidity of 6 to 10 cases per 100,000 inhabitants has been reported in heavily endemic areas, such as Vietnam and Thailand.

Travelers, military personnel, and others temporarily assigned to endemic areas may require immunization. Exposure to Japanese encephalitis virus has increased greatly with rapid economic development of the Pacific rim countries, and the large number of U.S. citizens visiting this region. The treatment of Japanese encephalitis is mainly supportive because antiviral drug chemotherapy has not been developed. In developed countries, the control of mosquito vectors or the immunization of host reservoirs has limited the spread of the virus, but these public health measures have been difficult to accomplish in developing countries.

An inactivated virus vaccine exists and has been used successfully to reduce the incidence of Japanese encephalitis in Japan, Taiwan, and Korea. Currently mass-produced and licensed in Japan, the vaccine has been tested under various experimental protocols. The vaccine is made by Biken and was licensed in the United States in late 1992. It also is distributed by Connaught Laboratories. The vaccine consists of partially purified, formalin-inactivated Japanese encephalitis virus that is propagated in mouse brain tissue. It requires a series of three to five injections to stimulate immunity.

A different, live-attenuated, vaccine (SA 14-14-2) has been developed and tested in China. It appears to be safe and effective in annual Chinese immunization programs involving millions of children. Efforts are underway to reconfirm safety and efficacy in carefully monitored trials in infants and children from 1 to 6 years of age, to secure international approval. A review of 13,000 vaccinated and control children in Chengdu Province, China, indicated low rates of acute systemic and local side effects, and no central nervous system infections were reported. The vaccine is produced in primary hamster kidney cells. Production issues remain a problem because this is not a widely accepted substrate for the production and licensure of vaccines in some countries, and the vaccine is not currently produced under good manufacturing practice conditions. Further research is also needed to determine the vaccine's thermostability, ability to revert to a more virulent form of the virus, efficacy in children with maternal antibody, and immunogenicity when used in combination with other vaccines.

NIAID currently funds several extramural and intramural projects studying basic virological and immunological aspects of flaviviruses. Some of the most promising molecular studies that might be applied to the development of an improved Japanese encephalitis vaccine focus on the development of full-length, infectious Japanese encephalitis cDNAs. Information from studies using this infectious clone has been combined with sequence data and immunological data to yield new insights into important antigenic regions on the Japanese encephalitis virion. Furthermore, NIH has supported the development of a chimeric vaccine using yellow fever vaccine as a vector carrying Japanese encephalitis coat proteins. Early clinical studies are very encouraging.

As mentioned above, further safety and efficacy studies are planned for the live SA 14-14-2. In addition, SA 14-14-2 is being molecularly modified, using infectious clones, to produce a vaccine that is highly stable to reversion.

Poxvirus vectors have been employed to deliver antigenic Japanese encephalitis proteins to humans in phase I trials. Further studies are needed, but these vectors induce cellular and antibody immunity against Japanese encephalitis.

Sources

Barrett, A. D. (1997). Japanese encephalitis and dengue vaccines. *Biologicals, 25*(1), 27-34.

Barrett, A. D. (1997). Yellow fever vaccines. *Biologicals, 25*(1), 17-25.

Chambers, T., Tsai, T., Pervikov, Y., & Monath, T. (1997). Vaccine development against dengue and Japanese encephalitis: Report of a World Health Organization meeting. *Vaccine, 15*(14), 1494-1502.

Halstead, S. B. (1996). Vaccines for Japanese encephalitis. *Lancet, 348*(9023), 341.

Shope, R., & Meegan, J. (1997). Arboviruses. In A. Evans & R. Kaslow (Eds.), *Viral infections of humans* (pp. 151-183). New York: Plenum Publishing Corporation.

World Health Organization. (1996). *State of the world's vaccines and immunization*. Geneva, Switzerland: WHO Press.

LYME DISEASE

Background

Lyme disease (borreliosis), which is caused by the tick-borne spirochete *Borrelia burgdorferi*, was first recognized as an infectious disease in 1975. It is the most prevalent tick-borne infectious disease in the United States. In 2000, 13,309 cases throughout the United States were reported to CDC. This represents an 18-percent decrease from the 16,273 cases reported in

1999. Decreases of 6 and 24 percent were reported in the New England States (4,361 versus 4,642) and mid-Atlantic States (6,770 versus 8,902), respectively. Within the New England States, increases were reported for New Hampshire (84 versus 27), Vermont (39 versus 26), Massachusetts (1,098 versus 787), and Rhode Island (590 versus 546), whereas a 21-percent decrease (2,550 versus 3,215) was reported for Connecticut. Within the mid-Atlantic States, another major endemic area, decreases of 8, 15, and 54 percent were reported for Upstate New York (3,916 versus 4,266), New Jersey (1,467 versus 1,719), and Pennsylvania (1,276 versus 1,719), respectively. There was a 27-percent decrease (423 versus 586) in cases reported for the East North Central States. Increases were reported for Ohio (89 versus 47) and Indiana (32 versus 21); however, there was a 41-percent decrease in the number of cases reported for Wisconsin (291 versus 407). An increase of 22 percent was reported for the West North Central States (495 versus 407), with a 39-percent increase in cases reported for Minnesota (393 versus 283). The data reported for these geographic areas of the United States represent 91 percent of all cases of Lyme disease reported to CDC by State public health agencies.

Ticks infected with *B. burgdorferi* often are co-infected with the agents of human granulocytic or human monocytic ehrlichiosis (HGE and HME, respectively), as well as with *Babesia microti*, a malaria-like parasite that causes babesiosis. Throughout the United States in 2000, 192 and 102 cases of HGE and HME, respectively, were reported to CDC. How co-infection influences the ability to detect Lyme disease or the severity of infection is not known.

Current Status of Research and Development

NIAID has supported an extramural research program on Lyme disease since 1985. The research grant portfolio has grown from 2 research grants in 1985 to more than 48 grants and contracts at present. It supports research on animal models of disease; microbial physiology; mechanisms of pathogenesis; mechanisms involved in the development of protective immunity; identification and characterization of virulence-associated antigens and their use as vaccines and diagnostic reagents; vectors, vector competence, and disease transmission mechanisms; therapeutic approaches for the treatment of acute and chronic infection; and the development of rapid, sensitive, and specific diagnostic tests for Lyme disease.

On December 21, 1998, the Food and Drug Administration (FDA) licensed LYMErix™ (SmithKline Beecham Biologicals), a new vaccine designed to block the transmission of Lyme disease by infected ticks. The major component of this vaccine is highly purified, recombinant outer surface protein A (OspA), an outer surface protein of *B. burgdorferi* that is produced in the midgut of infected ticks. Immunization with LYMErix™ stimulates the production of antibodies specific for OspA. When a tick takes a blood meal from an individual vaccinated with LYMErix™, it ingests these antibodies, which then bind to the surface of *B. burgdorferi* present in the midgut. As a result, *B. burgdorferi* is

either killed or prevented from migrating to the salivary glands of ticks where it can be transferred to humans to cause disease. Thus, LYMErix™ is considered to be a transmission-blocking vaccine. Since it was shown to be 80-percent effective in preventing borreliosis in humans 15 to 70 years of age, after three injections, LYMErix™ was recommended for use by those living in endemic areas where the risk of contracting Lyme disease is great.

Concerns were raised by patients and clinicians about associations between the vaccine and joint pain and swelling. This led the FDA to sponsor a public meeting in January 2001 to review the product's safety and update the advisory panel on complaints that LYMErix™ may be linked to an untreatable type of arthritis. At the time, the FDA considered the link between the vaccine and arthritis theoretical, but planned further study of dozens of reports from consumers who have arthritis or similar symptoms. In February 2002, the company pulled LYMErixÔ from the market, citing poor sales.

Separate studies, involving a total of 4,087 children from 4 to 18 years of age, also were conducted to assess the safety and immunogenicity of LYMErix™. The results showed that the administration of 30 mg of vaccine on a 0-, 1-, and 12-month schedule was well tolerated, safe, and immunogenic. In fact, the IgG antibody response in children 13 months after immunization was three times higher than that generated in the adult efficacy study; this suggests that the higher immune response in children should provide significant protection against Lyme disease.

Although OspA-based vaccines are effective in blocking the transmission of Lyme disease, NIAID also is supporting basic research to identify other vaccine candidates that, when combined with OspA, will provide even greater efficacy and perhaps longer lasting protective immunity. Among the candidates being considered are *in vivo*-expressed, Borrelia-specific, virulence-associated antigens that, unlike OspA, are capable of boosting the anamnestic immune response soon after infection. Study results indicate that *B. burgdorferi* decorin binding protein A (DbpA) elicits a sustained serum antibody response that is capable of inducing in experimental animals protective immunity against a wide range of needle-inoculated *B. burgdorferi sensu stricto* isolates. However, immunization with DbpA does not appear to protect against borreliosis transmitted by infected *Ixodes* ticks. This suggests that a DbpA-based vaccine may have limited utility, and that other potential candidate vaccines need to be examined and tested, especially under conditions that mimic the natural transmission of infection.

Sources

Centers for Disease Control and Prevention. (2000). Morbidity tables. *Morbidity and Mortality Weekly Report,* Week 52.

de Silva, A. M., Telford, S. R., III, Brunet, L. R., Barthold, S. W., & Fikrig, E. (1996). *Borrelia burgdorferi* OspA is an arthropod-specific transmission-blocking Lyme disease vaccine. *Journal of Experimental Medicine, 183,* 271-275.

Hagman, K. E., Yang, X., Wikel, S. K., Schoeler, G. B., Caimano, M. J., Radolf, J. D., & Norgard, M. V. (2000). Decorin-binding protein A (DbpA) of *Borrelia burgdorferi* is not protective when immunized mice are challenged via tick infestation and correlates with the lack of DbpA-expression by *B. burgdorferi*. *Infection and Immunity, 68,* 4759-4764.

Hanson, M. S., Cassatt, D. R., Guo, B. P., Patel, N. K., McCarthy, M. P., Dorward, D. W., & Hook, M. (1998). Active and passive immunity against *Borrelia burgdorferi* decorin binding protein A (DbpA) protects against infection. *Infection and Immunity, 66,* 2143-2153.

Sigal, L. H., Zahradnik, J. M., Lavin, P., Patella, S. J., Bryant, G., Haselby, R., Hilton, E., Kunkel, M., Adler-Klein, D., Doherty, T., Evans, J., Molloy, P. J., Seidner, A. L., Sabetta, J. R., Simon, H. J., Klempner, M. S., Mays, J., Marks, D., & Malawista, S. E. (1998). A vaccine consisting of recombinant *Borrelia burgdorferi* outer-surface protein A to prevent Lyme disease. Recombinant Outer-Surface Protein A Lyme Disease Vaccine Study Consortium. *New England Journal of Medicine, 339,* 216-222.

Sikand, V. K., Halsey, N., Krause, P. J., Sood, S. K., Geller, R., Van Hoecke, C., & Buscarino, C. P. (2001). Safety and immunogenicity of a recombinant *Borrelia burgdorferi* outer surface protein A vaccine against Lyme disease in healthy children and adolescents: A randomized controlled trial. *Pediatrics, 108,* 123-128.

Steere, A. C., Sikand, V. K., Meurice, F., Parenti, D. L., Fikrig, E., Schoen, R. T., Nowakowski, J., Schmid, C. H., Laukamp, S., Buscarino, C., & Krause, D. S. (1998). Vaccination against Lyme disease with recombinant *Borrelia burgdorferi* outer-surface lipoprotein A with adjuvant. Lyme Disease Vaccine Study Group. *New England Journal of Medicine, 339,* 209-215.

Thanassi, W. T., & Schoen, R. T. (2000). The Lyme disease vaccine: Conception, development, and implementation. *Annals of Internal Medicine, 132,* 661-668.

RABIES

Rabies continues to be a significant international health problem. Globally, attention has been drawn recently to potentially significant underreporting of rabies in developing countries. In these areas, a number of vaccines for human use, which vary in quality, are produced nationally and regionally, but postexposure treatment remains costly and often beyond the financial reach of those exposed. Moreover, such treatment must be administered properly, requiring product and delivery infrastructure. The need remains for economical, safe, and effective animal vaccines suitable for mass immunization of domestic animals and wildlife. In the United States, the continuing emergence of zoonotic rabies remains an expanding problem, especially in the raccoon population along the east coast. About a dozen human fatalities occur annually in the United States, and the number of postexposure treatments is rapidly increasing, with a substantial associated financial burden.

Research aimed to improve vaccines is underway with NIAID support. Vaccinia recombinants continue to be studied as an oral vaccine for wild animals, and there are attempts to develop a nucleic acid vaccine for possible oral administration. To date, large field trials of vaccinia recombinant wildlife vaccine have shown promise, but further studies should continue to better establish efficacy and carefully define safe, optimal application of the vaccine. Research on postexposure prophylaxis focuses on developing a one-shot, easily administered human vaccine and on safe, inexpensive, carefully defined rabies virus-specific immunoglobulins. Although not now available, an antiviral drug against rabies might be useful for postexposure prophylaxis.

Interestingly, in the United States and Canada, many recent human victims did not report a bite by a potentially rabid animal, or reported only limited exposure to bats. In many of these cases, the virus isolated was related to the strain found in silver-haired bats. It is thought that this bat is becoming an increasingly significant reservoir for rabies in the United States and that its bite often might go unnoticed. However, some health officials have questioned whether exposure might have occurred by inhalation of bat excretions. Although the guidelines for commencing postexposure treatment are well established for exposure to domestic animals, updated guidelines will have to be developed for exposure to wildlife, particularly bats. Recently, a bat-associated lyssavirus similar or identical to rabies has been identified in Australia, a previously rabies-free area.

Sources

Brown, C., & Szakacs, J. (1997). Rabies in New Hampshire and Vermont: An update. *Annals of Clinical and Laboratory Science, 27*(3), 216-223.

Centers for Disease Control and Prevention. (1997). Human rabies—Montana and Washington, 1997. *Morbidity and Mortality Weekly Report, 46*(33), 770-774.

Centers for Disease Control and Prevention. (1997). Update: Raccoon rabies epizootic—United States, 1996. *Morbidity and Mortality Weekly Report, 45*(51-52), 1117-1120.

Centers for Disease Control and Prevention. (2000). Human rabies—California, Georgia, Minnesota, New York, and Wisconsin, 2000. *Morbidity and Mortality Weekly Report, 49*(49), 1111-1115.

Centers for Disease Control and Prevention. (2000). Public health dispatch: Human rabies—Quebec, Canada, 2000. *Morbidity and Mortality Weekly Report, 49*(49), 1115-1116.

Dreesen, D. (1997). A global review of rabies vaccines for human use. *Vaccine, 15*(Suppl.), S2-S6.

Fu, Z. (1997). Rabies and rabies research: Past, present and future. *Vaccine, 15*(Suppl.), S20-S24.

Meslin, F. (1997). Global aspects of emerging and potential zoonoses: A WHO perspective. *Emerging Infectious Diseases, 3*(2), 223-228.

Rupprecht, C. E., Smith, J. S., Krebs, J. W., & Childs, J. E. (1997). Molecular epidemiology of rabies in the United States: Reemergence of a classical neurotropic agent. *Journal of Neurovirology, 3*(Suppl. 1), S52-S53.

World Health Organization. (1996). *State of the world's vaccines and immunization.* Geneva, Switzerland: WHO Press.

YELLOW FEVER

Yellow fever was first distinguished from other tropical febrile diseases during the 1647 to 1649 epidemics in the Americas. Since then, it has caused periodic epidemics in the Americas and Africa. The yellow fever virus is mosquito borne, and in humans produces a clinical disease that starts with the sudden onset of acute fever followed by a second phase of hepatorenal dysfunction and hemorrhage. Reported mortality rates vary widely from 20 to 80 percent of all cases.

During the latter half of the 20th century, yellow fever circulated in an endemic sylvatic cycle in the Americas, usually infecting up to 500 unvaccinated forest workers per year. In contrast, yellow fever in Africa periodically explodes from its endemic cycle to infect large numbers during major epidemics. The highly successful mosquito eradication campaigns of the early 20th century effectively eliminated urban yellow fever epidemics in South America and limited persistence of the virus to a monkey-mosquito cycle in jungle areas. However, the disease now appears to be slowly reemerging from the forest into those parts of South America where the vector *A. aegypti* has reinfested urban areas.

In the late 1980s, the total number of cases of yellow fever worldwide (with case fatality rates of about 50 percent) represented the greatest number reported to WHO during any 5-year period since 1948. Numerous studies showed that in Africa, only a small number of cases of yellow fever are reported. Ironically, 1988 marked the 50th anniversary of the development of the attenuated vaccine for yellow fever¾a safe and effective vaccine for this disease.

The 17D yellow fever vaccine was one of the first viral vaccines to be developed. It is a live-attenuated vaccine that is produced in eggs. After one injection, the vaccine induces protective immunity in more than 98 percent of vaccinees for a period of at least 10 years. In fact, protection may be lifelong because neutralizing antibodies have been detected as long as 40 years after immunization. The vaccine is one of the safest viral vaccines produced. Since 1965 alone, approximately 300 million doses of yellow fever vaccine have been administered. About 2 to 5 percent of individuals report mild headaches, myalgia, and low-grade fever after vaccination; less than 1 percent report altering their usual activities. The frequency of anaphylaxis attributed to yellow fever vaccine is approximately 1 in 130,000 vaccinees, and other severe illnesses attributed to yellow fever vaccination (including encephalitis, primarily in infants) are rare. From 1945 through 1989, only 17 cases of encephalitis associated with yellow fever immunization (1 fatal in a 3 year old) were reported worldwide. Because all but three of these cases occurred in children immunized at 4 months of age or younger, a review by a panel of experts recommended that the yellow fever vaccine not be given before 6 months of age.

However, recently there have been a series of reports of multiorgan system failure (MOSF) associated with yellow fever vaccination. Two Brazilian residents became ill after receiving 17D yellow fever vaccine administered during a 1999/2000 immunization campaign initiated in response to a local yellow fever epidemic. Between 1996 and 2001, five other persons became ill after receiving 17D-204 yellow fever vaccine administered for international travel. All seven persons became ill within 2 to 5 days of vaccination and required intensive care; six died. None had documented immunodeficiency. MOSF associated with yellow fever vaccination was not reported before 1996. The frequency of febrile MOSF after vaccination with 17D in the United States during 1990 to 1998 is now estimated at 1 in 400,000 doses.

Over the past 40 years, two vaccine-based control strategies have been attempted in Africa. The first consists of routine immunization, whereas the second involves emergency control measures that are implemented after the start of an outbreak. A routine, mandatory yellow fever immunization program was begun in the early 1940s in French West Africa; as a result, the recurring pattern of epidemics in West Africa has been interrupted. However, this strategy was abandoned in 1960 when a postoutbreak, fire-fighting type of emergency immunization and control strategy was adopted. Since then, there has been a series of epidemics of varying severity. In recent years, with the help of the WHO Expanded Programme on Immunization (EPI), more African countries have apparently, at least partially, incorporated the yellow fever vaccine into their immunization programs. Most give the yellow fever vaccine and measles vaccine to children at 9 months of age because the simultaneous administration of the vaccines has been shown to be acceptable. Recently, the Global Advisory Group for WHO-EPI reviewed the status of yellow fever and recommended that all 31 nations in the yellow fever endemic area incorporate the vaccine into their routine immunization programs.

In South America, yellow fever control strategies have been primarily based on reducing mosquito vectors by altering their breeding environment. Extensive studies on the maintenance of yellow fever virus have shown that the virus exists in two cycles: An urban cycle involving humans and *A. aegypti* mosquitoes, and a sylvatic or jungle cycle involving forest primates (principally monkeys) and forest canopy mosquitoes, with human infections tangential to the transmission cycle. In the Western Hemisphere, *A. aegypti* mosquitoes were the sole transmitters of urban yellow fever. In 1901, eradication efforts directed toward *A. aegypti* mosquitoes were launched under the direction of Dr. William Gorgas in Havana. These eradication efforts, with concomitant reduction of yellow fever, were extended throughout Central and South America in the early 1900s. The eradication program successfully broke the chain of urban *A. aegypti*-transmitted yellow fever. The eradication of the vector, and the subsequent reduction of urban yellow fever cases in the Americas, represents one of the world's most successful public health campaigns against an infectious disease. Unfortunately, *A. aegypti* has now reinfested most of South and Central America and occupies habitats just adjacent to the areas where endemic yellow fever transmission occurs. A major threat is that this species could transmit yellow fever in an urban cycle. The Pan American Health Organization (PAHO) is monitoring the need for incorporation of yellow fever immunization into the EPI programs in South America. Some authorities believe serious consideration should be given to expanding yellow fever immunization in South American EPI programs in an attempt to prevent the reemergence of urban yellow fever.

The EPI program provides an excellent way to deliver yellow fever vaccines to a larger population at a reduced cost; however, despite the fact that the current yellow fever vaccine is an excellent public health tool, further studies are needed to better define its role in controlling yellow fever. In the past, the amount of vaccine available has been a limitation. The number of surviving infants in the 1990s in the countries where yellow fever is a potential risk is approximately 18 million. Although the vaccine is made in a number of developing countries, including Senegal and Nigeria, only about 6 million doses are produced yearly in Africa. Newer technology, combined with efficient technology transfer, might help solve the problem of availability. The development of a cell culture-produced vaccine might result in increased vaccine production. One recent study of vaccine thermostability showed that further work on stabilizing the yellow fever vaccine is needed because only 5 of 12 manufactured lots met the WHO criteria for vaccine thermostability. More research is needed on the safety of combining this vaccine with other vaccines in a multiple-dose regimen for immunization.

NIAID currently funds several extramural and intramural projects studying basic virological and immunological aspects of flaviviruses. Some of the most promising molecular studies that might be applied to the development of an improved yellow fever vaccine focus on the development of a full-length, infectious yellow fever cDNA. Information from studies using this infectious clone has been combined with sequence data and immunological data to yield new insights into important antigenic regions on the yellow fever virion. It is hoped that this research will yield efficient and less costly ways to manufacture safe flavivirus vaccines. At a minimum, a clone-derived vaccine seed virus might reduce yellow fever vaccine production lot diversity, improve quality control, and reduce the need for vaccine safety testing in primates.

Sources

Barrett, A. D. (1997). Japanese encephalitis and dengue vaccines. *Biologicals, 25*(1), 27-34.

Barrett, A. D. (1997). Yellow fever vaccines. *Biologicals, 25*(1), 17-25.

Centers for Disease Control and Prevention. (2001). Notice to readers: Fever, jaundice, and multi-organ system failure associated with 17D derived yellow fever vaccination, 1996-2001. *Morbidity and Mortality Weekly Report, 50*(30), 643-644.

Chambers, T., Tsai, T., Pervikov, Y., & Monath, T. (1997). Vaccine development against dengue and Japanese encephalitis: Report of a World Health Organization meeting. *Vaccine, 15*(14), 1494-1502.

Robertson, S., Hull, B., Tomori, O., Bele, O., LeDuc, J., & Esteves, K. (1996). Yellow fever; a decade of re-emergence. *Journal of the American Medical Association, 276*(14), 1157-1162.

Shope, R., & Meegan, J. (1997). Arboviruses. In A. Evans & R. Kaslow (Eds.), *Viral infections of humans* (pp. 151-183). New York: Plenum Publishing Corporation.

World Health Organization. (1996). *State of the world's vaccines and immunization.* Geneva, Switzerland: WHO Press.

Yellow fever in 1994 and 1995. (1996). *Weekly Epidemiological Record, 71*(42), 313-318.

WEST NILE FEVER

The identification of West Nile virus (WNV) in New York in the summer of 1999 was the first time the mosquito-borne microbe had been detected in the Western Hemisphere. Until then, the virus had been found chiefly in Africa, Eastern Europe, the Middle East, and Asia. Since 1999, WNV has been reported in an ever-growing number of States within the United States. From 1999 to 2001, there were 149 confirmed cases of WNV in the United States, including 18 deaths. To date in 2002, the number of confirmed cases and deaths in the United States already exceed these numbers. Although infection with WNV usually causes only mild symptoms in humans, it can spread to the central nervous system and cause a potentially deadly brain inflammation called encephalitis, most common among the elderly. Currently, no treatment is available for WNV encephalitis, and no licensed vaccine exists to prevent the disease. Mosquito control has been the only available strategy to combat the rapid spread of this emerging disease, but effective spraying is difficult to carry out in urban areas.

Faced with the potential for a serious WNV epidemic, NIH-supported researchers started to develop a vaccine that protects against infection with the virus. Basic research on newly emerging microbes has enabled rapid progress in the development of a WNV vaccine. In addition, WNV vaccine development has benefited from the fact that WNV belongs to the group of viruses known as flaviviruses, which have many characteristics in common. These similarities have allowed scientists to build on earlier discoveries about other flaviviruses that are closely related to WNV, including Japanese encephalitis virus, St. Louis encephalitis virus, yellow fever virus, and dengue virus.

There has been great success controlling yellow fever and Japanese encephalitis with well-organized vaccination campaigns centered on an efficacious vaccine. Therefore, NIH encouraged similar WNV vaccine development programs.

Importantly, NIH-supported basic research studies discovered that hamsters, and to a lesser extent mice, were good models for West Nile disease. NIH-supported researchers at the University of Texas Medical Branch, Galveston, conducted a series of preliminary experiments to learn more precisely the degree of protection that candidate WNV and other licensed flavivirus vaccines might have against WNV. Researchers found that hamsters were completely protected by prototype WNV vaccines, and surprisingly, at least partially protected by Japanese encephalitis and yellow fever vaccines. Thus, this new model is an important resource that could be used in the development of WNV vaccines to test the efficacy of a new vaccine candidate (or a new antiviral medicine).

NIH is supporting a number of vaccine approaches. One of the earliest was started in 1999 when NIH funded a fast-track project to develop a candidate WNV vaccine with Acambis, Inc. Since then, scientists have developed a prototype vaccine that has shown promise in animal tests. The vaccine is constructed using vaccine licensed for preventing yellow fever (caused by another flavivirus) as the backbone. For WNV vaccine, researchers substituted the surface protein of WNV for the deleted yellow fever virus protein. This method of creating chimeric flavivirus vaccines is also being applied to developing a vaccine for dengue and Japanese encephalitis virus. The Acambis, Inc., vaccine has undergone preclinical evaluations in hamsters, mice, monkeys, and horses with encouraging results. The company is moving forward with phase I trials. Vaccine is now being pro-

duced and an investigational new drug application will be filed with the FDA. Trials are anticipated to begin in early 2003.

Other NIH scientists and collaborators from WRAIR capitalized on recent advances in recombinant DNA technology and previous research on another flavivirus—dengue virus—to produce a new candidate WNV vaccine. The NIH team already had tested successfully a strategy that used the new technology to replace key genes of different flaviviruses with those of dengue virus type 4 (DEN4). Unlike many flaviviruses, DEN4 does not cause disease in the brain. The resulting weakened, or attenuated, virus strains were safer for use in a vaccine but still protective. The NIH-WRAIR research team then used this strategy to combine genes from WNV and DEN4. This hybrid virus did not infect the brain, yet still stimulated a strong immune response with even a single dose. When tested in mice, the hybrid vaccine protected all animals against lethal WNV infection. The findings from these studies provide the basis for pursuing the development of a WNV vaccine. The next step for the NIH-WRAIR research team is to test the promising hybrid vaccine in monkeys in late 2002. Progress to vaccine trials in humans is expected to be rapid because one of the dengue viruses used to construct the hybrid virus already has been proven safe in people.

Early studies are also underway by other NIH-supported scientists on a DNA vaccine approach and a protein vaccine approach.

Sources

Monath, T. P. (2001). Prospects for development of a vaccine against the West Nile virus. *Annals of the New York Academy of Sciences, 951,* 1-12.

Pletnev, A. G., Putnak, R., Speicer, J., Wagar, E. J., & Vaughn, D. (2002). West Nile virus/dengue type 4 virus chimeras that are reduced in neurovirulence and peripheral virulence without loss of immunogenicity or protective efficacy. *Proceedings of the National Academy of Sciences, 99,* 3036-3041.

Tesh, R. B., Travassos da Rose, A. P. A., Guzman, H., Araujo, T. P., & Xiao, S. Y. (2002). Immunization with heterologous flaviviruses protective against fatal West Nile encephalitis. *Emerging Infectious Diseases, 8,* 245-251.

Xiao, S-Y, Guzman, H., Zhang, H., Travassos da Rosa, A. P. A., & Tesh, R. B. (2001). West Nile virus infection in the golden hamster (*Mesocricetus auratus*): A model for West Nile encephalitis. *Emerging Infectious Diseases, 7,* 714-721.

Viral Hepatitis

Viral Hepatitis

OVERVIEW

In spite of many advances impacting overall health worldwide, infection, disease, and death from hepatitis viruses continue into the 21st century. Twenty years ago, only three viral causes of acute and chronic hepatitis had been identified (hepatitis A, B, and D), with serologic assays in use to protect patients from exposure by transfusion. Even then, physicians were addressing unidentifiable infections as non-A non-B. Patients with non-A non-B were treated with interferon alpha (IFNa) therapy prior to the laudable discovery in 1988 by Chiron investigators of the principal cause of blood-borne, non-A non-B, hepatitis C. Unable to identify the virus directly, hepatitis C was genetically cloned out of the plasma of a non-A non-B patient. New technological advances had facilitated this and future non-A non-B discoveries.

Five distinct viruses are the known etiologic agents for hepatitis, leading to fatigue; jaundice; liver damage; and, in chronic cases, cirrhosis and even liver cancer. Hepatitis A is transmitted fecal-orally, and outbreaks of this acute infectious agent are common at daycare centers, nursing homes, and restaurants where inappropriate food handling might occur. Hepatitis B virus (HBV) and hepatitis C virus (HCV) are blood-borne agents and may cause chronic diseases. The infections produced by HBV are more likely to be symptomatic and to resolve spontaneously. The infections produced by HCV have a high chronicity rate at all ages and are far more likely to be asymptomatic, despite ongoing liver disease. Until recently, the only licensed therapy for either hepatitis B or hepatitis C was IFNa, which has low success rates for both diseases. Infection with hepatitis D virus (HDV) is dependent on co-infection with HBV, and may lead to life-threatening superinfections. Hepatitis E virus (HEV), like hepatitis A virus (HAV), is transmitted via the fecal-oral route and produces an acute illness associated with a high mortality rate in pregnant women. Hepatitis E is reported primarily in developing countries; however, the Centers for Disease Control and Prevention (CDC) has determined by serologic screenings that more than 1 percent of the U.S. population has been exposed to hepatitis E.

In addition to these agents, there are some other viruses associated with hepatitis that have been identified. Hepatitis G virus (HGV) [or GB virus C (GBV-C)] is a flavivirus, related to HCV. It is a blood-borne agent that produces chronic carriage, but to date it has not been associated with a specific disease. Another similar virus, transfusion transmitted virus (TTV), is found in about 7 percent of healthy blood, as well as in patients with hepatitis as a co-infection. It is assumed to be transmitted via the fecal-oral route and has yet to be associated with a specific disease. An additional virus, SEN-V, has been isolated from a patient with acquired immunodeficiency syndrome (AIDS), and does appear to produce hepatitis.

Several notable advances have been made in the structural biology of hepatitis viruses. The structure of the core protein of hepatitis B, a molecule that does not crystallize and was therefore incapable of being studied by x-ray crystallography, was determined by electron cryomicroscopy. Two groups have published reports on the x-ray structure of the hepatitis C nonstructural NS3 protease, which is important for viral replication and is a target for antivirals. At least five companies are presently working on inhibitors for the HCV protease. Finally, researchers identified the structure of the helicase of hepatitis C, an enzyme that is needed to uncoil the viral RNA and allow it to make a copy of itself for reproduction.

A novel tissue culture hepatitis C model, replicating only the nonstructural proteins in high numbers, may allow testing of targeted antivirals. The transgenic potato hepatitis B vaccine is in clinical trials. Due to possible associated adverse events, the safety of licensed hepatitis B vaccines for neonates is also under scrutiny. Meanwhile, the identification of a new hepatitis virus may explain remaining non-A-E,G chronic infections.

HEPATITIS A

HAV accounts for about 55 percent of acute hepatitis cases in the United States, with the highest incidence in the Southwest. There are approximately 132,000 cases per year, with elevated rates among Native Americans, Hispanics, people in low socioeconomic levels, and people practicing risky lifestyle behaviors. Rates in males are 20-percent higher than in females, and prevalence of exposure (antibody to HAV) ranges from 11 percent in persons less than 5 years of age to 74 percent in persons more than 50 years of age. Most of the symptomatic disease is seen in 10- to 30-year-old patients. Person-to-person contact, or sexual contact with a person infected with HAV, accounts for most transmissions; but there is a viremic phase during acute infections when blood-borne transmission is possible. Asymptomatic infection is common below the age of 2, but becomes less common with increasing age. Fulminant disease may be fatal, and accounts for 70 to 80 deaths per year among those between the ages of 30 and 49. Work-loss costs associated with acute HAV infection in the United States are $200 million (1991) each year.

Natural immunity levels in the United States have undergone a significant decline since 1980, and are currently in the 21- to 33-percent range. Two formalin-killed, licensed HAV vaccines are available for adults and children more than 2 years of age—HavrixÒ (SmithKline Beecham Biologicals) and VaqtaÒ (Merck & Co., Inc.). HavrixÒ and VaqtaÒ contain inactivated viral particles

(HM175 and CR326F strains, respectively) produced in infected human diploid fibroblasts. Although hepatitis A outbreaks occur globally, the vaccine was initially marketed as a traveler's vaccine. Areas in the United States where HAV outbreaks commonly occur are also targeted. The licensing in May 2001 of a new combination HAV/HBV vaccine called TwinrixÒ by GlaxoSmithKline offers a highly protective vaccine with fewer injections for those 18 years of age and older. Hepatitis A and B vaccines are strongly recommended for patients with hepatitis C, to prevent harsher disease burdens.

HEPATITIS B

HBV infections kill 4,000 to 5,000 Americans each year, and 1 million people worldwide. Approximately 300 million people worldwide have chronic hepatitis B infections, with endemic areas primarily in Asia and Africa. HBV is highly contagious [100 times more contagious than human immunodeficiency virus (HIV)] and, like HAV, is capable of producing fulminant disease. It is highly transmissible from HBV-positive mothers to their newborns.

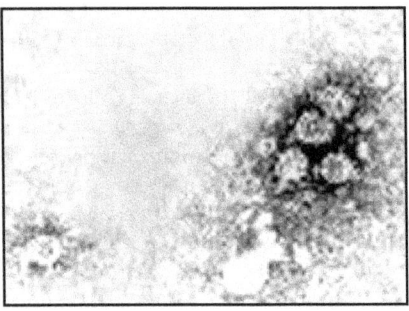

Hepatitis B Virus

About 25 percent of infected adults become chronic carriers, and 20 percent of those patients develop cirrhosis or liver cancer. Perinatal infection of infants has a much higher chronicity rate of 70 percent, resulting in a higher rate of subsequent cirrhosis and liver cancer. Each year, an estimated 20,000 infants are born to hepatitis B surface antigen-positive women in the United States. From 200,000 to 300,000 new HBV infections have been reported in the United States annually for the past decade. Annually, hepatitis B accounts for 60,000 hospitalizations and 5,000 deaths, for a total yearly cost of $800 million, excluding the cost of transplantation for end-stage liver disease. It is estimated that there are 1 million to 1.25 million chronic carriers of HBV in the United States.

Vaccines were developed for hepatitis B, a chronic blood-borne and highly transmissible virus, starting in 1981 with the licensing of a plasma-derived vaccine called HepatavaxÒ. Infants born to hepatitis B-positive mothers were immunized at birth to prevent transmission during birth. An added benefit was that vaccination against hepatitis B also protected against superinfection with HDV. Although HepatavaxÒ was highly protective against hepatitis B, improved recombinant vaccines promoting antibodies to the outer envelope protein of the virus were licensed— Recombivax HBÒ by Merck, Sharp & Dohme (June 1986) and Energix-BÒ by SmithKline Beecham Biologicals (August 1989). Both vaccines use a three-dose regimen at 0, 1, and 6 months.

Initially, no plan was enacted to target at-risk populations, but that changed when the Government promoted universal childhood HBV vaccination.

As of 10 years ago, most infants in developed countries begin their HBV immunizations at birth. Success of this policy has seen dramatic reductions in transmission to children in high-risk populations, such as in Taiwan, where there is a large burden of disease with chronic hepatitis B. Cancer incidence in 6- to 9-year-olds also dropped from 0.52 percent to 0.13 percent. A study of high-risk Taiwanese infants demonstrated that antibody levels remained high for at least 10 years, suggesting that booster doses would not be needed.

There have been delays and setbacks in universal immunization in the United States and abroad due to concerns about side effects and possible overexposure to a mercury-based preservative. In July 1999, the Association of American Physicians and Surgeons called for an immediate moratorium on mandatory hepatitis B vaccines for schoolchildren, pending further research on serious side effects. In the same month, the American Academy of Pediatrics issued precautionary recommendations to delay initiation of hepatitis B vaccination in healthy newborns due to possible ill effects of early exposure to the common vaccine preservative thimerosol. The level of HBV vaccination in infants fell significantly as a result of these concerns, and thimerosol is being removed from childhood vaccines.

HEPATITIS C

Infection with HCV accounts for about 12 percent of the acute viral hepatitis in the United States. Approximately 35,000 cases occur annually (declining over the past decade from 180,000), with about 85 percent of those infected becoming chronic carriers, at a total yearly cost of $600 million, excluding transplants. Most carriers are asymptomatic. Many cases of hepatitis C can be attributed to the 1 million blood transfusions administered before 1990, from which an estimated 290,000 Americans became infected. A look-back study is currently alerting these patients to the potential risk. Most cases of HCV infection occur among young adults (especially injecting drug users); although among adults more than 40 years of age, HCV is often the most common cause of acute hepatitis. Sexual transmission may account for as many as 20 percent of the cases. No risk factor can be identified for 10 to 30 percent of HCV carriers. Each year there are 8,000 to 10,000 deaths and 1,000 transplantations due to HCV infections. The current estimate, based on random serologic screenings of more than 21,000 serum samples, is that 3.9 million Americans are chronically infected with HCV—1.8 percent of the population— with higher rates among African Americans (8 to 10 percent), who are also more refractory to current therapies. Hemodialysis patients and hemophiliacs are at exceptionally high risk, and noninvasive person-to-person transmission has been documented. The World Health Organization (WHO) estimates that 3 percent of the world's population has been infected, and that there are 170 million chronic carriers at risk of developing liver cirrhosis and/or liver cancer.

Several investigators have reported a relatively high efficiency vertical transmission of HCV from mothers who were co-infected with HIV. Other major studies in the United States and Europe have failed to demonstrate transmission from HCV-positive mothers. Risk factors for transmission, which is assumed to occur *in utero,* include a high HCV RNA level in the mother, and the presence of specific HCV variants. Results of a study of infants born to HCV-infected mothers demonstrated biochemical features of liver damage (ALT abnormalities) during the first 12 months of life, although HCV-associated liver disease is likely to be mild throughout infancy and childhood. Multivariate analyses of risk factors for cirrhosis and/or liver cancer with HCV infections demonstrated that increased age, male gender, and excessive alcohol consumption were all important factors. Additional risk factors for cancer were hepatitis B antibody positivity and HCV genotype. There was no relationship between the development of liver cancer and serum HCV levels.

Although HCV is the leading cause of chronic viral hepatitis in the United States, a vaccine has been difficult to develop because of extensive genetic and possibly antigenic diversity among the different strains. New variants known as quasi-species arise quickly and frequently, thus allowing escape from neutralizing antibodies and cytotoxic T lymphocytes. Amino acid changes frequently observed in a region of about 27 amino acids, termed the hypervariable region 1 (HVR1), which is located at the amino terminus of the hepatitis C envelope protein E2, are postulated to lead to this viral escape from neutralizing antibodies. The identification of this most variable region of HCV, the HVR1, as a critical neutralization domain poses a major challenge for the development of a broadly reactive vaccine against HCV. Early vaccine studies in chimpanzees using recombinant envelope glycoproteins showed limited protection upon challenge with the same virus. DNA vaccines are now being tested in chimpanzees, using envelope as well as core protein constructs. Virus-like particles (VLPs) made up of structural HCV proteins have been produced successfully in insect cells and may serve as a potential vaccine model. Ribozymes, catalytic RNA molecules that bind specifically to target RNA by an antisense mechanism, are also being tested as a possible strategy for the treatment of HCV infection.

Tissue culture models or small animal models of infection are needed to study the infection process and for testing drugs and vaccines. Currently, a tissue culture model of a portion of the HCV genome is the best characterized HCV model, but an infection model would be more useful. The chimpanzee remains the only HCV infection animal model. Also, there are no good correlates of immunity. Even though infection by HCV generates antibodies, none of these are capable of resolving or neutralizing the infection. A vaccine, to be successful, will need to launch strong antibody responses as well as cytotoxic T lymphocyte and T helper lymphocyte responses. In addition, HCV is characterized by constant immune evasion by continuous development of variant HCV species. HCV, like many RNA viruses, generates a lot of mutations, thus making a moving target for vaccine design. There are 6 HCV genotypes and more than 100 sub-types.

Potential HCV vaccine candidates that are currently under development include recombinant proteins (principally, the structural proteins such as the viral core protein or the two viral envelope glycoproteins), recombinant viruses, DNA constructs, synthetic peptides, and VLPs. Various vaccine candidates have been shown to generate antibody-producing and cellular immune responses in animals, primarily in mice. However, the efficacy of most vaccine candidates in protecting against HCV has not been tested because the chimpanzee, the only animal other than humans that is susceptible to HCV, is endangered, is not readily available, requires special facilities, and is very expensive.

Hepatitis D

The prevalence of HDV infection does not parallel that of HBV, although it is dependent on HBV for its transmission. It is highest in those individuals with repeated percutaneous exposures, including intravenous drug users and hemophiliacs. Perinatal transmission is rarely reported (as yet undocumented in the United States). An estimated 70,000 people (4 percent of HBV cases) in the United States have chronic hepatitis D. There are 7,500 infections each year, and about 1,000 people die annually of HDV infections. There are three genetically different types: Type 1 is found worldwide, type 2 in Southeast Asia, and type 3 in northern South America. Vaccination against HBV prevents infection by HDV. As yet, there are no proven therapies for co-infection with HBV and HDV.

Hepatitis E

Like hepatitis A, hepatitis E is transmitted fecal-orally, causing acute hepatitis principally seen in young adults in Asian or African countries. Surprisingly, about 2 percent of the global population carries antibodies to hepatitis E. It is considered a zoonotic disease in that it is commonly found in pigs, rats, sheep, monkeys, cattle, and ducks. The actual isolation of the virus from patient stools occurred in 1990. It was subsequently cloned and sequenced with the immunogenic ORF2 peptide being developed for vaccines. Successful passive and active immunization was demonstrated against hepatitis E challenge in monkeys, and currently a couple of vaccines are in phase II clinical trials in endemic regions.

HEV infections are rare in the United States, but do pose a risk to persons who travel overseas to endemic areas. CDC developed a mosaic protein enzyme immunoassay that, based on antibody titers, showed a 3-percent rate of recent exposure to HEV in a cohort of randomly screened patients, none of whom had traveled abroad, in four geographic areas of the United States. A 1.2-percent rate of previous exposure among the U.S. population was also determined. There is a high seroprevalence among renal transplantation and hemophilia patient populations.

In National Institute of Allergy and Infectious Diseases (NIAID) studies conducted at the National Institutes of Health (NIH), cynomolgus monkeys were partially or completely protected against infection with HEV by passive and active immunization. Convalescent serum was used for the passive immunization, and a recombinant 55-kilodalton open-reading frame 2 protein known to induce antibody formation was used for the active immunization. These results pointed the way toward development of a vaccine, but so far none has been licensed.

HEPATITIS G OR HEPATITIS GB VIRUS-C

Much progress has been made in analyzing, sequencing, serotyping, and determining the prevalence of the blood-borne HGV and GBV-C. Discovered by Genelabs and Abbott Laboratories, respectively, these two viruses are now assumed to be different isolates of the same virus and are distantly related to another flavivirus, HCV (only 25-percent homology). Studies of stored serum specimens show that these viruses are not new. Their identification has awaited new methods of detection. They are endemic worldwide, though their potential for disease production remains unclear, as most carriers are asymptomatic. Cases of fulminant hepatitis have been linked to these agents; however, they are not generally considered to be a cause of non-A-E hepatitis. Multiple strains of HGV/GBV-C have been found in dialysis patients, and the virus is common in transplantation settings. It is found in 10 percent of injecting drug users. HGV/GBV-C infection has often been associated with co-infection with certain strains of HCV (types 1a, 1b, and 3), but this additional infection does not seem to affect the patient.

OTHER HEPATITIS VIRUSES

Four percent of acute cases of hepatitis are currently classified as non-A-E,G. A few years ago, a novel fecal-orally spread form of hepatitis was named hepatitis F by a French team of researchers. No subsequent publications have appeared about hepatitis F virus (HFV), but a second publication did refer to a novel hepatitis agent being detected from a screening of HEV-infected sera from an epidemic in the Andaman Islands.

TTV, a non-enveloped DNA virus discovered initially in a patient with hepatitis, appears to be following a similar path as HGV/GBV-C. It is still too early to determine whether it is a direct cause of hepatitis or merely a confounding co-infection.

Using an unusual "degeneration" technique for screening, researchers in Italy have isolated a potential hepatitis agent from the blood of immunosuppressed HIV patients. The new virus that was isolated was called SEN-V after the patient from whom it came. Extensive verification under code, as yet ongoing, found SEN-V in a high percentage of previously unclassified hepatitis patients and in low numbers of healthy controls. The data are premature, but promising.

Appendices

Appendix A

Original Jordan Report

National Institute of Allergy and Infectious Diseases

ACCELERATED DEVELOPMENT OF NEW VACCINES

In the fall of 1980, the Secretary of the Department of Health and Human Services accepted the recommendation of the HHS Steering Committee for the Development of a Health Research Strategy that an NIAID proposal for the "Accelerated Development of New Vaccines" be added as one of four new initiatives to 11 prior initiatives identified in December 1979. The 15 initiatives then constituted the Department's proposed initiatives for FY 81. The purpose of the NIAID initiative is to develop within DHHS a clearly-identified, coordinated, and recognized approach to the further conquest of vaccine-preventable disease. The incentive for an expanded effort lies in new knowledge and processes emerging from recombinant DNA and hybridoma technology and in the better understanding of the workings of the immune system. The goal of the initiative is to expedite the availability of needed vaccines by selecting a few candidate vaccines for extra research and development efforts. Studies are in progress on more than 50 vaccine antigens for over 30 different bacterial, viral, and parasitic diseases, the majority of these studies being dependent on investigator-initiated projects. With the assistance of existing advisory committees and "state-of-the-art" reviews by workshops, and in coordination with the HHS Interagency Group to Monitor Vaccine Development, Production and Usage, and with enhanced and collaboration with industry, efforts will be made to bring a few selected, high priority candidate vaccines into use several years earlier than might otherwise be the case.

The first step toward implementation of the Institute's initiative was taken in the fall of 1981 when the professional staff of MIDP met for a three-day review of the status of NIAID's vaccine development program, and reached a consensus as to those vaccines that should be assigned priority for accelerated development. Following review and discussion of over 30 agents or groups of agents, excluding influenza, the staff updated three developmental listings: (1) development completed; ready for expanded clinical trials; (2) encouraging progress made; further development needed; and (3) early development; basic studies in progress. Concurrently, the agents were placed in three categories for phased, sequential study: (1) diseases for which safe, effective vaccines do not now exist, but that result in high morbidity, mortality or socio-economic costs in the U.S. population in general; (2) diseases of importance to special subsets of the U.S. population; and (3) diseases of importance to less technologically advanced nations.

The diseases were next ranked according to priority of need in the U.S. and developing countries, and then ranked according to technical feasibility and the prospects for accelerated development using new and emerging technology. A consensus was reached as to how these rankings should be integrated. On this basis, MIDP staff assigned priority to ten agents or agent pairs, five for use in the U.S. and five for use in developing countries, as follows:

	For U.S.			International
1.	Haemophilus influenzae,		1.	Malaria
2	Gonococcal		2	Typhoid / E. coli
3.	Parainfluenza/RSV		3.	Leprosy
4.	Pertussis (improved)		4.	Streptococcal, Group A
5.	Rotavirus		5.	Shigella

Priority has yet to be assigned to limited use vaccines for special populations.

The proposed initiative called for a review of potential vaccine-preventable diseases from the standpoint of socio-economic and medical needs and for an assessment of the cost/benefit ratios of vaccines for each of these diseases. In the fall of 1982, the Institute of Medicine was asked to undertake this review and evaluation so as to assist NIAID in setting priorities for development and to develop for

NIAID a new model system for the decision-making process that can be applied to the setting of priorities in the future. To date (November 1982), workshops have reviewed three of the five high priority domestic candidates: improved pertussis, Haemophilus influenzae, and the parainfluenza/respiratory syncytial viruses. A workshop on gonococcal vaccine is planned for FY 1983.

A table summarizing the status of the NIAID vaccine development effort as of October 1982 is provided as Attachment 1. Brief descriptions of progress in the development of some of the more promising vaccines are included in Attachment 2.

BACTERIAL VACCINES (cont.)

10/1/82

Agent	Type of Vaccine	Number of Preparations Available	Animal Model Studies		Human Trials	
			Antigenicity	Efficacy	Antigenicity	Efficacy
Pseudomonas	Polysaccharide	7	IP	IP	P	P
	LPS (heptavalent)	1	IP	IP	IP	IP
	Cell wall extract	1	IP	IP	IP	IP
RMSF	Inactivated (whole organism)	1	IP	IP	C	C
	Cell component preparation	1	IP	IP	DR	DR
Streptococcus Group A	M protein synthetic peptides (some preparations linked to polylysine or tetanus toxiod carriers)	9	IP	IP	DR	DR
Streptococcus Group B	Polysaccharide	6	C	IP	IP	DR
	Polysaccharide-protein complex	2	C	IP	IP	DR
Streptococcus pneumoniae	14-valent polysaccharide	1	NA	NA	IP*	NA
Vibrio cholerae	Inactivated					
	Oral (El Tor-Inaba-Ogawa, Phenol-alcohol)	1	C	C	C	IP
	B Subunit	1	C	C	C	NTBD
	Whole cell + B subunit	1	C	IP	C	P
	Paracholeragenoid	1	C	C	C	P
	Flagella Sheath	1	C	C	DR	DR
	Outer membrane Proteins	3	C	NTBD	DR	DR
	Lectin -protease	1	C	NTBD	R	DR
	Attenuated					
	B+A – Texas Star	1	C	C	C	C
	B+A – Baltimore Bullet	1	IP	IP	DR	DR
	B+A – Mechalonis Strain	1	IP	IP	DR	DR

FUNGAL VACCINES

10/1/82

Agent	Type of Vaccine	Number of Preparations Available	Animal Model Studies		Human Trials	
			Antigenicity	Efficacy	Antigenicity	Efficacy
Coccidioides imitis	Mycelia cell wall antigen	1	IP	IP	P	P
	Spherule cell wall antigen	1	IP	IP	P	P
Malaria	Gametes	1 (live organisms)	IP	IP	DR	DR
	Asexual strategy	4 (irradiated merozoites) (killed merozoites) (merozoite/schizont antigen) (sporozoite antigen)	IP	IP	DR	DR
Schistosoma	Irradiated larva stages	1	IP	IP	DR	DR
	Non-specific immune stimulation	(?)	IP	IP	DR	DR
Toxoplasma	Attenuated strains	(?)	IP	IP	DR	DR
Trypanosoma	Cell surface glycoprotein	Numerous variant derived preparations	IP	DR	DR	DR
Leishmania	Promastigote membrane antigens	(?)	IP	DR	DR	DR

VIRAL VACCINES

10/1/82

Agent	Type of Vaccine	Number of Preparations Available	Animal Model Studies		Human Trials	
			Antigenicity	Efficacy	Antigenicity	Efficacy
Cytomegalovirus	Attenuated	1	C	C	IP	NTBD
Hepatitis B	Subunit, inactivated	6	C(2)	C(2)	C(4)	IP(2)
	Polypeptide, chemically synthesized	1	IP	P	DR	DR
Hepatitis A	Attenuated	2	IP	IP	NA	NA
Influenza A & B	Subunit	2	C(6) IP(2)	P(2)	C(2)	NTBD
	Attenuated (ts and cold-adapted)	6	C(10) IP(6) P(5)	C(1)	C(7) IP(2) P(7)	P(4)
	Inactivated (whole virus) Licensed	0	NA	NA	0	P(1)
Parainfluenza Virus 3	Subunit	IP	NA	NA	NA	NA
Rabies	Killed, whole virus	1	C	C	C	C
Rotavirus	Live, human strain					
	WA	1	C	C	IP	DR
	D	1	P	P	DR	DR
	DSI	1	P	P	DR	DR

Varicella Attenuated 1 C NA C IP

C = Completed
IP = In Progress
P = Planned

NTBD = Needs to be Done
NA = Not Applicable
( ) = Number of Preparations under Test

DR = Depends on Results of Current Studies

National Institute of Allergy and Infectious Diseases

STATUS OF PROGRESS IN DEVELOPMENT OF SOME NEW VACCINES

******

BACTERIAL VACCINES

Cholera
Need to mimic natural infection. Oral immunization necessary.

1. Purified cholera toxid – no protection.

2. Inactivated whole cell: Transient protection

3. Inactivated

    (a) Whole vibrio plus purified B subunit of toxin molecule (Svennerholm and Holmgren). Safe and antigenic in volunteers. Ready for field trial after proof of efficacy in volunteers.

    (b) Procholeragenoid (Pierce and Germanier) stable, high molecular weight aggregate produced by heating cholera toxin to 65°C.

        Safe and protective in dogs.

        Volunteer studies of procholeragenoid combined with inactivated whole vibrios are being planned.

4. Attenuated

    (a) Texas Star SR (Honda and Finkelstein)

        Attenuated mutant of an El Tor Ogawa strain obtained by nitrosoquanidine mutagenesis. Identity of genetic lesion not known.

        Stable clone that produces ample amounts of B subunit, the antigenic, binding portion responsible for immunogenicity but produces only small amounts of A subunit, the active portion of the toxin molecule that activates adenylate cyclase.

        Induced antitoxin or vibriocidal antibodies in 93% of 68 volunteers. Protected against challenge with virulent El Tor Ogawa and Inaba.

        But caused mild diarrhea in 24% of vaccines.

    (b) Genetic engineering being used to produce a better A minus, B plus vaccine candidate strain. Genes that produce the toxic A subunit in the toxin molecule have been replaced with a plasmid containing a modified or inactive gene; genes for making five proteins of B subunit retained.

(c) An A minus, B minus strain is to be tested in the spring on 1983.

Entertoxigenic E. Coli
Two toxins; heat stable (ST) and heat labile (LT); some strains have both; some only one.

ST   Sta and Stb; neither antigenic without adjuvant

LT   Antigenic; anti-toxin immunity not principal protective mechanism; gene that codes for this toxin has been cloned.

Sta   -LT Cross linked toxin vaccine protects rats against ST and LT-producing E. coli

Colonization factors (pili or fimbriae)

CFAI and CPAII – 25% of strains; no identified pili – 75% of strains.

Complete amino acid sequence of the CFAI fimbrial protein (as well as that of the porcine organism, K88) has been elucidated. Computerized algorithms have been used to predict the potential antigenic determinants, envisaging the design of synthetic vaccines.

Gonococcal

Two types of immunogens are under study:

Pili (now renamed fimbriae) antigen to induce local antibody to block attachment of gonococci.

Principal Outer Membrane Protein (now renamed Protein I) antigen to induce protective serum antibody and prevent dissemination of gonococci.

Results obtained to date (Buchanan) are as follows:

Fimbrial Antigen:

Shown to be safe in dosages of 220 mcg: induced good antibody titers (ELISA) in volunteers (62 total) mean antibody levels of 20 mcg/ml. Antibody persistence was prolonged when aluminum adjuvants used.

After cleavage by cyanogen bromide, largest fragment (101 amino acids long) – called CNBrI. Used as an antigen to elicit higher antibody levels. Proved to be safe in dosages up to 600 mcg in volunteers (total of 24). Mean antibody level of 1.87 mcg/ml (ELISA).

The antibody raised to CNBrI antigens showed attachment – inhibiting and opsonic activity; activity was maximal against fimbriated gonococci of same serotype. Antibody to fimbrial antigens barely detectable in local secretions (unlikely to have functional activity here). There were low levels of cross reactivity to heterologous fimbriae. Systemic immunization with this antigen is not likely to prevent gonorrheal infection at mucosal sites.

Note: Similar results have reported by the U.S. Army (WRAIR) for the Army-developed pili candidate vaccine, following urethral challenge with heterologous and homologous strains of immunized volunteers.

Protein I

Purified protein I candidate vaccine contains antigens (epitopes) that are recognized by monoclonal antibodies with bactericidal activity for the gonococcus.

It can be safely given to volunteers in dosages of 100 mcg/serotype, and is immunogenic. The predominant antibodies induced recognize the trimeric form of each serotype of the Protein I molecule.

Immunization produces enhanced bactericidal activity against gonococci.

Eight lots of Protein I candidate vaccine prepared by Buchanan and used to immunize the total of 82 volunteers.

Lot 12, a trivalent preparation of serotypes 1, 5 and 9

Lot 14, a pentavalent preparation of serotypes 1, 5, 7, 8 and 9.

Estimates are that pentavalent vaccine, if it protects against these serotypes, will protect recipients against approximately 95% of U.S. strains of gonococci causing pelvic inflammatory disease.

Each of these candidate vaccines contains 100 mcg of each serotype.

Serum antibody responses (ELISA) showed good responses; mean levels for each serotype ranged from 0.24 to 0.75 mcg/ml ten weeks post immunization.

Data from monoclonal antibody studies strongly indicate that serotype-specific antibodies are bactericidal.

Hemophilus influenzae

Purified capsular polysaccharide, polyribose ribosyl phosphate; is a T independent antigen; need to make T dependent.

Conjugate vaccines under study; to elicit T-cell dependent response and, thus, immunologic memory.

1.   Office of Biologics

        Derivatize polysaccharide with adipic acid dihydrazide.

        Bind to protein with cayanogen bromide.

                Proteins used: tetanus toxoid; hemocyanin

                Also PRP-tetanus conjugate plus DTP

        Best results in rhesus monkeys with PRP-tetanus toxid conjugate

Even better if add pneumococcal 6A-tetanus toxid conjugate.

2.   Lederle

PRP plus whole pertussis cell (discontinued)

PRP plus DTP – under study; promising

3.   Connaught

Derivatized diphtheria toxoid with adipic acid dihydrazide and linked to PRP via cayanogen bromide.
      Induces antibody response in rabbits

4.   University of Rochester

PRP + CMR-197; prepared by conjugating via amination oligosaccharides obtained from PRP with cross reactive mutant (CMR-197) of <u>Corynebacterium</u> <u>diptheriae</u>. This mutant produces a non-toxic protein immunologically similar to diphtheria toxin. Induced good antibody response in animals; human studies beginning.

5.   Several Investigators are studying outer membrane proteins

(a). 5 or 6 major ones

antibodies to two in convalescent sera; also to minor proteins 100,000 and 39,000 dalton proteins seem most important.

(b). P2 protective in infant rat model

(c). 39,000 dalton protein

antigenic in rats and humans

monoclonal AB protected against homologous challenge in infant rat.

(d). Possible approach: couple with PRP as vaccine

6. Two trials have shown polysaccharide alone to be effective in prevention of meningitis in children over 18 months of age. Immunization of children at this age could prevent up to 50% of <u>H</u>. <u>influenzae</u> disease.

<u>Leprosy</u>:

Two glycolipid antigens specific to <u>Mycobacterium</u> <u>leprae</u> have been characterized as triglycosyl phenolic phthicerol diesters with trisaccharide chains specific to <u>M</u>. <u>leprae</u>. Glycolipid I, found in abundance in the bacillus and in infected tissue, reacts specifically with sera from leprosy patients. Its use as a skin test antigen should facilitate epidemiological studies, including the identification of susceptible. It is likely to be an essential component of any vaccine.

Pertussis (improved)

There is a need for a less reactogenic vaccine that is as effective as the present whole cell one.

The Japanese (Nahase and Doi) reported the preparation of a partially purified acellular vaccine. Sato and investigators of the U.S. Office of Biologics have studied the two major subunits considered to be protective antigens. Both are hemagglutinins.

1. Leucocytosis Promoting Factor Hemagglutinin (LPF-HA) is also called Leucocytosis Promoting Toxin (LPT) or simply "Pertussis Toxin" because of its many effects:

(a) Lymphocytosis

(b) Stimulates insulin secretion (islet cell activation)

(c) Sensitizes to histamine

(d) Mitogen

(e) Adjuvant (IgE specific)

(f) Activates cyclic AMP

(g) Elevates brain cyclic GMP

LPF-HA appears as spherical structures 6nm in diameter by electron microscopy.

Sato and associates have recently reported the separation of LPF-HA into five subunits with molecular weights of 25,000, 21,000, 20,000, 12,000, and 10,000. OB/NCDB investigators have identified four subunits.

1. Filamentous hemagglutinin (FHA) appears as fine filaments about 2 nm in diameter and 40-100 nm in length on electron microscopy. Its hemagglutinating activity is 5-7 times greater than LPF, but it lacks the other biologic activities of LPF.

In the intracerebral mouse protection model, the current measure of potency, LPF-HA protects while FHA does not. Both protect against an aerosol challenge. When either antigen is used to immunize the mother, the newborn are protected, although when used for direct passive protection, anti-LPF protects and anti-FHA does not.

An acellular vaccine has been in used in Japan since 1981. LPF-HA and FHA are the major components, but account for only 50% of the total protein in the preparation. One goal is to purify and concentrate the two "essential" antigens and develop precise assays of their quantitation. Another is to further characterize the subunits of LPF-HA and to confirm the recent observations of Sato and colleagues that the protein responsible for most of the toxic manifestations can be separated for the protective antigen.

Shigella

Plasmid genes coding for protective antigen of S. sonnei have been inserted into S. typhi ty21a (Formal).

Mutant stable; protects mice against challenge with either Salmonella typhi or

S. sonnei

May be possible to construct and "all purpose" oral, attenuated typhoid-dysentery vaccine consisting of "protective" antigens of S. sonnei, S. flexnerii 2 and 3, and S. dysenteriae 1, each in a K12 E. coli host and combined to give a multivalent preparation.

Streptococcal, Group B

Vaccines are under development (Kasper and Swenson) for the prevention of neonatal infections caused by four types of Group B streptococci, Ia, Ib, II, and III. Two distinct syndromes have been recognized: early onset disease (primarily pneumonia and bacteremia) and late onset disease (primarily meningitis).

The primary objective is to immunize pregnant women at risk of delivering infected infants to provide high titer maternal antibody trans-placentally to the neonate. A second approach would be to immunize human volunteers to obtain hyperimmune globulin for passive immunization after delivery.

Structural analyses have been completed on all four GBS type-specific polysaccharides. All contain galactose, glucose, glucosamine and sialic acid, but in different molar ratios. Siatlic acid occurs as a terminal sugar on a side chain; it exerts important conformational control in antibody elicited in response to the antigen.

Phase I studies have been conducted with types Ia, II and III polysaccharides. Over 85% of volunteers with pre-existing antibody levels greater than 2 mcg/ml (RABA and ELISA) respond to immunization with significant boost in antibody levels. Individuals with less than 2 mcg/ml pre-existing antibody levels have lesser post-immunization responses.

GBS Type Ibc protein antigen is under study as a possible adjunct to polysaccharide candidate vaccines of GBS types III, II, and Ia.

GBS polysaccharide type III is nearing completion of development as a candidate vaccine; this type accounts for 95% of neonatal infection.

Antibody to these polysaccharide vaccines correlates well with bactericidal assays as measured by opsono-phagocytic assays.

Specific and quantitative opsonic activity of immune sera showed good correlation between opsonic activity and assay of antigen concentration as measured by ELISA. Immune sera contained only IgG class.

ELISA assays were developed for GBS types Ia, II, and III antigens. All showed excellent linear responses; the O.D. values correlated with nanograms of antibody as bound by quantitative precipitin tests.

Examples of serum antibody responses following immunization with GBS candidate vaccines:

-   60 volunteers immunized with GBS type III antigen; 6 wk. antibody mean titer of 40 mcg/ml (ELISA) were elicited following immunization with 50 mcg antigen.

-   80 volunteers immunized with GBS type II antigen; 6 wk. antibody mean titer of 29 mcg/ml were (ELISA) elicited following immunization with 50 mcg GBS type II antigen.

-   80 volunteers immunized with GBS type Ia antigen; 6 wk. Antibody mean titer of 16 mcg/ml were elicited following immunization with 50 mcg of GBS type Ia antigen. This antigen is not as immunogenic as types II and III GBS antigens. Methods for improvement in immunogenic potency of this antigen are under investigation.

Combined antigen preparations, containing 50 mcg of each GBS antigen preparation, are under investigation as multivalent candidates vaccines.

Typhoid

Live, oral, attenuated vaccine; a double mutant. Ty21a.

Developed by Swiss Serum and Vaccine Institute (Germanier), and now licensed in Switzerland.

Strain lacks the enzyme UDP-glactose-4 epimerase, and the activity of two other enzymes - galactokinase and galactose-1-phosphate-uridyl-transferase - is reduced. It is incapable of utilizing galactose after this sugar enters the bacterium. Galactose accumulates and kills cell in 3-5 days.

But organism proliferates in bowel to sufficient numbers to immunize.

A field trial of this live oral vaccine administered in three doses of lyophilized vaccine with bicarbonate to Egyptian children showed a 95% protection rate after three years of observation.

One dose of vaccine in an enteric coated capsule was shown to immunize volunteers equally well.

A field trial of this vaccine is now in progress in Chile using one or two doses of enteric coated capsules.

PARASITIC VACCINES

Malaria

Antibodies specific for Plasmodium falciparum sporozoites are detected in more than 90% of West African adults, whereas most samples from children have low or negative reactions. A sporozoite vaccine would ideally induce immunity in children, eliminating the long period required for the development of anti-sporozoite antibodies under natural conditions. Irradiated sporozoite vaccines have induced active immunity in mice (P. berghei and men (P. falciparum and P. vivax). A vaccine containing the relevant sporozoite antigen, perhaps a few or even a single epitope, now seems feasible since monoclonal antibodies can be utilized to purify and characterize sporozoite antigens.

One such antigen of Plasmodium berghei, Pb44, is a differentiation antigen involved in a unique, presumably essential, function associated with mature sporozoites. Incubation of sporozoites in vitro with antibodies to Pb44 abolished their infectivity; antibodies to P. berghei sporozoite surface antigen block the entry of sporozoites into cultured cells and confer complete passive protection on recipient mice. Similar studies with P. knowlesi and P. cynomolgi have identified surface circumsporozoite (CS) antigens that induce protective monoclonal antibodies, with molecular weights of 42 (P.k.) and 48 (P.c) kilodaltons. The key antigens of P. falciparum have molecular weights of 80, 67, and 58 kilodaltons, with the latter showing the greatest immunoprecipitin reactivity with sera from volunteers.

The challenge now is to apply new technology to the development of a P. falciparum vaccine for man, i.e., purification of the sporozoite antigen, extraction of mRNA coding for this antigen, sequencing and synthesis of the essential peptides, and administration with a safe and effective adjuvant. Experimental vaccines also are being developed using other extracellular stages of the parasite-merozoites and gametes.

VIRAL VACCINES

Cytomegalovirus

There are two candidate strains of CMV being tested for attenuation and use as vaccines.

1. AD-169 (Elek and Stern)

2. Towne-125 (Plotkin); its DNA is 90% homologous with AD-169.

    Being tested in seronegative patients with end-stage renal disease who are candidates for kidney transplantation and are at risk of being infected by CMV from the donor kidney. There is some indication, based on small numbers, that survival is greater in vaccines.

Hepatitis A

Successful cultivation of the virus, particularly direct isolation in cell culture, has provided antigen for an inactivated vaccine. Continuous passage is being used to develop attenuated strains that are now being tested as candidates for a live vaccine.

Human hepatitis A virus was attenuated in virulence for marmosets (Provost et al.; Merck) by passage in FRhK6 and human diploid lung fibroblast cell culture. Some variants were over attenuated. Those marmosets which responded to attenuated virus were immune to challenge with virulent virus. Antibody stimulated by the vaccine equated with protection.

The HM-175 strain of HAV, recovered from the stool of a patient with type A hepatitis in Melbourne, Australia, was isolated directly in primary African green monkey kidney, a cell substrate suitable for vaccine development (Purcell et al.; NIAID). Tissue culture-passaged virus was fully infectious for chimpanzees but did not produce biochemical evidence of hepatitis. Similarly, hepatitis A viral antigen could not be detected in liver biopsies, and little or no viral antigen could be detected in acute phase stool samples. In addition, there is preliminary evidence that the tissue culture-attenuated HAV has very limited potential for horizontal transmission, at least in chimpanzees.

It is quite likely that HAV with a proper degree of attenuation for man can be selected from the various tissue culture-passaged strains currently available.

<u>Hepatitis B</u>

Current vaccines consist of inactivated highly purified 22-nm particles of surface antigen (HBsAg) of hepatitis B virus (HBV). They are safe and effective, but costly to produce. The genetic engineering of DNA recombinant technology and other molecular manipulations are being used in the search for equally effective second and third generation vaccines. This has required purification and characterization of the subunits of HBsAg.

Two major subunits: one non-glycosylated, one glycosylated.

> Molecular weights of 25,000 and 30,000. It is the large subunit that contains carbohydrate; otherwise, two subunits may be same, since they have similar amino acid sequence.

> Subunits purified by preparative polyacrylamide gel electrophoresis shown to be immunogenic in mice and guinea pigs.

> Pool of P25-GP30, 4 doses of 50 micrograms each, induced anti-HBs and protection in chimpanzees.

> Denaturing effect of SDS and mercaptoethanol circumvented by solubilizing 22-nm particles with Triton x-100.

> Dimers of P25-GP30 purified by lectin affinity chromatography; upon removal of detergent by ultra filtration in sucrose gradients, aggregates - micelles - free of lipoprotein formed. These shown to be immunogenic, particularly when alum-adsorbed (Zuckermann).

Such preparations still very expensive. Alternate approaches:

HBsAg from hepatoma cell lines. There are at least two such lines - Alexander and Wistar B3. But both of these lines would be classified as "malignant" and material derived from them would have the potential of transforming normal cells.

Cloning of HBV DNA in prokaryotic cells (<u>E. coli</u> and <u>B. subtilis</u>). The antigen is not released in particulate form, and this approach has not been useful.

Cloning of HBV DNA in eukaryotic cells to produce HBsAg (mouse LM, Hela and African green monkey cells). The latter have the advantage of being a suitable vaccine substrate. In this instance (Moriarty and Gerin) inserted less than the whole genome - 1450 base pairs - in AGMK cells using a defective SV40 vector. The 22 nm particles excreted in the culture medium were antigenic in small animals and chimpanzees. The one chimp available for challenge was protected.

Investigators at Merck (Valenzuela) inserted even a smaller piece of the genome - 830 base pairs - into yeast. Since the particles are not released, the yeast must be lysed. This yields 17 nm, non-glycosylated particles. These also have been shown to be antigenic in small animals and chimps.

<u>Synthetic Peptide Vaccine</u>

Work being done by at least four groups: (Dressman and Hollinger; Lerner et al.; Hopp and Prince; Veyas).

The search for appropriate polypeptides has been assisted by recombinant DNA technology that has supplied the entire nucleotide sequence (and therefore the entire amino acid sequence of the HBsAg gene and by computer programs that have identified the most hydrophilic (and therefore external) portions of the HBsAg molecule. Such hydrophilic regions have also proven to be the most variable in amino acid sequence, suggesting that these regions contain the antigenic domains that define subtype specificity. Other regions appear to contain antigenic domains that are mutually exclusive but that are identified as the group-reactive a specificity. Thus, multiple a domains appear to exist, and it is not clear at present which of these elicit antibody that protects against type B hepatitis.

As an example, cloning of HBV DNA genome made it possible for investigators at Baylor to establish the amino acid sequence of P25.

Peptides were synthesized to reproduce this sequence.

Linear peptides may be poor immunogens. As learned with synthetic antigen for foot and mouth disease virus, antigenic determinants of proteins are confirmational rather than linear.

Peptides cyclized by introduction of disulfide bond between cysteine residues at amino acid positions 124 and 137 (Hollinger).

Two cyclic peptides created, and peptide 1 with mw of 2219, and 5 fewer amino acid residues than peptide 2, selected for study.

Peptides linked by carbodiimide reaction through the amino terminal lysine group to tetanus toxoid, a carrier protein more suitable than Freund's adjuvant.

Major response in mice was to anti a group specificity. Thus the group a epitope is associated with peptide 1.

Immunization and challenge of chimpanzees are planned. However, a problem is the unpredictable immunogenicity of synthetic polypeptides; synthetic polypeptides of foot-and-mouth disease virus appear to be highly immunogenic, whereas those of HBV appear to be less so in preliminary experiments in chimpanzees. It is likely that new knowledge about adjuvants suitable for use with polypeptides must be acquired before widespread use of synthetic polypeptides for vaccine development will become a reality. Should the synthetic antigen induce protective antibodies, it has been estimated that the source material for the vaccine would cost seven cents a dose.

Influenza

Prior to the initiative for the Accelerated Development of New Vaccines, NIAID had made a major commitment to influenza research, including the development of improved vaccines. Two current approaches to new influenza vaccines are summarized here for the sake of completeness.

Live, Attenuated Vaccines

The segmented genome of influenza A has facilitated the segregation and characterization of individual genes. Two genes code for the antigenic surface glycoproteins, the hemagglutinin (HA) and neuraminidase (NA); six genes code for nonsurface proteins. The most promising current approach involves the use of a donor virus [A/Ann/Arbor/6/60 (H2N2)] adapted to growth at a temperature (cold adapted; ca) that does not support efficient replication of wild virus. Reassortant viruses have been produced (Maasab et al.) by mating the ca donor with new influenza A viruses. Attenuation and stability of reassortants have been achieved when all nonsurface viral protein genes have been received from the ca donor and the HA and NA genes from the wild-type variant. Vaccines derived by genetic reassortment of contemporary wild-type A influenza viruses and the A/Ann Arbor cold-adapted master strain have been extensively tested. In the last year, six vaccine clones have been prepared as vaccine pools and are currently being tested for safety, antigenicity, reactogenicity and efficacy. Influenza B influenza vaccines attenuated in this way are presently in an early stage of development.

Other approaches to attenuation include the use of reassortants produced by mating restricted avian virus with a virulent human influenza A virus (Murphy), and by the construction of stable deletion mutations. This latter type of genetic engineering cannot be performed with RNA, so the RNA viral genomes must first be transmitted into DNA and then the manipulated DNA with the desired deletion transcribed into an RNA form that can be transferred back into an infectious virus (Lai and Chanock).

Synthetic Vaccines

Four antigenic sites on the three-dimensional structure of the hemagglutinin of influenza A viruses have been identified (Wiley, Wilson, and Skekel). Now that amino acid sequences of the hemagglutinin of a new variant can be determined, peptides can be synthesized for use as vaccine antigens. As with other synthetic polypeptides, this will require adjuvants suitable for human use.

Poliomyelitis

Now that an improved IPV is available, greater attention is being focused on cases associated with the administration of OPV. The occurrence of such cases, although few in number, is a reason to seek totally avirulent, yet immunogenic, strains of the three polio virus types. This may now be possible, although trials to establish absolute safety will be extremely difficult.

Investigators at MIT (Racaniello and Baltimore) used reverse transcriptase to make complementary DNA using poliovirus RNA as a model. A plasmid containing this complementary DNA was found to infect human (Hela) and monkey (CY-1) cells and bring about the development of intact poliovirus particles.

This was the first demonstration that cloned DNA derived from the RNA genome of a lytic animal virus can be infectious. Since a cDNA copy of an RNA virus can initiate the infectious process, the investigators propose that it should be possible to specifically mutagenize the cloned DNA and generate mutants with defects in any part of the genome, including mutants incapable of virulence or of reversion to virulence.

Provided such mutants are still immunogenic, vaccines made with them would retain all of the advantages of OPV over IPV, including less cost.

Rabies

Two cell culture grown inactivated rabies virus vaccines have recently been licensed in the U.S. Because of their greater antigenicity, fewer doses are required for post-exposure prophylaxis, and small intradermal doses can be used for pre-exposure prophylaxis.

A cheaper vaccine may be developed using rabies virus glycoprotein.

    a.   Virus codes for glycoprotein containing 524 amino acids.

    b.   Gene that codes for this glycoprotein has been clones, but signal that allows expression has not been identified.

    c.   Monoclonal antibodies have detected antigenic variations and demonstrated that glycoprotein possesses four antigenic sites on each molecule. These sites differ in position and reactivity among strains.

Rotavirus

There are at least four serotypes.

Have now been grown in cell culture; selected strains to be tested for attenuation.

Virus has segmented genome.

Calf derived rotavirus protects calves against challenge with human rotavirus.

One approach: immunize children against human rotavirus disease using calf virus if latter induces clinical immunity without inducing illness.

Also, through co-cultivation, replace human gene segments with bovine or simian gene segments to produce either viruses that are easier to cultivate or that can be used as an attenuated oral vaccine.

Another approach: clone genes that specify protective antigens in K12 E. coli; may immunize without risk of spread.

Varicella

Oka strain developed by Takahashi; vaccines produced by RIT (Belgium) and Merck (U.S.)

Serologic tests developed that permit assessment of immunogenicity and detection of reinfection.

Viral markers identified that distinguish vaccine strain from wild strain.

Clinical trials now underway in leukemic children at high risk of severe disease and in normal children.

Preliminary results indicate protection against household exposure. In one study, 40% of leukemic children lost antibody after 6 to 12 months, but it is suggested that a skin test is all that is needed to boost the level.

No cases of herpes zoster have been seen in the U.S. as yet (approximately 3 years).

William S. Jordan, Jr., M.D./NIAID/NIH   November 1982

Appendix B

Task Force on Safer Childhood Vaccines: Final Report and Recommendations

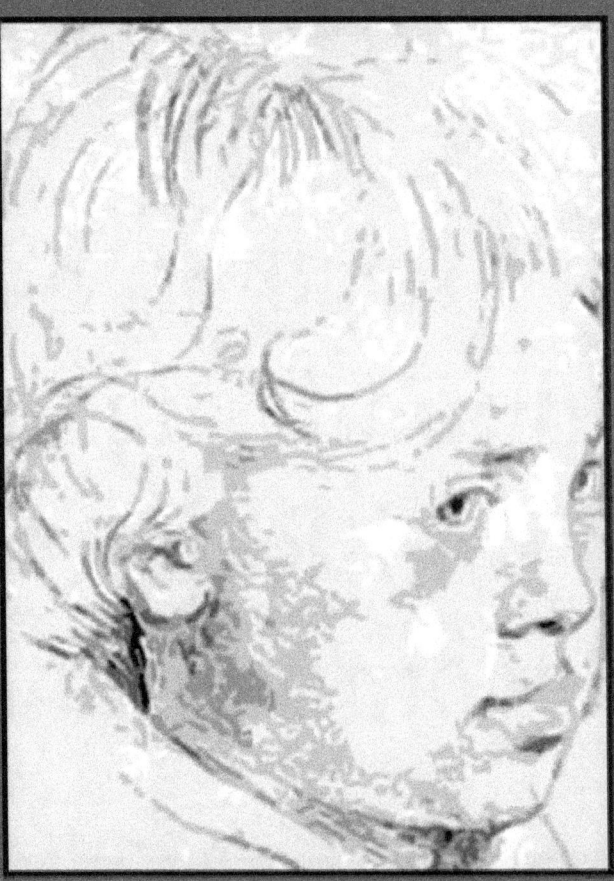

Task Force on Safer Childhood Vaccines

Final Report and Recommendations

National Institute of Allergy and Infectious Diseases

National Institutes of Health

Executive Summary

As we prepare to enter the 21st century, the promise of vaccines has never been greater. If this promise is to be fully realized, vaccines must not only be effective in the prevention of diseases—they must also be safe. Recent reviews by the Institute of Medicine have identified many gaps and limitations, however, in current knowledge of vaccine safety (Howson et al., 1991; Stratton et al., 1994). The Task Force on Safer Childhood Vaccines (TFSCV or the Task Force) was established by the Secretary of Health and Human Services at the direction of Congress, with the sole purpose of examining vaccine safety and making recommendations to the Secretary to ensure development of safer childhood vaccines and improve licensing, manufacturing, processing, testing, labeling, warning, use instructions, distribution, storage, administration, field surveillance, adverse reaction reporting, recall of reactogenic lots or batches, and research on vaccines. This report summarizes the findings and recommendations of the Task Force.

The Task Force comprised representatives from several Public Health Service agencies: National Institutes of Health; Food and Drug Administration; Centers for Disease Control and Prevention; National Vaccine Injury Compensation Program; Office of the General Counsel, Department of Health and Human Services; and National Vaccine Program Office. As with any committee activity, a number of individuals have participated in discussions that resulted in the creation of this report (see acknowledgements).

There are many reasons why examining the safety of childhood vaccines is a critical task and, therefore, mandated by law, but several reasons were emphasized by the Task Force.

The first is a paradox inherent in the very success of vaccines and immunization programs. Concerns about vaccine safety become increasingly prominent when effective use of vaccines in a population reduces the incidence of the target diseases. Yet, since few diseases are eradicable, only immunization programs that maintain public confidence in vaccines can prevent tragic recurrence of disease, as demonstrated by outbreaks of pertussis in several countries during the 1980s. The second reason is that even under conditions of epidemic or endemic transmission, any given individual in the population may escape infection and disease. Vaccination is still essential, however, to protect the population from the spread of disease. Finally, vaccines, unlike therapeutic interventions, are given to healthy individuals. Consequently, the risks associated with any vaccine must be minimal, and vaccines must be extraordinarily safe.

Since 1990, the Public Health Service has created much of the infrastructure necessary to reduce gaps in current knowledge about the safety of vaccines, as identified by the Institute of Medicine, but the process is still incomplete. Safety issues regarding already licensed vaccines have become of paramount importance to the success and stability of immunization programs, vaccine companies, and public support for these activities. At the same time, advances in basic biomedical research and the accelerating pace of the revolution in biotechnology will make a large array of new vaccines possible. The continued improvement and assurance of vaccine safety are as much a research priority as the development of vaccines for the diseases that continue to affect humankind.

Although a number of vaccine-preventable diseases, such as poliomyelitis, may be controlled and even eliminated globally, others, such as pertussis, tetanus, or diphtheria, are not candidates for eradication. Therefore, vaccination against these diseases must be continued to protect each new cohort of infants, both in the United States and worldwide. The perception of risks due to reports of adverse events will also continue indefinitely. Therefore, systems required to ensure vaccine safety must be maintained. Given new technologies for the development, production, manufacture, regulation, and administration of vaccines, the vaccine safety network for the United States must be enhanced to provide appropriate evaluation of new candidates. To ensure continued public acceptance of vaccines, close monitoring of potential adverse events and adverse reactions, adequate scientific evaluation of hypothesized associations, and appropriate responses to newly identified risks of vaccines, including research and targeted development of new technologies and vaccines, are critical.

The recommendations of the Task Force arise from broad review and evaluation spanning the activities and responsible agencies required to ensure vaccine safety. These recommendations, developed to address gaps and ensure the continuing safety of vaccines, are summarized below:

1. **Assess and address national concerns about the risks and benefits of vaccines in order to enhance the education of the public, families, and health care professionals.**

   As development of vaccines to fight diseases progresses, the assessment of risks and benefits of this intervention has changed, as few health care providers or parents may have seen a case of a vaccine-preventable disease. We need to know more about how to communicate what is known and what is not known about true and perceived risk (Evans et al., 1997). Furthermore, it is extraordinarily difficult to obtain spontaneous report-

ing of adverse events after immunization without a presumption of potential causality. Education must appropriately target the public, families, and health care professionals in order to assure optimal prevention with vaccines. The Task Force made the following recommendations:

A) Identify the public's and health care professionals' concerns, attitudes, and knowledge about immunization and the benefits and risks of vaccination.

B) Develop appropriate interventions to enhance knowledge of vaccines and their benefits and risks, reporting of adverse events, and immunization programs and their public health impact.

2. **Strengthen the national capability to conduct research and development needed to promote the licensure of safer vaccines.**

   Vaccine research and development are driven both by scientific advances and by the need to control and prevent disease. Finally, when an effective and safe vaccine is available, the perception or association of true adverse events must be high indeed to support the costly development (approximately $200 million) of a new vaccine. Technological barriers, however, may confound the process. For example, recombinant hepatitis B vaccines that did not confer the potential risk of transmission of other infections were developed less than a decade after the licensure of serum-derived vaccine. However, the development of safer acellular pertussis vaccines, a complex task that has required new technologies not available 10 years ago, has been a much slower process. To promote the development of safer vaccines, the Task Force made the following recommendations:

A) Where an association is demonstrated between an adverse event and vaccination, ensure that these findings will lead to relevant research and vaccine improvements.

i)   Initiate appropriate regulatory review and action.

ii) Conduct studies of the biologic basis for vaccine adverse events.

iii) Develop, where feasible, epidemiologic and biologic markers or tests that would be useful to evaluate, predict, or determine risk groups for adverse events.

iv) Use, wherever possible, vaccines that have been modified or improved to avoid adverse events.

B) Consider new assays to detect potential mediators of adverse events, laboratory correlates of vaccine safety and efficacy, and evaluation of the safety of novel methods to enhance immunogenicity and vaccine delivery technologies and improve the thermostability of vaccines.

C) Foster the active participation of industry and increase public-private collaboration in development of safer vaccines of public health priority.

D) Encourage research and development leading to production of "limited-use vaccines" of potential public health importance through public support of research and development and strengthened interaction with industry. The development of vaccines for limited populations poses special challenges to the development of a safety profile.

3. **Strengthen the national capability to conduct surveillance of vaccine-preventable diseases and to evaluate potential adverse events and vaccine efficacy.**

Safe use of a vaccine to control disease requires continuous monitoring for the disease as well as for known and potential adverse events following vaccine administration. This type of monitoring makes it possible to answer the following vital public health questions: Is the disease effectively controlled or has something (the vaccine, the human host, or the environment) changed? Has the risk/benefit evaluation altered? Does the use or composition of the vaccine need to be modified in response to different conditions? Are changes in national immunization policies regarding mandated childhood vaccines warranted?

Historically, for both methodological and logistical reasons, effective surveillance for adverse events after licensure has been difficult to maintain. Since 1990, the Public Health Service has initiated major improvements in its ability to conduct both passive and active surveillance for adverse events. Continued support for these projects is critical for adequate monitoring of the present and future safety of vaccines in the United States. To reduce gaps in vaccine surveillance efforts, the Task Force made the following recommendations:

A) Integrate government postlicensure surveillance activities to enhance evaluation of available information, identify gaps, and reduce duplication of effort, with emphasis on the following areas:

i)   Develop new methods and approaches for postlicensure evaluation of the safety and efficacy of vaccines and vaccine uses and ensure that appropriate studies are conducted.

a) Prospectively evaluate vaccine safety and efficacy in large populations, including adults, to help identify the association of vaccination with serious but uncommon adverse events. Develop methodology for investigating causality of rare events in vaccine recipients, especially in highly immunized populations.

b) Develop novel methods and approaches for the detection and evaluation of adverse events associated with new vaccines or new uses of vaccines to supplement systems such as Vaccine Adverse Events Reporting System. Identify and incorporate into the current system other U.S. and international agencies or survey systems that collect information relevant to the evaluation of adverse events.

ii) Identify differences in rates of adverse events associated with the simultaneous or combined administration of vaccines.

B) Ensure the adequacy of clinical data to support new recommendations for vaccine use, and when appropriate, conduct studies to address safety considerations.

C) Improve the coordination and sharing of data concerning standards, adverse event reports, and analyses with other national control and epidemiologic authorities, including the World Health Organization (regulatory harmonization). The United States should participate in the development of an international network to monitor vaccine safety, taking advantage of the differences and similarities in the vaccines used and in national health care structures.

D) Encourage industry participation in the collection and analysis of data to address

both prelicensure and postlicensure vaccine safety.

i) Review industry's role and responsibilities in collection, receipt, followup, and analysis of received adverse event reports.

ii) In consultation with vaccine manufacturers, develop procedures to optimize collection of complete data and analysis of reports by product category, product-specific data by company, and product interaction with other co-administered vaccines.

4. **The Task Force recommends that the Interagency Vaccine Group (IAVG), composed of representatives from agencies involved in vaccine research, development, evaluation, regulation, and immunization, be charged with the ongoing responsibility of ensuring that appropriate vaccine safety activities are carried out. The IAVG would be expected to seek routine technical consultation from an expert external advisory body.**

The Task Force identified the roles and responsibilities of Federal agencies, vaccine companies, health care providers, the research community, and parents in ensuring that vaccines are safe. Experience over the past century teaches that the activities of each group are linked to the activities of the other groups, making both coordination and communication essential to vaccine safety. Furthermore, the group charged with this responsibility must be able to focus on safety. In accordance with the original mandate to integrate the Nation's vaccine efforts, the National Vaccine Program Office could serve as the secretariat for this group and the entity to ensure action toward emergent vaccine safety needs. The

Task Force defined the IAVG's role as follows:

A) The IAVG would monitor the vaccine safety activities of the various agencies and work to improve interagency communication. It would also facilitate and monitor progress on the investigation and evaluation of reports of serious or frequent adverse events.

   i)   Evaluate data relevant to vaccine safety, which may currently be scattered among various agencies and manufacturers.

   ii)   Ensure periodic reviews of the safety of licensed vaccines and their recommended immunization schedules. If appropriate, propose studies to address areas where additional data may be informative or supportive, such as in special target groups or programs.

   iii)   Ensure effective communication among existing advisory committees that focus on vaccines and immunization, including specifically the Advisory Commission on Childhood Vaccines, the Advisory Committee on Immunization Practices, the National Vaccine Advisory Committee, and the Vaccines and Related Biological Products Advisory Committee.

B) The IAVG would be expected to seek routine technical consultation from an expert external advisory body.

The Task Force is committed to the concept that the public health is best served by the continued pursuit of safer and more effective vaccines and by the safe use of existing vaccines through improvements in the immunization schedule and delivery of vaccines. The recommendations presented in this report are congruent with the Nation's immunization and vaccine goals presented in the U.S. National Vaccine Plan in 1994.

Appendix C

Status of Vaccine Research and Development 2002

Status of Vaccine Research and Development 2002

Target Agent	Vaccine	Basic R&D	Preclinical	Phase I	Phase II	Phase III
Ancyclostoma duodenale	Recombinant protein	+	+			
Bacillus anthracis	Recombinant subunit	+	+			
Bordetella pertussis	B. pertussis surface protein expressed by vector (e.g., *Salmonella* and *Vibrio cholerae*)	+	+			
	Purified PT vaccine-acellular	+	+	+	+	+
	Recombinant PT vaccine-acellular	+	+	+	+	
	Purified PT and FHA-acellular	+	+	+	+	+
	Purified PT, FHA, pertactin, and agglutinogens 2 & 3-acellular	+	+	+	+	+
	Purified PT, FHA, pertactin-acellular	+	+	+	+	+
	Recombinant PT, FHA, pertactin-acellular	+	+	+	+	+
	PT peptides-CRM conjugates	+	+			
	Purified adenylate cyclase	+	+			
	DTP-Hib conjugate	+	+	+	+	+
	DTP-Hib conjugate-HBV	+	+	+	+	+
	DTP-IPV	+	+	+	+	
	DTP-Hib conjugate-IPV-HBV	+	+	+	+	
	DTaP-Hib conjugate-HBV	+	+	+	+	
	DTaP-IPV-monovalent aP	+	+	+	+	
	DTaP-Hib conjugate-IPV-HBV-bivalent and trivalent aP	+	+	+	+	
	DTaP-Hib	+	+	+	+	+
	DTaP-Hib conjugate-IPV	+	+	+	+	
Blastomyces dermatitidis	Purified yeast cell proteins (e.g., WI-1)	+	+			
	Recombinant proteins (e.g., WI-1)	+				
	WI-1 DWA	+	+			
	Live-attenuated strain	+	+			
Borrelia burgdorferi	Recombinant Osp A	+	+	+	+	+
	Osp A-based DNA vaccine	+	+			
	BCG-expressed Osp A	+	+			
	Purified Osp B, Osp C	+	+	+		
	Osp C (14 valent)	+	+	+	+	
	DbpA	+				
	DbpB	+				
Brugia malayi	Purified parasite antigens (paramyosin, etc.)	+	+			
Calicivirus	Norwalk VLPs in transgenic potato	+	+	+		
	Norwalk VLPs orally delivered	+	+			
Campylobacter jejuni	Inactivated whole cell with mutant E. coli labile toxin (mLT) adjuvant, oral vaccine	+	+	+		
	Whole cell (intact)	+	+	+	+	
Chlamydia pneumoniae	Purified, major outer membrane protein, heat shock protein	+				
	Outer membrane protein-based DWA vaccine	+				

Target Agent	Vaccine	Basic R&D	Preclinical	Phase I	Phase II	Phase III
Clostridium difficile	Formalin-inactivated toxins A and B	+	+	+		
Clostridium tetani	Recombinant toxin	+	+			
	Salmonella vector	+	+	+		
	Microencapsulation	+	+			
	Transcutaneous immunization	+	+			
Candida albicans	Cell surface oligomannosyl epitope	+	+			
Chikungunya virus	Live, attenuated	+	+	+	+	
Coccidioides immitis	Formalin-killed spherules	+	+	+	+	+
	Recombinant protein for Ag2, rAg2 (PRAg2)	+	+			
	Spherule homogenate (27kxg)	+	+			
	C-ASWS (Ag2)	+	+			
	Urease (recombinant and cDNA) (rURE)	+	+			
	Spherule outer wall glycoprotein (SOWgp)	+	+			
Corynebacterium diphtheriae	Recombinant toxin	+	+			
	Salmonella vector	+	+	+		
	Transcutaneous immunization	+	+			
Coxiella burnetti	Formalin inactivated	+	+	+	+	
Cryptococcus neoformans	Partially purified capsular polysaccharide	+	+			
	Glycoconjugate of capsular polysaccharide with tetanus toxoid	+	+	+		
Cytomegalovirus (CMV)	Live, attenuated strains (conventional)	+	+	+	+	
	Live, attenuated strains (engineered)	+	+			
	Glycoprotein subunit vaccine	+	+	+	+	
	Multiprotein subunit vaccine	+				
	Nucleic acid (DNA) vaccines	+	+			
	Canarypox vectored	+	+	+		
Dengue virus	Purified rDNA-expressed viral proteins	+	+			
	Infectious clone	+	+			
	Chimeric virus	+	+			
	Inactivated whole virus particle	+	+	+		
	Vaccinia vector (live)	+	+			
	Vaccinia subunit	+	+			
	Baculovirus subunit	+	+			
	Synthetic peptide	+	+			
	Micelle/ISCOM	+	+			
	Yeast subunit	+	+			
	Recombinant envelope (baculovirus and Drosophila expression systems)	+	+			
	Live, attenuated dengue virus (monovalent)	+	+	+	+	
	Live, attenuated dengue virus (combined quadrivalent)	+	+	+		

Target Agent	Vaccine	Basic R&D	Preclinical	Phase I	Phase II	Phase III
Entamoeba histolytica	Yeast subunit	+	+			
	Recombinant galactose-binding protein	+	+			
	Galactose-binding proteins expressed in *Salmonella*	+	+			
Enterohemorrhagic	Nontoxic mutant toxins	+	+			
Escherichia coli	Intimin	+				
(EHEC) [Shiga	LPS conjugates	+	+			
toxin-producing	Intimin expression in plants	+				
E. coli (STEC)]	Stx-1 beta-subunit *in Vibrio cholerae* vector	+	+			
Enterotoxigenic	Killed cells and beta-subunit of cholera toxin	+	+	+	+	
Escherichia coli	Nontoxigenic ETEC derivative, live, attenuated	+	+	+	+	
ETEC	*Salmonella* and *Shigella* vectored CFAs	+	+			
	Subunit synthetic toxoid (ST) and B subunit of heat-labile toxin (LT)	+	+			
	LTB expressed in potatoes	+	+	+		
	CFA II microencapsulated	+	+			
Epstein-Barr virus	Glycoprotein subunit (gp350)	+	+	+		
(EBV)	Vaccinia recombinant virus expressing gp350	+	+	+		
	Peptide induction of CTL	+	+	+		
Escherichia coli (urinary tract)	Anti-FimH adhesin	+	+			
*Filoviridae (*Ebola)	Recombinant subunit	+	+			
	Replicons	+	+			
Francisella tularensis	Live, attenuated	+	+	+	+	
Group A streptococcus	Glycoconjugate Group A polysaccharide with tetanus toxoid	+	+			
	M protein, multivalent type-specific epitopes	+	+	+		
	M protein conserved epitope expressed in a commensal vector (*S. gordonii)*	+	+			
	M Protein conserved epitope in combination with M serotype epitopes	+	+			
	Cysteine protease	+	+			
	C5a peptidase	+	+			
	Fibronectin-binding protein Sfb1	+	+			
	Streptococcal pyrogenic exotoxins	+	+			
Group B streptococcus	Glycoconjugate vaccines of type Ia, Ib, II, III, and V polysaccharides linked to carrier proteins	+	+	+	+	
Haemophilus ducreyi	Major outer membrane protein	+	+			
	Hemolysin/cytotoxin	+	+			
	Hemoglobin receptor	+	+			
Haemophilus influenzae (nontypeable)	Recombinant protein subunit containing either P1, P2, or P6 proteins to serve as carriers in	+	+			

Target Agent	Vaccine	Basic R&D	Preclinical	Phase I	Phase II	Phase III
Haemophilus influenzae	Subunit lipoprotein D (nonacylated)	+	+	+		
(nontypeable)	Subunit detoxified lipooligosaccharide conjugate to tetanus toxoid	+	+			
	Subunit detoxified lipooligosaccharide conjugated to HMW protein from *H. influenzae* (nontypeable)	+	+			
	OMP HiN47	+	+	+	+	
	Pili (HifE)	+	+			
Haemophilus influenzae	Glycoconjugate of Hib PRP with CRM197	+	+	+	+	+
type b (Hib)	Glycoconjugate of Hib PRP with diphtheria toxoid	+	+	+	+	+
	Glycoconjugate of Hib PRP with tetanus toxoid	+	+	+	+	+
	Hib-IPV-HBV	+	+	+	+	+
	Glycoconjugate of Hib PRP with meningococcal type B outer membrane protein	+	+	+	+	+
	Glyconjugate Hib with meningococcal type A and/or C	+	+	+		
Hantaan virus	Vaccinia vector	+	+	+	+	
	Recombinant subunit	+				
	RNA replicons	+	+			
Helicobacter pylori	Recombinant *H. pylori* urease and cholera toxin-oral vaccine	+	+	+		
	H. pylori antigens and mutant CT or LT	+	+	+		
	Killed whole cells	+	+			
	Salmonella vectored *H. pylori* antigens	+	+			
Hepatitis A virus	Inactivated HAV particles	+	+	+	+	+
(HAV)	Live, attenuated HAV	+	+	+	+	+
	Virosome-formulated inactivated HAV	+	+	+	+	+
	Viral proteins expressed by vectors (baculovirus or vaccinia virus)	+	+			
Hepatitis B virus	HBV core protein expressed by rDNA	+	+			
(HBV)	HBV proteins expressed in yeast cells by rDNA	+	+	+	+	+
	Salmonella vector	+	+	+		
	Variants	+	+			
	Generation of cytotoxic T lymphocytes	+	+	+	+	
	DNA vaccines	+	+			
	rDNA, plants	+	+	+		
Combined HAV/HBV vaccine	Combined inactivated components	+	+	+	+	+
Hepatitis C virus (HCV)	rDNA-expressed surface proteins and epitopes	+	+			
	Generation of cytotoxic T lymphocytes	+	+			
	Nucleocapsid	+	+			
	DNA vaccines	+	+			
Hepatitis D virus	Synthetic peptides	+	+			
(HDV)	Baculovirus	+				
Hepatitis E virus (HEV)	Expressed proteins	+	+	+	+	

Target Agent	Vaccine	Basic R&D	Preclinical	Phase I	Phase II	Phase III
Herpes simplex virus types 1 and 2 (continued)	Heteroconjugate recombinant protein, T cell ligands with HSV-associated peptides	+	+			
	Vaccinia-vectored proteins glycoproteins	+	+			
Histoplasma capsulatum	Purified yeast cell proteins (e.g., His-62)	+	+			
capsulatum	Recombinant proteins (e.g., His 62, H antigen, hsp-70)	+	+			
Human immunodeficiency virus, HIV-1	See Appendix F					
Human immunodeficiency virus, HIV-2	Inactivated HIV-1	+	+			
	Live, attenuated HIV-2	+	+			
	rgp 125 or 130 (purified from virion)	+	+			
	rgp 160 (insect cells)	+	+			
	Highly attenuated, vaccinia HIV-2 gag-pol-env	+	+			
	Vaccinia HIV-2 env	+	+			
	Canarypox HIV-2 gag-pol-env	+	+			
	Salmonella HIV-2 env, gag	+	+			
Human papillomavirus (HPV)	Capsid protein	+	+			
	TA-HPV (live recombinant vaccinia) E6 and E7 (from HPV-16, and HPV-18)	+	+	+	+	
	TA-GN recombinant protein L2 and E7 (from HPV-6)	+	+	+	+	
	MEDI-501 recombinant VLP L1 from HPV-11	+	+	+		
	Quadrivalent recombinant VLP L1 (from HPV-6, HPV-11, HPV-16, and HPV-18)	+	+			
	DNA vaccine	+	+			
	LAMP-E7 (from HPV-16)	+	+			
Influenza virus	Cold-adapted lilve, attenuated	+	+	+	+	+
	Purified viral HA subunit	+	+	+		
	Liposome containing viral HA	+	+	+	+	
	Purified CTL specific peptides	+	+	+		
	Microencapsulated inactivated vaccine	+	+	+		
	Purified, inactivated viral neuraminidase	+	+	+		
	Baculovirus expressed recombinant HA subunit	+	+	+	+	
	Baculovirus expressed nucleoprotein	+	+	+		
	Transfection with nucleic acid (DNA) plasmid expressing HA subunit	+	+			
	Inactivated viral vaccines with novel adjuvants	+	+	+	+	
Japanese encephalitis virus	Whole, inactivated virus particles	+	+	+	+	+
	Infectious clone	+	+			
	Purified DNA expressed protein	+	+			
	Live attenuated virus	+	+	+	+	
	Vaccinia vector (live)	+	+	+		
	Chimeric virus	+	+	+		

Target Agent	Vaccine	Basic R&D	Preclinical	Phase I	Phase II	Phase III
Leishmania major	Attenuated or killed whole parasites	+	+	+	+	+
	Deletion mutagenized, attenuated parasite	+	+			
Multiple Leishmania spp.	Leishmanial surface antigens (gp63, 46 kD, and lipophosphoglycan)	+	+			
Measles virus	rDNA HA and fusion proteins	+	+			
	ISCOM	+	+			
	Live, attenuated	+	+	+	+	+
	High-titer live (multiple strains)	+	+	+	+	+
	Poxvirus vector (live)	+	+	+		
Moraxella catarrhalis	High molecular weight, outer membrane proteins CD, E, B1, and LBP for use in conjugate vaccines	+	+			
	Detoxified LOS conjugated to either tetanus toxoid or high MW proteins from nontypeable *H. influenzae*	+	+			
Mycobacterium leprae	BCG plus purified M. leprae antigens (35 kD)	+				
	Recombinant antigens in BCG	+	+			
	Live BCG expressing *M. leprae* antigens	+	+			
	BCG plus heat-killed *M. leprae*	+	+	+	+	+
	Heat-killed, purified *M. leprae*	+	+	+	+	+
	Mycobacterium w	+	+	+	+	+
	BCG	+	+	+	+	+
	ICRG	+	+	+	+	+
	Mycobacterium habana	+	+	+		
	Vaccinia virus vector expressing mycobacterial antigen	+	+			
Mycobacterium tuberculosis	BCG plus purified *M. tuberculosis* antigens	+	+			
	T-cell reactive immunogens	+	+			
	Recombinant antigens in BCG	+	+			
	M. vaccae	+	+	+	+	
	Recombinant antigens in *M. vaccae*	+	+			
	M. tuberculosis culture filtrate proteins (CFP)	+	+			
	M. tuberculosis culture filtrate proteins and cytokines	+	+			
	Mycolic acids	+	+			
	BCG with CFP "boost"	+	+			
	Dendritic cells pulsed with for-met peptides	+	+			
	Transfected EL-4 cells	+	+			
	Recombinant *Salmonella* constructs	+	+			
	M. smegmatis expressing *M. tb* antigens	+				
	rBCG expressing cytokines	+	+			
	Auxotrophic mutant BCG	+	+			
	DNA vaccines	+	+			
	Auxotrophic mutant *Mycobacterium tuberculosis*	+	+			
	Live *Mycobacterium microti*	+	+			
Mycoplasma pneumoniae	Recombinant membrane-associated proteins	+	+			
	Purified outer membrane protein	+	+			
	Inactivated (heat-killed) oral vaccine	+	+	+		

Target Agent	Vaccine	Basic R&D	Preclinical	Phase I	Phase II	Phase III
Neisseria gonorrheae	LPS anti-idiotype	+	+			
	Whole cells	+	+			
Neisseria meningitidis (Group A)	Glycoconjugate with tetanus toxoid	+	+			
	Group A LOS	+				
Neisseria meningitidis (Group B)	Native outer membrane vesicle (NOMV)-intranasal route	+	+	+		
	OMP-dLPS liposome	+	+			
	Recombinant PorA outer membrane protein in liposomes	+	+			
	Outer membrane vesicles (OMVs), high MW proteins, and C polysaccharide	+	+	+	+	+
	Hexvalent PorA outer membrane vesicle vaccine	+	+	+	+	
	Outer membrane vesicles (deoxycholate extracted)	+	+	+	+	+
	Recombinant transferrin binding protein (TBP1 and TBP2)	+	+			
	Recombinant low MW (NspA) outer membrane protein	+	+			
	Glycoconjugate modified polysaccharide with recombinant PorB protein	+	+			
	LOS micelle-based vaccine	+				
Neisseria meningitidis (Group C)	Glycoconjugate with tetanus toxoid	+	+	+	+	+
Neisseria meningitides A and C	Glycoconjugate A and C with CRM197	+	+	+	+	
	Glycoconjugate A and C with DT	+	+	+		
Neisseria meningitides A, B, and C	Combination glycoconjugate with recombinant PorB	+	+			
Neisseria meningitides A, B, C, and W-135	Glycoconjugate with DT	+	+	+		
Onchocerca volvulus	Recombinant proteins	+	+			
Paracoccidioides brasiliensis	Purified yeast cell proteins	+	+			
	Recombinant proteins	+	+			
	Synthetic peptide or multipeptide construction (P10, MAP-10)	+	+			
	DNA plasmid with gp43 gene	+	+			
Parainfluenza virus	Cold-adapted PIV3 attenuated virus	+	+	+	+	
	Purified HN and F protein subunit vaccine	+	+			
	Bovine attenuated PIV3 vaccine	+	+	+	+	
Plasmodium falciparum	Circumsporozoite antigen-based peptide or recombinant protein	+	+	+	+	
	Circumsporozoite antigen expressed in various vectors	+	+	+		
	Circumsporozoite antigen-based DNA vaccine	+	+	+		
	Noncircumsporozoite, pre-erythrocytic antigen-based constructs	+	+			
	Merozoite surface protein-1 (MSP-1) based recombinant protein	+	+	+		
	Non-MSP-1 asexual blood stage	+	+			

Target Agent	Vaccine	Basic R&D	Preclinical	Phase I	Phase II	Phase III
Plasmodium falciparum	Multivalent viral vector-based combination vaccines incorporating different stage-specific antigens (e.g., NYVAC Pf7)	+	+	+	+	
	Subunit (RTS, S)	+	+	+	+	
	DNA-based combination vaccines incorporating different stage-specific antigens	+	+			
	Combination vaccines incorporating different stage-specific antigens (e.g., SPf 66)	+	+	+	+	+
Plasmodium vivax	Circumsporozoite antigen-based peptide or recombinant protein	+	+	+		
	Asexual erythrocytic antigens	+	+			
Poliovirus	Reversion-stable attenuated OPV	+				
	Live (nonreverting)	+	+			
	Chimeric virus	+	+			
Pseudomonas aeruginosa	Purified bacterial proteins, including flagellar Ag, LPS-O, porins, several inactivated bacterial toxins, and high MW polysaccharide antigen and glycoconjugate	+	+	+		
	Inactivated whole bacteria-oral preparation	+	+	+		
	Synthetic peptides	+	+	+		
Pseudomonas (Burkholderia) cepacia	Purified bacterial proteins, LPS	+				
Pythium insidiosum	Sonicated hyphal antigens	+	+			
	Culture filtrate antigens	+	+			
	Purified proteins (e.g., 28, 30, 32 kD)	+	+			
Rabies virus	rDNA vaccinia virus recombinant for use in sylvatic rabies (veterinary vaccine)	+	+	+	+	+
	Inactivated mammalian brain	+	+	+	+	+
	Inactivated cell culture	+	+	+	+	+
Respiratory Syncytial virus (RSV)	Live, attenuated *ts* and/or *ca* strains	+	+	+	+	
	Purified F protein subunit vaccine	+	+	+	+	
	G protein expressed vaccine	+	+	+	+	
	rRSVA2 live attenuated strains	+	+	+		
Rickettsia rickettsii	Subunit vaccine containing major surface proteins (155 and 120 kD)	+	+			
Rift Valley Fever virus	Inactivated	+	+	+	+	
	Live, attenuated	+	+	+		
Rotavirus	Attenuated human rotavirus (cold-adapted)	+	+	+		
	Salmonella expressing VP4, VP7, or both	+	+			
	Attenuated bovine/human virus reassortants (WC3)	+	+	+	+	+
	Human nursery strains	+	+	+	+	
	Purified rotavirus proteins rDNA-derived virus-like particles (VLPs)	+	+			

Target Agent	Vaccine	Basic R&D	Preclinical	Phase I	Phase II	Phase III
Rotavirus (continued)	Vaccina virus recombinant expressing					
	VP4, VP7, or both	+	+			
	DNA vaccines	+	+			
Rubella Virus	Live, attenuated	+	+	+	+	+
	Infectious clone	+				
	Synthetic peptide	+				
Salmonella typhi	Vi carbohydrate	+	+	+	+	+
	Vi carbohydrate	+	+	+	+	
	Live, attenuated Ty21a vaccine	+	+	+	+	+
	Live, attenuated auxotrophic mutants	+	+	+	+	
Schistosoma mansoni	Purified larval antigens	+	+			
Schistosoma haematobium, Schistosoma japonicum	Recombinant larval antigens	+	+			
Shigella dysenteriae	Live auxotrophic, attenuated mutants	+	+	+		
	Polysaccharide-protein conjugate	+	+	+	+	
Shigella flexneri	*E. coli* hybrids	+	+	+	+	
	Polysaccharide-protein conjugate	+	+	+	+	
	Live, attenuated oral vaccines	+	+	+	+	
	LPS proteosome (intranasal)	+	+			
Shigella sonnei	Live, attenuated (WRSS1) oral vaccine	+	+			
	LPS proteosome (intranasal)	+	+			
	Polysaccharide-protein conjugate	+	+	+	+	
	Nucleoprotein	+	+			
Staphylococcus aureus	Type 5/Type capsular polysaccharide (CPS) conjugate with *Pseudomonas aeruginosa* recombinant exoprotein A	+	+	+	+	
Staphylococcal entertoxin B	Recombinant toxin	+	+			
Streptococcus pneumoniae	Glycoconjugate vaccine (1,4, 5, 6B, 9N, 14, 18C, 19F, 23F) conjugated to meningococcal B OMP	+	+	+		+
	Glycoconjugate vaccine (1, 3, 4, 5, 6B, 7F, 9V, 14, 18C, 19F, 23F) conjugated to CRM197	+	+			
	Glycoconjugate vaccine (3, 4, 6B, 9V, 14, 18C, 19F, 23F) conjugated to either tetanus toxoid or diphtheria toxoid	+	+	+	+	
	Glycoconjugate vaccine (6B, 14, 19, 23F) conjugated to tetanus toxoid	+	+	+	+	
	Glycoconjugate vaccine (4, 6B, 9V, 14, 18C, 19F, 23F) conjugated to CRM197	+	+	+	+	+
	Glycoconjugate vaccine (1, 4, 5, 6B, 9V, 14, 18C, 19F, 23F) conjugated to CRM197	+	+	+	+	+
	23-valent licensed vaccine with novel adjuvants (Quil A, QS21, MPL)	+	+	+		
	Glycoconjugate multivalent vaccine with novel adjuvants (e.g., MPL)	+	+	+		
	PspA	+	+	+		
	PsaA	+	+			
	Pneumolysin	+	+			

Target Agent	Vaccine	Basic R&D	Preclinical	Phase I	Phase II	Phase III
Streptococcus pneumoniae (continued)	Autolysin	+	+			
	Neuraminidase	+	+			
	Glycoconjugate vaccine (11-valent) linked to nontypeable H. influenzae OMP	+	+	+	+	
	Glycoconjugate vaccine (1, 3, 4, 5, 6B, 7F, 9V, 14, 18C, 19F, 23F) linked to either tetanus or diphtheria toxoid carrier	+	+	+	+	
	Phospholcholine	+	+			
	Synthetic peptide epitopes and capsular polysaccharide combined	+	+			
	Genetic fusions (PspA-IL2 and PspA-GM-CSF)	+	+			
	CpG motifs cross-linked with 7-valent pneumococcal vaccine	+	+			
Tick-borne	DNA vaccine	+	+			
Encephalitis virus	Inactivated, alum adjuvant	+	+	+	+	
Toxoplasma gondii	Recombinant parasite surface protein (p30)	+	+			
	Live, attenuated parasites	+	+			
	Parasite surface protein expressed in viral vector	+	+			
Treponema pallidum	Surface lipoproteins	+	+			
	Anti-idiotype/fibronectin	+	+			
Trypanosoma cruzi	Recombinant peptide	+	+			
Varicella zoster virus	Live, attenuated vaccine	+	+	+	+	+
	Subunit, glycoproteins	+				
	Vaccinia-vectored glycoprotein	+				
Venezuelan equine	Inactivated, whole virus particles	+	+	+	+	
Encephalitis	Live, attenuated virus strain (TC-83)	+	+	+	+	
	Infectious clones	+	+			
Vibrio cholerae	Killed bacteria plus toxin B subunit	+	+	+	+	+
	Live, recombinant O1	+	+	+	+	+
	Live, recombinant O139	+	+	+	+	
	Conjugate lipopolysaccharide (LPS)	+	+			
Yellow Fever virus	Live attenuated	+	+	+	+	+
	Infectious clone	+	+			
Western equine encephalitis virus	Inactivated, whole virus particles	+	+	+	+	
Yersinia pestis	Recombinant subunit	+	+			

Appendix D

Vaccines Currently Licensed in the United States

Division of Vaccines and Related Products Applications

Office of Vaccines Research and Review, Center for Biologics Evaluation and Research (CBER)

Vaccines Currently Licensed in the United States
June 2001

Code	Product Name	Trade Name	License Date	License No.	Establishment
HF-01	Acellular Pertussis Vaccine Concentrate (For Further Manufacturing Use)	No Trade Name	17-Dec-91	1146-001	Takeda Chemical Industries, Ltd.
HF-01	Acellular Pertussis Vaccine Concentrate (For Further Manufacturing Use)	No Trade Name	20-Aug-92	1156-001	Research Foundation for Microbial Diseases of Osaka University
CY-23	Adenovirus Vaccine, Live, Oral, Type 4	No Trade Name	01-Jul-80	0003-001	Wyeth Laboratories, Inc.[1]
CY-24	Adenovirus Vaccine, Live, Oral, Type 7	No Trade Name	01-Jul-80	0003-001	Wyeth Laboratories, Inc.[1]
HC-31	Anthrax Vaccine Adsorbed	No Trade Name	04-Nov-70	1260-001	BioPort Corporation[2]
HC-32	BCG Vaccine	No Trade Name	10-Jan-95	0956-005	Organon Teknika Corporation
HC-32	BCG Vaccine (Reissued)	Mycobax®	09-Oct-98	1280-001	Aventis Pasteur, Ltd.[3]
HC-33	Cholera Vaccine	No Trade Name	16-Jul-52	0003-001	Wyeth Laboratories, Inc.[1]
IY-03	Diphtheria & Tetanus Toxoids Adsorbed	No Trade Name	29-Jul-70	0017-001	Lederle Lab. Div., Amer. Cyanamid Co.
IY-03	Diphtheria & Tetanus Toxoids Adsorbed	No Trade Name	27-Aug-70	1260-001	BioPort Corporation[2]
IY-03	Diphtheria & Tetanus Toxoids Adsorbed	No Trade Name	11-Sep-70	0003-001	Wyeth Laboratories, Inc.[1]
IY-03	Diphtheria & Tetanus Toxoids Adsorbed	No Trade Name	18-Sep-84	1277-001	Aventis Pasteur, Inc.[4]
IY-03	Diphtheria & Tetanus Toxoids Adsorbed	No Trade Name	11-Apr-97	1280-001	Aventis Pasteur, Ltd.[3]
IY-13	Diphtheria & Tetanus Toxoids & Acellular Pertussis Vaccine Adsorbed	Acel-Imune®	17-Dec-91	0017-001	Lederle Lab. Div., American Cyanamid Co.
IY-13	Diphtheria & Tetanus Toxoids & Acellular Pertussis Vaccine Adsorbed	Tripedia®	20-Aug-92	1277-001	Aventis Pasteur, Inc.[4]
IY-13	Diphtheria & Tetanus Toxoids & Acellular Pertussis Vaccine Adsorbed	Infanrix®	29-Jan-97	1090-001	SmithKline Beecham Biologicals
IY-13	Diphtheria & Tetanus Toxoids & Acellular Pertussis Vaccine Adsorbed	Certiva®	29-Jul-98	1254-001	North American Vaccine, Inc.

Division of Vaccines and Related Products Applications

Office of Vaccines Research and Review, Center for Biologics Evaluation and Research (CBER)

Vaccines Currently Licensed in the United States
June 2001 (continued)

Code	Product Name	Trade Name	License Date	License No.	Establishment
IY-05	Diphtheria & Tetanus Toxoids & Pertussis Vaccine Adsorbed	No Trade Name	27-Aug-70	1260-001	BioPort Corporation[2]
IY-05	Diphtheria & Tetanus Toxoids & Pertussis Vaccine Adsorbed	No Trade Name	11-Sep-70	0003-001	Wyeth Laboratories, Inc.[1]
IY-05	Diphtheria & Tetanus Toxoids & Pertussis Vaccine Adsorbed	No Trade Name	03-Jan-78	1277-001	Aventis Pasteur, Inc.[4]
BY-02	Diphtheria Toxoid Adsorbed	No Trade Name	27-Aug-70	1260-001	BioPort Corporation[2]
HC-46	Haemophilus b Conjugate Vaccine (Diphtheria Toxoid Conjugate)	ProHIBiT®	22-Dec-87	1277-001	Aventis Pasteur, Inc.[4]
HC-47	Haemophilus b Conjugate Vaccine (Diphtheria CRM197 Protein Conjugate)	HibTITER®	06-Dec-94	0017-004	Lederle Lab. Div., American Cyanamid Co.
HC-48	Haemophilus b Conjugate Vaccine (Meningococcal Protein Conjugate)	PedvaxHIB®	20-Dec-89	0002-001	Merck & Co., Inc.
HC-50	Haemophilus b Conjugate Vaccine (Tetanus Toxoid Conjugate)	ActHIB® OmniHIB®	30-Mar-93	1279-001	Aventis Pasteur, S.A.[5]
IY-16	Haemophilus b Conjugate Vaccine (Meningococcal Protein Conjugate) & Hepatitis B Vaccine (Recombinant)	Comvax®	02-Oct-96	0002-001	Merck & Co., Inc.
HC-45	Haemophilus b Polysaccharide Vaccine	HibVAX®	20-Dec-85	1277-001	Aventis Pasteur, Inc.[4]
CY-29	Hepatitis A Vaccine, Inactivated	Havrix®	22-Feb-95	1090-001	SmithKline Beecham Biologicals
CY-29	Hepatitis A Vaccine, Inactivated	VAQTA®	29-Mar-96	0002-001	Merck & Co., Inc.
CM-01	Hepatitis A Inactivated and Hepatitis B (Recombinant) Vaccine	TWINRIX®	11-May-01	1090-001	SmithKline Beecham Biologicals
CM-25	Hepatitis B Vaccine (Recombinant)	Recombivax HB®	23-Jul-86	0002-001	Merck & Co., Inc.
CM-25	Hepatitis B Vaccine (Recombinant)	Engerix-B®	28-Aug-89	1090-001	SmithKline Beecham Biologicals

Division of Vaccines and Related Products Applications

Office of Vaccines Research and Review, Center for Biologics Evaluation and Research (CBER)

Vaccines Currently Licensed in the United States
June 2001 (continued)

Code	Product Name	Trade Name	License Date	License No.	Establishment
CY-02	Influenza Virus Vaccine	Flu-Immune®	07-Dec-45	0017-001	Lederle Lab. Div., American Cyanamid Co.
CY-02	Influenza Virus Vaccine	Fluvirin®	12-Aug-88	1262-001	Medeva Pharma, Ltd.[6]
CY-02	Influenza Virus Vaccine, Trivalent, Types A and B	Fluogen®	26-Nov-45	1241-001	Parkedale Pharmaceuticals, Inc.[7]
CY-02	Influenza Virus Vaccine, Trivalent, Types A and B	FluShield®	13-Dec-61	0003-001	Wyeth Laboratories, Inc.[1]
CY-02	Influenza Virus Vaccine, Trivalent, Types A and B	Fluzone®	03-Jan-78	1277-001	Aventis Pasteur, Inc.[4]
CY-30	Japanese Encephalitis Virus Vaccine Inactivated	JE-Vax®	10-Dec-92	1156-001	Research Foundation for Microbial Diseases of Osaka University
HC-53	Lyme Disease Vaccine (Recombinant OspA)	LYMErix®	21-Dec-98	1090-001	SmithKline Beecham Biologicals
CY-03	Measles Virus Vaccine, Live	Attenuvax®	26-Nov-68	0002-001	Merck & Co., Inc.
CY-22	Measles and Mumps Virus Vaccine, Live	M-M-Vax®	18-Jul-73	0002-001	Merck & Co., Inc.
CY-04	Measles, Mumps, and Rubella Virus Vaccine, Live	M-M-R®II	22-Apr-71	0002-001	Merck & Co., Inc.
HC-40	Meningococcal Polysaccharide Vaccine, Group A	Menomune®-A	03-Jan-78	1277-001	Aventis Pasteur, Inc.[4]
HC-39	Meningococcal Polysaccharide Vaccine, Group C	Menomune®-C	03-Jan-78	1277-001	Aventis Pasteur, Inc.[4]
HC-41	Meningococcal Polysaccharide Vaccine, Groups A and C Combined	Menomune®-A/C	03-Jan-78	1277-001	Aventis Pasteur, Inc.[4]
HC-44	Meningococcal Polysaccharide Vaccine, Groups A, C, Y and W-135 Combined	Menomune®-A/C /Y/W-135	23-Nov-81	1277-001	Aventis Pasteur, Inc.[4]
CY-08	Mumps Virus Vaccine Live	Mumpsvax®	28-Dec-67	0002-001	Merck & Co., Inc.
HC-35	Pertussis Vaccine Adsorbed	No Trade Name	12-Oct-67	1260-001	BioPort Corporation[2]

Division of Vaccines and Related Products Applications
Office of Vaccines Research and Review, Center for Biologics Evaluation and Research (CBER)
Vaccines Currently Licensed in the United States
June 2001 (continued)

Code	Product Name	Trade Name	License Date	License No.	Establishment
HC-36	Plague Vaccine	No Trade Name	05-Oct-94	0308-002	Greer Laboratories, Inc.
HC-42	Pneumococcal Vaccine, Polyvalent	Pneumovax® 23	21-Nov-77	0002-001	Merck & Co., Inc.
HC-42	Pneumococcal Vaccine, Polyvalent	Pnu-Imune® 23	15-Aug-79	0017-001	Lederle Lab. Div., American Cyanamid Co.
HC-55	Pneumococcal 7-valent Conjugate Vaccine (Diphtheria CRM197 Protein)	Prevnar™	17-Feb-00	0017-001	Lederle Lab. Div., American Cyanamid Co.
CY-28	Poliovirus Vaccine Inactivated (Human Diploid Cell)	Poliovax®	20-Nov-87	1280-001	Aventis Pasteur, Ltd.[3]
CY-09	Poliovirus Vaccine Inactivated (Monkey Kidney Cell)	IPOL®	21-Dec-90	1279-001	Aventis Pasteur, S.A.[5]
CY-11	Poliovirus Vaccine Live Oral Trivalent (Sabin Strains Types 1, 2 and 3)	Orimune®	25-Jun-63	0017-001	Lederle Lab. Div., American Cyanamid Co.
CY-12	Poliovirus Vaccine Live Oral Type I	No Trade Name	27-Mar-62	0017-001	Lederle Lab. Div., American Cyanamid Co.
CY-13	Poliovirus Vaccine Live Oral Type II	No Trade Name	27-Mar-62	0017-001	Lederle Lab. Div., American Cyanamid Co.
CY-14	Poliovirus Vaccine Live Oral Type III	No Trade Name	27-Mar-62	0017-001	Lederle Lab. Div., American Cyanamid Co.
CY-15	Rabies Vaccine	Imovax® Rabies	09-Jun-80	1279-001	Aventis Pasteur, S.A.[5]
CY-15	Rabies Vaccine	Rabie-Vax®	27-Dec-91	1280-001	Aventis Pasteur, Ltd.[3]
CY-15	Rabies Vaccine	RabAvert®	20-Oct-97	1222-001	Chiron Behring GmbH & Co.
CY-27	Rabies Vaccine Adsorbed	No Trade Name	18-Mar-88	1260-001	BioPort Corporation[2]
CY-31	Rotavirus Vaccine Live, Oral, Tetravalent[8]	RotaShield®	31-Aug-98	0003-001	Wyeth Laboratories, Inc.[1]
CY-18	Rubella Virus Vaccine Live	Meruvax®	09-Jun-69	0002-001	Merck & Co., Inc.
CY-19	Smallpox Vaccine	Dryvax®	19-May-44	0003-001	Wyeth Laboratories, Inc.[1]
IV-10	Tetanus & Diphtheria Toxoids Adsorbed for Adult Use	No Trade Name	27-Jul-70	0064-001	Massachusetts Public Health Biologic Lab.

Division of Vaccines and Related Products Applications

Office of Vaccines Research and Review, Center for Biologics Evaluation and Research (CBER)

Vaccines Currently Licensed in the United States
June 2001 (continued)

Code	Product Name	Trade Name	License Date	License No.	Establishment
TY-10	Tetanus & Diphtheria Toxoids Adsorbed for Adult Use	No Trade Name	29-Jul-70	0017-001	Lederle Lab. Div., American Cyanamid Co.
TY-10	Tetanus & Diphtheria Toxoids Adsorbed for Adult Use	No Trade Name	11-Sep-70	0003-001	Wyeth Laboratories, Inc.[1]
TY-10	Tetanus & Diphtheria Toxoids Adsorbed for Adult Use	No Trade Name	03-Jan-78	1277-001	Aventis Pasteur, Inc.[4]
BY-05	Tetanus Toxoid	No Trade Name	14-Jan-43	1280-001	Aventis Pasteur, Ltd.[3]
BY-05	Tetanus Toxoid	No Trade Name	19-May-44	0003-001	Wyeth Laboratories, Inc.[1]
BY-05	Tetanus Toxoid	No Trade Name	03-Jan-78	1277-001	Aventis Pasteur, Inc.[4]
BY-06	Tetanus Toxoid Adsorbed	No Trade Name	29-Jul-70	0017-001	Lederle Lab. Div., American Cyanamid Co.
BY-06	Tetanus Toxoid Adsorbed	No Trade Name	29-Jul-70	0064-001	Massachusetts Public Health Biologic Lab.
BY-06	Tetanus Toxoid Adsorbed	No Trade Name	27-Aug-70	1260-001	Bioport Corporation[2]
BY-06	Tetanus Toxoid Adsorbed	No Trade Name	11-Sep-70	0003-001	Wyeth Laboratories, Inc.[1]
BY-06	Tetanus Toxoid Adsorbed	Te Anatoxal Berna®	11-Dec-70	0021-001	Swiss Serum and Vaccine Institute Berne[9]
BY-06	Tetanus Toxoid Adsorbed	No Trade Name	03-Jan-78	1277-001	Aventis Pasteur, Inc.[4]
HC-38	Typhoid Vaccine	No Trade Name	16-Jul-52	0003-001	Wyeth Laboratories, Inc.[1]
HC-49	Typhoid Vaccine Live Oral Ty21a	Vivotif Berna®	15-Dec-89	0021-001	Swiss Serum and Vaccine Institute Berne[9]
HC-51	Typhoid Vi Polysaccharide Vaccine	Typhim Vi®	28-Nov-94	1279-001	Aventis Pasteur, S.A.[5]
CY-26	Varicella Virus Vaccine Live	Varivax®	17-Mar-95	0002-001	Merck & Co., Inc.
CY-21	Yellow Fever Vaccine	YF-Vax®	03-Jan-78	1277-001	Aventis Pasteur, Inc.[4]

Footnotes

1. Wyeth Laboratories, Inc., is the new corporate name for Wyeth-Ayerst, Inc., effective July 1, 1980.
2. BioPort Corporation acquired product ownership on November 12, 1998, from the Michigan Biologic Products Institute, formerly under the Michigan Department of Public Health.
3. Aventis Pasteur, Ltd., obtained product ownership from Connaught Laboratories, Ltd., effective February 24, 2000.
4. Aventis Pasteur, Inc., obtained product ownership from Connaught Laboratories, Inc., effective December 9, 1999.
5. Aventis Pasteur, S.A., is the new corporate name for Pasteur Mérieux Sérums et Vaccins, S.A., effective February 4, 2000.
6. Medeva Pharma, Ltd., obtained product ownership from Evans Medical, Ltd., effective November 3, 1998.
7. ParkeDale Pharmaceuticals, Inc., is the new corporate product owner name for Parke-Davis, Div. of Warner-Lambert Co., effective April 20, 1998.
8. Wyeth Lederle Vaccines announced that RotaShield® is withdrawn from the market, effective October 15, 1999.
9. Berna Products Corp. is the subsidiary in North America for Swiss Serum and Vaccine Institute Berne.

Appendix E

HIV Vaccine Candidates in Clinical Trials December 2001

HIV Vaccine Candidates in Clinical Trials
December 2001

Type of Vaccine	Vaccine	HIV Subtype	Developer/Manufacturer	Conducting Trial	Status
Subunit	AIDSVAX MN™	B	VaxGen	NIAID's HVTN	Phase II Caribbean, South America (with vCP1452)
	AIDSVAX B/B™	B	VaxGen	VaxGen	Phase II United States (with vCP1452)
	AIDSVAX B/B™	B	VaxGen	VaxGen	Phase III North America, Europe
	AIDSVAX B/E™	B and E	VaxGen	VaxGen	Phase III Thailand
	AIDSVAX B/B™	B	VaxGen	NIAID's HVTN	Phase II United States (with vCP 1452)
	AIDSVAX B/E™	B and E	VaxGen	WRAIR	Phase II Thailand (with vCP1521)
	rgp 120 CM235/SF-2	B and E	Chiron	WRAIR	Phase I/II Thailand (with vCP1521)
	rgp 160 THO23/LAI-DID	E and B	Aventis Pasteur	WRAIR	Phase I/II Thailand (with vCP1521)
DNA	Gag DNA	B	Merck	Merck	Phase I United States
	VRC 4302; gag-pol fusion DNA	B	Vaccine Research Center	NIAID	Phase I United States
	Mulit-epitope + gag	A	Cobra Pharmaceuticals	OXAVI, KAVI, IAVI	Phase I United Kingdom, Kenya
Live Vector	vCP 1452	B	Aventis Pasteur	NIAID's HVTN	Phase II United States, Caribbean, South America (with AIDSVAX MN™)
	vCP 1521	E and B	Aventis Pasteur	WRAIR	Phase I/II Thailand (with gp120 CM235/SF-2 or rpg 160 THO23/LAI-DID)
	vCP205 (dendritic cells)	B	Aventis Pasteur	WRAIR	Phase I United States
	PolyEnv1 vaccinia	B	St. Jude Children's Research Hospital	St. Jude Children's Research Hospital	Phase I United States
	Adenovirus-gag	B	Merck	Merck	Phase I United States
	MVA-mulit-epitope + gag	A	Impfstoffwerk Dessau-Tornau GmbH (IDT)	OXAVI, KAVI, IAVI	Phase I United Kingdom, Kenya
Peptide	LIP05	B	Aventis Pasteur	ANRS	Phase I France
	LIP06T	B	Aventis Pasteur	ANRS	Phase I France

ANRS, French National Agency for Research on AIDS; HIV, human immunodeficiency virus; HVTN, HIV Vaccine Trials Network; IAVI, International AIDS Vaccine Initiative; KAVI, Kenya AIDS Vaccine Initiative; NIAID, National Institute of Allergy and Infectious Diseases; OXAVI, Oxford AIDS Vaccine Initiative; WRAIR, Walter Reed Army Institute of Research

Appendix F

HIV Vaccine Candidates in Preclinical Development December 2001

HIV Vaccine Candidates in Preclinical Development
December 2001

Vaccine*	HIV Subtype	Preclinical Partners**
Adeno-associated virus expressing multiple genes	C	Targeted Genetics, Ohio State University, IAVI
Adenovirus expressing multiple genes (replicating)	B	NCI
ALVAC expressing multiple genes	A	Aventis Pasteur
DNA and nonreplicating adenovirus expressing multiple genes	B	Merck
DNA and nonreplicating adenovirus expressing multiple genes	B	NIAID Vaccine Research Center
DNA and MVA expressing multiple genes	B, A/G	Emory University, NIAID, CDC
MVA expressing multiple genes	A, D	WRAIR
DNA, Sindbis replicons expressing multiple genes, novel recombinant envelope proteins	B, C	Chiron, NIAID
DNA expressing multiple HIV genes, DNA expressing cytokine gene and peptide boost	B	Wyeth-Lederle, NIAID
DNA and fowlpox expressing multiple HIV genes and cytokine	B, E	University of New South Wales, NIAID
DNA–env and envelope protein	Multiple	ABL, NIAID
Gp120 and regulatory proteins	B	GlaxoSmithKline
MVA expressing multiple genes, including CCR5-using envelope	B, C	Therion, University of Massachusetts, NIAID, IAVI
MVA, NYVAC, DNA, Semiliki Forest Virus expressing multiple genes and envelope protein	C	EuroVac, Aventis Pasteur
Salmonella expressing multiple genes	A, A/G, B	IHV, IAVI, NIAID
Vaccinia-env and envelope proteins	Multiple	St. Jude Children's Research Hospital, NIAID
VEE-gag	C	AlphaVAX, IAVI, NIAID
VEE expressing multiple genes (replicons)	C	AlphaVAX, NIAID, WRAIR, IAVI

*CCR5, CC chemokine receptor 5; HIV, human immunodeficiency virus; MVA, modified vaccinia Ankara; NYVAC, attenuated vaccinia virus; VEE, Venezuelan equine encephalitis virus; VLP, virus-like particles. **ABL, Advanced BioScience Laboratories; CDC, Centers for Disease Control and Prevention; EuroVac, consortium of 21 laboratories in 8 European countries funded by the European Union; IAVI, International AIDS Vaccine Initiative; IHV, Institute of Human Virology; NCI, National Cancer Institute; NIAID, National Institute of Allergy and Infectious Diseases; WRAIR, Walter Reed Army Institute of Research.

Appendix G

Recommended U.S. Childhood Immunization Schedule

Recommended Childhood Immunization Schedule
United States, 2002

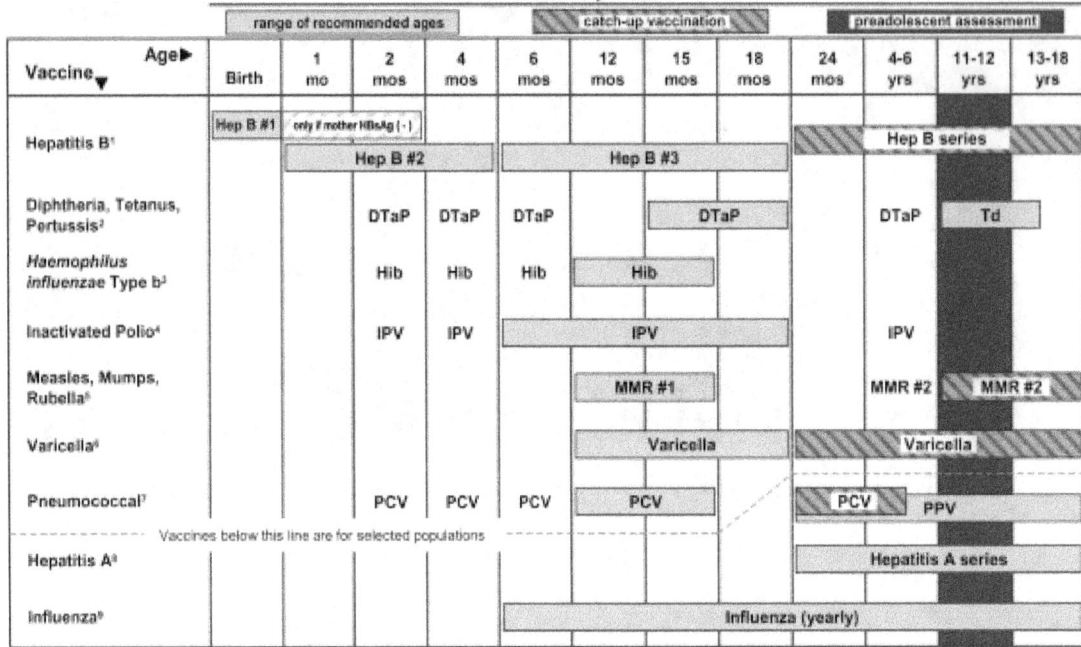

	range of recommended ages				catch-up vaccination					preadolescent assessment		
Age ▶ Vaccine ▼	Birth	1 mo	2 mos	4 mos	6 mos	12 mos	15 mos	18 mos	24 mos	4-6 yrs	11-12 yrs	13-18 yrs
Hepatitis B[1]	Hep B #1 only if mother HBsAg (-)		Hep B #2			Hep B #3				Hep B series		
Diphtheria, Tetanus, Pertussis[2]			DTaP	DTaP	DTaP		DTaP			DTaP	Td	
Haemophilus influenzae Type b[3]			Hib	Hib	Hib	Hib						
Inactivated Polio[4]			IPV	IPV		IPV				IPV		
Measles, Mumps, Rubella[5]						MMR #1				MMR #2	MMR #2	
Varicella[6]						Varicella					Varicella	
Pneumococcal[7]			PCV	PCV	PCV	PCV			PCV	PPV		
Hepatitis A[8]										Hepatitis A series		
Influenza[9]						Influenza (yearly)						

Vaccines below this line are for selected populations

This schedule indicates the recommended ages for routine administration of currently licensed childhood vaccines, as of December 1, 2001, for children through age 18 years. Any dose not given at the recommended age should be given at any subsequent visit when indicated and feasible. ▒ Indicates age groups that warrant special effort to administer those vaccines not previously given. Additional vaccines may be licensed and recommended during the year. Licensed combination vaccines may be used whenever any components of the combination are indicated and the vaccine's other components are not contraindicated. Providers should consult the manufacturers' package inserts for detailed recommendations.

1. Hepatitis B vaccine (Hep B). All infants should receive the first dose of hepatitis B vaccine soon after birth and before hospital discharge; the first dose may also be given by age 2 months if the infant's mother is HBsAg-negative. Only monovalent hepatitis B vaccine can be used for the birth dose. Monovalent or combination vaccine containing Hep B may be used to complete the series; four doses of vaccine may be administered if combination vaccine is used. The second dose should be given at least 4 weeks after the first dose, except for Hib-containing vaccine which cannot be administered before age 6 weeks. The third dose should be given at least 16 weeks after the first dose and at least 8 weeks after the second dose. The last dose in the vaccination series (third or fourth dose) should not be administered before age 6 months.

Infants born to HBsAg-positive mothers should receive hepatitis B vaccine and 0.5 mL hepatitis B immune globulin (HBIG) within 12 hours of birth at separate sites. The second dose is recommended at age 1-2 months and the vaccination series should be completed (third or fourth dose) at age 6 months.

Infants born to mothers whose HBsAg status is unknown should receive the first dose of the hepatitis B vaccine series within 12 hours of birth. Maternal blood should be drawn at the time of delivery to determine the mother's HBsAg status; if the HBsAg test is positive, the infant should receive HBIG as soon as possible (no later than age 1 week).

2. Diphtheria and tetanus toxoids and acellular pertussis vaccine (DTaP). The fourth dose of DTaP may be administered as early as age 12 months, provided 6 months have elapsed since the third dose and the child is unlikely to return at age 15-18 months. **Tetanus and diphtheria toxoids (Td)** is recommended at age 11-12 years if at least 5 years have elapsed since the last dose of tetanus and diphtheria toxoid-containing vaccine. Subsequent routine Td boosters are recommended every 10 years.

3. Haemophilus influenzae type b (Hib) conjugate vaccine. Three Hib conjugate vaccines are licensed for infant use. If PRP-OMP (PedvaxHIB® or ComVax® [Merck]) is administered at ages 2 and 4 months, a dose at age 6 months is not required. DTaP/Hib combination products should not be used for primary immunization in infants at ages 2, 4 or 6 months, but can be used as boosters following any Hib vaccine.

4. Inactivated polio vaccine (IPV). An all-IPV schedule is recommended for routine childhood polio vaccination in the United States. All children should receive four doses of IPV at ages 2 months, 4 months, 6-18 months, and 4-6 years.

5. Measles, mumps, and rubella vaccine (MMR). The second dose of MMR is recommended routinely at age 4-6 years but may be administered during any visit, provided at least 4 weeks have elapsed since the first dose and that both doses are administered beginning at or after age 12 months. Those who have not previously received the second dose should complete the schedule by the 11-12 year old visit.

6. Varicella vaccine. Varicella vaccine is recommended at any visit at or after age 12 months for susceptible children, i.e. those who lack a reliable history of chickenpox. Susceptible persons aged $\geq$ 13 years should receive two doses, given at least 4 weeks apart.

7. Pneumococcal vaccine. The heptavalent **pneumococcal conjugate vaccine (PCV)** is recommended for all children age 2-23 months. It is also recommended for certain children age 24-59 months. **Pneumococcal polysaccharide vaccine (PPV)** is recommended in addition to PCV for certain high-risk groups. See MMWR 2000;49(RR-9);1-35.

8. Hepatitis A vaccine. Hepatitis A vaccine is recommended for use in selected states and regions, and for certain high-risk groups; consult your local public health authority. See MMWR 1999;48(RR-12);1-37.

9. Influenza vaccine. Influenza vaccine is recommended annually for children age $\geq$ 6 months with certain risk factors (including but not limited to asthma, cardiac disease, sickle cell disease, HIV, diabetes; see MMWR 2001;50(RR-4);1-44), and can be administered to all others wishing to obtain immunity. Children aged $\leq$12 years should receive vaccine in a dosage appropriate for their age (0.25 mL if age 6-35 months or 0.5 mL if aged $\geq$ 3 years). Children aged $\leq$ 8 years who are receiving influenza vaccine for the first time should receive two doses separated by at least 4 weeks.

For additional information about vaccines, vaccine supply, and contraindications for immunization, please visit the National Immunization Program Website at www.cdc.gov/nip or call the National Immunization Hotline at 800-232-2522 (English) or 800-232-0233 (Spanish).

Approved by the Advisory Committee on Immunization Practices (www.cdc.gov/nip/acip), the **American Academy of Pediatrics** (www.aap.org), and the **American Academy of Family Physicians** (www.aafp.org).

Appendix H

Recommended U.S. Adult Immunization Schedule

2/4/2002	SUMMARY OF ADOLESCENT/ADULT IMMUNIZATION RECOMMENDATIONS			
Agent	Indications	Primary Schedule	Contraindications	Comments
Tetanus and Diphtheria Toxoids Combined (Td)	All adults All adolescents should be assessed at 11-12 or 14-16 years of age and immunized if no dose was received during the previous 5 years.	Two doses 4-8 weeks apart, third dose 6-12 months after the second. No need to repeat doses if the schedule is interrupted. Dose: 0.5 mL intramuscular (IM) Booster: At 10 year intervals throughout life.	Neurologic or severe hypersensitivity reaction to prior dose.	WOUND MANAGEMENT: Patients with three or more previous tetanus toxoid doses: (a) give Td for clean, minor wounds only if more than 10 years since last dose; (b) for other wounds, give Td if over 5 years since last dose. Patients with less than 3 or unknown number of prior tetanus toxoid doses; give Td for clean, minor wounds and Td and TIG (Tetanus Immune Globulin) for other wounds.
Influenza Vaccine	a. Adults 50 years of age and older. b. Residents of nursing homes or other facilities for patients with chronic medical conditions. c. Persons ≥6 months of age with chronic cardiovascular or pulmonary disorders, including asthma. d. Persons ≥6 months of age with chronic metabolic diseases (including diabetes), renal dysfunction, hemoglobinopathies, immunosuppressive or immunodeficiency disorders. e. Women in their 2nd or 3rd trimester of pregnancy during influenza season. f. Persons 6 mo-18 years of age receiving long-term aspirin therapy. g. Groups, including household members and care givers, who can infect high risk persons.	Dose: 0.5 mL intramuscular (IM) Given annually each fall and winter.	Anaphylactic allergy to eggs. Acute febrile illness.	Depending on season and destination, persons traveling to foreign countries should consider vaccination. Any person ≥ 6 months of age who wishes to reduce the likelihood of becoming ill with influenza should be vaccinated. Avoiding subsequent vaccination of persons known to have developed GBS within 6 weeks of a previous vaccination seems prudent; however, for most persons with a GBS history who are at high risk for severe complications, many experts believe the established benefits of vaccination justify yearly vaccination.
Pneumococcal Polysaccharide Vaccine (PPV)	a. Adults 65 years of age and older. b. Persons ≥ 2 years with chronic cardiovascular or pulmonary disorders including congestive heart failure, diabetes mellitus, chronic liver disease, alcoholism, CSF leaks, cardiomyopathy, COPD or emphysema. c. Persons ≥ 2 years with splenic dysfunction or asplenia, hematologic malignancy, multiple myeloma, renal failure, organ transplantation or immunosuppressive conditions, including HIV infection. d. Alaskan Natives and certain American Indian populations.	One dose for most people* Dose: 0.5 mL intramuscular (IM) or subcutaneous (SC) *Persons vaccinated prior to age 65 should be vaccinated at age 65 if 5 or more years have passed since the first dose. For all persons with functional or anatomic asplenia, transplant patients, patients with chronic kidney disease, immunosuppressed or immunodeficient persons, and others at highest risk of fatal infection, a second dose should be given- at least 5 years after first dose.	The safety of PPV during the first trimester of pregnancy has not been evaluated. The manufacturer's package insert should be reviewed for additional information.	If elective splenectomy or immunosuppressive therapy is planned, give vaccine 2 weeks ahead, if possible. When indicated, vaccine should be administered to patients with unknown vaccination status. All residents of nursing homes and other long-term care facilities should have their vaccination status assessed and documented.
Measles and Mumps Vaccines**	a. Adults born after 1956 without written documentation of immunization on or after the first birthday. b. Health care personnel born after 1956 who are at risk of exposure to patients with measles should have documentation of two doses of vaccine on or after the first birthday or of measles seropositivity. c. HIV-infected persons without severe immunosuppression. d. Travelers to foreign countries. e. Persons entering postsecondary educational institutions (e.g., college).	At least one dose. (Two doses of measles-containing vaccine if in college, in health care profession or traveling to a foreign country with second dose at least 1 month after the first). Dose: 0.5 mL subcutaneous (SC)	a. Immunosuppressive therapy or immunodeficiency including HIV-infected persons with severe immunosuppression. b. Anaphylactic allergy to neomycin. c. Pregnancy. d. Immune globulin preparation or blood/blood product received in preceding 3-11 months. e. Untreated, active TB.	Women should be asked if they are pregnant before receiving vaccine, and advised to avoid pregnancy for 28 days after immunization.
Rubella Vaccine**	a. Persons (especially women) without written documentation of immunization on or after the first birthday or of seropositivity. b. Health care personnel who are at risk of exposure to patients with rubella and who may have contact with pregnant patients should have at least one dose.	One dose. Dose: 0.5 mL subcutaneous (SC)	Same as for measles and mumps vaccines.	Women should be asked if they are pregnant before receiving vaccine, and advised to avoid pregnancy for 28 days after immunization.

2/4/2002	SUMMARY OF ADOLESCENT/ADULT IMMUNIZATION RECOMMENDATIONS			
Agent	**Indications**	**Primary Schedule**	**Contraindications**	**Comments**
Hepatitis B Vaccine	a. Persons with occupational risk of exposure to blood or blood-contaminated body fluids. b. Clients and staff of institutions for the developmentally disabled. c. Hemodialysis patients. d. Recipients of clotting-factor concentrates. e. Household contacts and sex partners of those chronically infected with HBV. f. Family members of adoptees from countries where HBV infection is endemic, if adoptees are HBsAg+. g. Certain international travelers. h. Injecting drug users. i. Men who have sex with men. j. Heterosexual men and women with multiple sex partners or recent episode of a sexually transmitted disease. k. Inmates of long-term correctional facilities. l. All unvaccinated adolescents.	Three doses: second dose 1-2 months after the first, third dose 4-6 months after the first. No need to start series over if schedule interrupted. Can start series with one manufacturer's vaccine and finish with another. Dose (Adult): intramuscular (IM) Recombivax HB®: 10 : g/1.0 mL (green cap) Engerix-B®: 20 : g/1.0mL (orange cap) Dose (Adolescents 11-19 years): intramuscular (IM) Recombivax HB®: 5 : g/0.5 mL (yellow cap) Engerix-B®: 10 : g/0.5 mL (light blue cap) Two doses (Only for Adolescents 11-15 years): intramuscular (IM), 4-6 months apart. Restricted to Recombivax HB®: 10 : g/1.0 mL (green cap) Booster: None presently recommended.	Anaphylactic allergy to yeast.	a. Persons with serologic markers of prior or continuing hepatitis B virus infection do not need immunization. b. For hemodialysis patients and other immunodeficient or immunosuppressed patients, vaccine dosage is doubled or special preparation is used. c. *Pregnant women should be sero-screened for HBsAg and, if positive, their infants should be given post-exposure prophylaxis beginning at birth.* d. Post-exposure prophylaxis: consult ACIP recommendations, or state or local immunization program.
Poliovirus Vaccine: IPV - Inactivated Vaccine; OPV - Oral (live) Vaccine	Routine vaccination of those ≥18 years of age residing in the U.S. is not necessary. Vaccination is recommended for the following high-risk adults: a. Travelers to areas or countries where poliomyelitis is epidemic or endemic. b. Members of communities or specific population groups with disease caused by wild polioviruses. c. Laboratory workers who handle specimens that may contain polioviruses. d. Health care workers who have close contact with patients who may be excreting wild polioviruses. e. Unvaccinated adults whose children will be receiving OPV.	Unimmunized adolescents/adults: IPV is recommended - two doses at 4-8 week intervals, third dose 6-12 months after second (can be as soon as 2 months) Dose: 0.5 mL subcutaneous (SC) or intramuscular (IM). Partially immunized adolescents/adults: Complete primary series with IPV (IPV schedule shown above). OPV is no longer recommended for use in the United States.	IPV: Anaphylactic reaction following previous dose or to streptomycin, polymyxin B, or neomycin.	In instances of potential exposure to wild poliovirus, adults who have had a primary series of OPV or IPV may be given 1 more dose of IPV. Although no adverse effects have been documented, vaccination of pregnant women should be avoided. However, if immediate protection is required, pregnant women may be given IPV in accordance with the recommended schedule for adults.
Varicella Vaccine	a. Persons of any age without a reliable history of varicella disease or vaccination, or who are seronegative for varicella. b. Susceptible adolescents and adults living in households with children. c. All susceptible health care workers. d. Susceptible family contacts of immunocompromised persons. e. Susceptible persons in the following groups who are at high risk for exposure: - persons who live or work in environments in which transmission of varicella is likely (e.g., teachers of young children, day care employees, residents and staff in institutional settings) or can occur (e.g., college students, inmates and staff of correctional institutions, military personnel) - nonpregnant women of childbearing age - international travelers	For persons <13 years of age, one dose. For persons 13 years of age and older, two doses separated by 4-8 weeks. If >8 weeks elapse following the first dose, the second dose can be administered without restarting the schedule. Dose: 0.5 mL subcutaneous (SC)	a. Anaphylactic allergy to gelatin or neomycin. b. Untreated, active TB. c. Immunosuppressive therapy or immunodeficiency (including HIV infection). d. Family history of congenital or hereditary immunodeficiency in first-degree relatives, unless the immune competence of the recipient has been clinically substantiated or verified by a laboratory. e. Immune globulin preparation or blood/blood product received in preceding 5 months. f. Pregnancy.	Women should be asked if they are pregnant before receiving varicella vaccine, and advised to avoid pregnancy for one month following each dose of vaccine.
Hepatitis A Vaccine	a. Persons traveling to or working in countries with high or intermediate endemicity of infection. b. Men who have sex with men. c. Injecting and non-injecting illegal drug users. d. Persons who work with HAV-infected primates or with HAV in a research laboratory setting. e. Persons with chronic liver disease. f. Persons with clotting-factor disorders. g. Consider food handlers, where determined to be cost-effective by health authorities or employers.	HAVRIX®: Two doses, separated by 6-12 months. Adults (19 years of age and older) - Dose: 1.0 mL intramuscular (IM). Persons 2-18 years of age: Dose: 0.5 mL (IM). VAQTA®: Adults (19 years of age and older): Two doses, separated by 6 months. Dose: 1.0 mL intramuscular (IM); Persons 2-18 years of age: Two doses, separated by 6-18 months; Dose: 0.5 mL (IM)	A history of hypersensitivity to alum or the preservative 2-phenoxyethanol	The safety of hepatitis A vaccine during pregnancy has not been determined, though the theoretical risk to the developing fetus is expected to be low. The risk of vaccination should be weighed against the risk of hepatitis A in women who may be at high risk of exposure to HAV.

Adapted from the recommendations of the Advisory Committee on Immunization Practices (ACIP).
Foreign travel and less commonly used vaccines such as typhoid, rabies, and meningococcal are not included.

**These vaccines can be given in the combined form measles-mumps-rubella (MMR). Persons already immune to one or more components can still receive MMR.

Appendix I

Web Sites

WEB SITES

Government Agency Web Sites:

National Immunization Program, Centers for Disease Control and Prevention
http://www.cdc.gov/nip/default htm

National Vaccine Program Office, Centers for Disease Control and Prevention
http://www.cdc.gov/od/nvpo/

Center for Biologics Evaluation and Research, Food and Drug Administration
http://www.fda.gov/cber/index.html

Bureau of Health Professions, Health Resources and Services Administration
http://bhpr hrsa.gov/

Division of Microbiology and Infectious Diseases

National Institute of Allergy and Infectious Diseases, National Institutes of Health
http://www niaid.nih.gov/dmid/vaccines/

Other Web Sites*:

World Health Organization (WHO)
http://www.who.int/health_topics/vaccines/en/
This site's section on vaccine safety educates visitors on current immunization issues and how vaccines are developed and distributed. It displays immunization statistics, maps, and charts. The site also describes the Global Alliance for Vaccines and Immunization (GAVI). WHO's perspective is global and the site's content is also available in Spanish and French.

Global Alliance for Vaccines and Immunization (GAVI)
http://www.VaccineAlliance.org
This site provides up-to-date information about GAVI and the Global Fund for Children's Vaccines.

Children's Vaccine Program
http://www.ChildrensVaccine.org
The resources section of the site offers many free materials, including advocacy-related publications and information on diseases and vaccines.

Immunization Action Coalition
http://www.immunize.org
This site offers information and materials on a wide variety of diseases and vaccines. It is available in English and other languages.

Media/Materials Clearinghouse at Johns Hopkins University
http://www.jhuccp.org/mmc/immune/
This site provides access to a wealth of immunization materials, posters, videos, photographs, and literature. Many immunization education materials are available from sources outside the United States.

Vaccine Page
http://www.vaccines.org
This site provides the latest vaccine news and links to high-quality vaccine sites.

National Network for Immunization Information (NNii)
http://www.immunizationinfo.org
This site is designed to provide healthcare professionals, the media, policymakers, and the public with up-to-date, science-based information on immunizations. The site features a searchable database of information on diseases prevented through immunization; a listing of all State vaccination requirements; and thrice-weekly *Immunization Newsbriefs*, which highlight vaccine issues in the news. It also includes background on vaccine development and vaccine safety, guidelines for how to evaluate health information on the Internet, and an image gallery of the effects of vaccine-preventable diseases. The NNii Resource Kit, *Communicating With Patients About Immunization*, is also available here in downloadable PDF format.

Every Child By Two (ECBT)
http://www.ecbt.org
This site contains information about the Every Child By Two early immunization campaign, but also has information for providers and parents. The content includes a newsletter with current information on immunization issues, and an electronic version of CDC's *Parents' Guide to Childhood Immunization*, which discusses individual vaccines and topics such as keeping immunization records.

DMID, NIAID, and NIH are not responsible for the content of these Web sites.